ADVANCES IN NEUROLOGY

Volume 46

Advances in Neurology

Advances in Neurology
Volume 46

Intensive Neurodiagnostic Monitoring

Editor

Robert J. Gumnit, M.D.

Director
Minnesota Comprehensive Epilepsy Program
and Professor of Neurology
University of Minnesota
Minneapolis, Minnesota

Raven Press ■ New York

Raven Press, 1185 Avenue of the Americas, New York, New York 10036

Made in the United States of America

Library of Congress Cataloging-in-Publication Data

Intensive neurodiagnostic monitoring.

(Advances in neurology ; vol. 46)
Based on the International Conference on Intensive Neurodiagnostic Monitoring, held as a satellite conference to the Annual Meeting of the American Epilepsy Society in San Francisco.
Includes bibliographies and index.
1. Epilepsy—Diagnosis—Congresses. 2. Convulsions—Diagnosis—Congresses. 3. Electroencephalography—Congresses. I. Gumnit, Robert J. II. International Conference on Intensive Neurodiagnostic Monitoring (1984 : San Francisco, Calif.) III. American Epilepsy Society. Meeting (1984 : San Francisco, Calif.) IV. Series: Advances in neurology ; v. 46. [DNLM: 1. Electroencephalography—methods—congresses. 2. Monitoring, Physiologic—methods—congresses. W1 AD684H v. 46 / WL 150 I553 1984]
RC321.A276 vol. 46 616.8 s 86-17918
[RC373] [616.8′047547]
ISBN 0-88167-232-7

The material contained in this volume was submitted as previously unpublished material, except in the instances in which credit has been given to the source from which some of the illustrative material was derived.

Great care has been taken to maintain the accuracy of the information contained in the volume. However, Raven Press cannot be held responsible for errors or for any consequences arising from the use of the information contained herein.

9 8 7 6 5 4 3 2 1

Advances in Neurology Series

Vol. 46: Intensive Neurodiagnostic Monitoring
R. J. Gumnit, editor. 336 pp., 1987.

Vol. 45: Parkinson's Disease
M. D. Yahr and K. J. Bergmann, editors. 640 pp., 1986.

Vol. 44: Basic Mechanisms of the Epilepsies: Molecular and Cellular Approaches
A. V. Delgado-Esueta, A. A. Ward, Jr., D. M. Woodbury, and R. J. Porter, editors. 1,120 pp., 1986.

Vol. 43: Myoclonus
S. Fahn, C. D. Marsden, and M. H. Van Woert, editors. 752 pp., 1986.

Vol. 42: Progress in Aphasiology
F. Clifford Rose, editor. 384 pp., 1984.

Vol. 41: The Olivopontocerebellar Atrophies
R. C. Duvoisin and A. Plaitakis, editors. 304 pp., 1984.

Vol. 40: Parkinson-Specific Motor and Mental Disorders, Role of the Pallidum: Pathophysiological, Biochemical, and Therapeutic Aspects
R. G. Hassler and J. F. Christ, editors. 601 pp., 1984.

Vol. 39: Motor Control Mechanisms in Health and Disease
J. E. Desmedt, editor. 1,224 pp., 1983.

Vol. 38: The Dementias
R. Mayeux and W. G. Rosen, editors. 288 pp., 1983.

Vol. 37: Experimental Therapeutics of Movement Disorders
S. Fahn, D. B. Calne, and I. Shoulson, editors. 339 pp., 1983.

Vol. 36: Human Motor Neuron Diseases
L. P. Rowland, editor. 592 pp., 1982.

Vol. 35: Giles de la Tourette Syndrome
A. J. Friedhoff and T. N. Chase, editors. 476 pp., 1982.

Vol. 34: Status Epilepticus: Mechanisms of Brain Damage and Treatment
A. V. Delgado-Escueta, C. G. Wasterlain, D. M. Treiman, and R. J. Porter, editors. 579 pp., 1983.

Vol. 33: Headache: Physiopathological and Clinical Concepts
M. Critchley, A. Friedman, S. Gorini, and F. Sicuteri, editors. 417 pp., 1982.

Vol. 32: Clinical Applications of Evoked Potentials in Neurology
J. Courjon, F. Mauguiere, and M. Revol, editors. 592 pp., 1982.

Vol. 31: Demyelinating Diseases: Basic and Clinical Electrophysiology
S. Waxman and J. Murdoch Ritchie, editors. 544 pp., 1981.

Vol. 30: Diagnosis and Treatment of Brain Ischemia
A. L. Carney and E. M. Anderson, editors. 424 pp., 1981.

Vol. 29: Neurofibromatosis
V. M. Riccardi and J. J. Mulvihill, editors. 288 pp., 1981.

Vol. 28: Brain Edema
J. Cervós-Navarro and R. Ferszt, editors. 539 pp., 1980.

Vol. 27: Antiepileptic Drugs: Mechanisms of Action
G. H. Glaser, J. K. Penry, and D. M. Woodbury, editors. 728 pp., 1980.

Vol. 26: Cerebral Hypoxia and Its Consequences
S. Fahn, J. N. Davis, and L. P. Rowland, editors. 454 pp., 1979.

Vol. 25: Cerebrovascular Disorders and Stroke
M. Goldstein, L. Bolis, C. Fieschi, S. Gorini, and C. H. Millikan, editors. 412 pp., 1979.

Vol. 24: The Extrapyramidal System and Its Disorders
L. J. Poirier, T. L. Sourkes, and P. Bédard, editors. 552 pp., 1979.

Vol. 23: Huntington's Chorea
T. N. Chase, N. S. Wexler, and A. Barbeau, editors. 864 pp., 1979.

Vol. 22: Complications of Nervous System Trauma
R. A. Thompson and J. R. Green, editors. 454 pp., 1979.

Vol. 21: The Inherited Ataxias: Biochemical, Viral, and Pathological Studies
R. A. Kark, R. Rosenberg, and L. Schut, editors. 450 pp., 1978.

Vol. 20: Pathology of Cerebrospinal Microcirculation
J. Cervós-Navarro, E. Betz, G. Ebhardt, R. Ferszt, and R. Wüllenweber, editors. 636 pp., 1978.

Vol. 19: Neurological Epidemiology: Principles and Clinical Applications
Bruce S. Schoenberg, editor. 672 pp., 1978.

Vol. 18: Hemi-Inattention and Hemisphere Specialization
E. A. Weinstein and R. P. Friedland, editors. 176 pp., 1977.

Vol. 17: Treatment of Neuromuscular Diseases
R. C. Griggs and R. T. Moxley, editors. 370 pp., 1977.

Vol. 16: Stroke
R. A. Thompson and J. R. Green, editors. 250 pp., 1977.

Vol. 15: Neoplasia in the Central Nervous System
R. A. Thompson and J. R. Green, editors. 394 pp., 1976.

Vol. 14: Dystonia
R. Eldridge and S. Fahn, editors. 510 pp., 1976.

Vol. 13: Current Reviews
W. J. Friedlander, editor. 400 pp., 1975.

Vol. 12: Physiology and Pathology of Dendrites
G. W. Kreutzberg, editor. 524 pp., 1975.

Vol. 11: Complex Partial Seizures and Their Treatment
J. K. Penry and D. D. Daly, editors. 486 pp., 1975.

Vol. 10: Primate Models of Neurological Disorders
B. S. Meldrum and C. D. Marsden, editors. 270 pp., 1975.

Vol. 9: Dopaminergic Mechanisms
D. B. Calne, T. N. Chase, and A. Barbeau, editors. 452 pp., 1975.

Vol. 8: Neurosurgical Management of the Epilepsies
D. P. Purpura, J. K. Penry, and R. D. Walter, editors. 370 pp., 1975.

Vol. 7: Current Reviews of Higher Nervous System Dysfunction
W. J. Friedlander, editor. 202 pp., 1975.

Vol. 6: Infectious Diseases of the Central Nervous System
R. A. Thompson and J. R. Green, editors. 402 pp., 1974.

Vol. 5: Second Canadian-American Conference on Parkinson's Disease
F. McDowell and A. Barbeau, editors. 526 pp., 1974.

Vol. 4: International Symposium on Pain
J. J. Bonica, editor. 858 pp., 1974.

Vol. 3: Progress in the Treatment of Parkinsonism
D. B. Calne, editor. 402 pp., 1973.

Vol. 2: The Treatment of Parkinsonism—The Role of DOPA Decarboxylase Inhibitors
M. D. Yahr, editor. 304 pp., 1973.

Vol. 1: Huntington's Chorea, 1872–1972
A. Barbeau, T. N. Chase, and G. W. Paulson, editors. 902 pp., 1973.

Preface

Intensive neurodiagnostic monitoring is a rapidly expanding field which includes combined video/EEG recording, cable- and radio-EEG telemetry, (portable) ambulatory cassette-recorded EEG, and the use of depth electrodes. It began in an experimental fashion in the 1950s. Fifteen years ago the Epilepsy Advisory Committee of the National Institute of Neurological and Communicable Disorders and Stroke (NINCDS) concluded that efforts to refine these techniques into clinically useful tools should begin. We have now arrived at the point where the indications for such efforts should be formalized, techniques and terminology standardized, and key research questions identified.

Episodic events are very difficult for physicians to diagnose and treat. For the most part one must depend on history and indirect evidence, unless the physician is fortunate enough to actually witness and adequately record the event. This rarely happens because most of these events do not occur frequently each day. Thus, the problem of obtaining good data with which to make a proper diagnosis of an episodic event is an important one for modern medicine. The challenge to obtain good information about events that present episodically is not unique to any one specialty. However, it is particularly common in two major areas: cardiology and neurology. Malfunctions of one system are frequently mistaken for the other.

Cardiology has done well in dealing with its particular problems because medicine and physiology have a better grasp of the fundamental aspects of the relationship between the electrical activity of the heart and the behavior of the pump. Since cardiac function is repetitious and the electrical activity is simpler, it is easier to analyze. Good instrumentation has been developed, for example, Holter monitoring with computer analysis.

The solutions are less well developed in malfunctions of the central nervous system. Data have been gathered in three major areas: seizures; "dizziness" which may involve seizures, vertigo, or cardiac problems; and other episodic disturbances of behavior. The techniques for making these observations have proliferated and the literature is large and confusing. At the same time, the general neurological community is ignorant of many of the new advances and does not truly understand the implications for improved diagnosis and treatment.

For many common and uncomplicated problems the history that a physician obtains and a routine interictal EEG recording are quite sufficient to make a diagnosis. However, the data gathered from carefully controlled studies of the treatment of intractable seizures indicate that more complex cases require intensive neurodiagnostic monitoring. The same situation holds true in the treatment of patients in whom the diagnosis of seizures is in doubt, for example, when it is not clear whether the problem is of CNS or cardiac origin, or if there is the question of psychogenic seizures.

This volume will be of interest to neurologists, internists, pediatricians, and others with a special interest in epilepsy and other causes of sudden, intermittent disturbances of consciousness. Electroencephalographers, EEG technologists, nurses, and psychologists will have a wealth of useful technical information.

Terminology

Many different words have been used to describe the same equipment and techniques by various authors. In the Editor's opinion, the general field can be called "intensive neurodiagnostic monitoring." Monitoring in some contexts, for example, postcoronary care units, may mean as little as a 24-hour/day display of the ECG with an automatic alarm system. The term intensive neurodiagnostic monitoring refers to close observation with the ability to review, at leisure, episodic events. The term intensive is added to separate it from the casual, routine checking for major rhythm disturbances that is often called ECG monitoring.

Although the word may sound a bit awkward, "neurodiagnostic" is very descriptive. It implies the technique is being used to look at changes of activity within the nervous system or at events that may affect the nervous system; and the term "diagnostic" carries with it the implication that this is something actively used in diagnosis of disease, and hence is part of an active treatment process. In much the same way that departments of radiology used to call themselves "departments of imaging," so many new techniques that have been grafted onto electroencephalography require us to take a broader perspective of what neurologists and electroencephalographers do.

Conventional EEG is performed with a technologist at an EEG machine, the patient connected by means of electrodes and wires, and the brain waves recorded for approximately 30 min. This technique has proven useful for over 50 years. For many common problems it is satisfactory for a technologist to record the EEG and for the physician to arrive later and interpret the test at some convenient time, often after the technologist has gone home. This is not the case in intensive neurodiagnostic monitoring. The techniques are too complex, the amount of material gathered is too great, and the cost is too high to permit this casual approach. All of the techniques described in this volume require extensive involvement by highly specialized technologists and physicians.

Video/EEG is the term used to denote a situation in which at least ten channels of EEG are simultaneously recorded with a video picture of the patient. The two must be closely time-synchronized, or the information is not useful. It is best if both a close-up of the face and a full body view of the patient be included using split-screen techniques. In actual fact, most institutions specializing in patients with intractable seizures or epilepsy surgery have the ability to superimpose EEG upon a full figure and facial close-up in order to allow for the most precise electroclinical correlations. Adequate video/EEG cannot be obtained where only the EEG is recorded (whether on paper or on tape), or where a close time synchronization does not exist between the videotape and the EEG record. Video/EEG may be performed for brief periods, or 24 hr/day, with one technologist continuously observing one patient, or in an automated suite where several patients are observed continuously. The indications and costs for these varied degrees of intensiveness vary accordingly.

The equipment may be set up in a special recording suite. This is optimum for the close investigation of patients in whom surgery is contemplated or for patients with highly complicated seizure problems. Specialized suites imply the presence of specially trained technologists in constant attendance. Portable equipment can also be used. Athough more convenient in some respects, the lack of a technologist in constant attendance may lead to important data being missed. Both types of units are commercially available. Automatic detection devices have been described but are not yet commercially available. Their main usefulness is to assist the technologist/EEG team to focus their attention on important events.

With telemetered EEG, a patient may be provided greater freedom to move about if special precautions are taken to minimize artifact and improve signal reliability. The patient may be connected to the EEG machine by means of a cable or by radiotransmitter. In either case the opportunity then presents itself for prolonged recording of the patient under more natural conditions. We refer to these procedures as "cable telemetry" or radiotelemetry," or simply "telemetered EEG." In day-to-day parlance the patient is said to be "on telemetry." This simple phrase does not do justice to the complexity of equipment, personnel, and operating systems that are required.

Even greater freedom of movement is possible if the patient wears a small cassette tape recorder to which has been attached a miniaturized EEG machine and specialized circuitry for the recording of up to sixteen channels of data. This almost miraculous advance in miniaturization opens new diagnostic possibilities. We refer to this as "ambulatory cassette-recorded EEG," which in many laboratories is abbreviated to ACR or PCR (portable cassette recorder). There are now three commercial manufacturers of such equipment. Under these circumstances, referring to the equipment by a specific manufacturer's name is inappropriate. "Ambulatory cassette recording" is preferable to "portable cassette recording" since the former term recognizes the ability of the patient to move freely while recordings are taking place. "Portable" implies that the equipment is movable from one location to the other, but that it is not necessarily ambulatory.

Another major area of terminology that has become confusing is the problem of "epileptic seizures" and "nonepileptic seizures." The term epileptic seizure refers to a sudden change in the electrical activity of the brain, usually accompanied by subjective or objective changes in behavior. Nonepileptic seizures are sudden changes of objective or subjective behavior which do not have at their root an independent sudden change in the electrical activity of the brain. Nonepileptic seizures can be divided into physiological non-CNS events, such as syncope, cardiac standstill, etc., and psychogenic seizures.

"Psychogenic seizures" is a broad term covering many different diagnostic categories. It includes malingering, sudden episodic events related to conversion reactions, misinterpretation of normal physiological stimuli, and behavioral changes secondary to psychological conflict.

The term "pseudoseizures" is not recommended because of lack of clarity of denotation and lack of general acceptance in the medical community. It tends to damn an important area of medical research and treatment by implying that somehow psychogenic seizures are not "real," and do not need treatment, or are something to be weeded out before we can deal with the real thing.

The term "hysterical epilepsy" has a long history. However, it implies different etiologies in different psychiatric systems, and refers only to a small portion of the broad spectrum of psychogenic seizures. It also tends to be used derisively by some physicians.

The International Conference on Intensive Neurodiagnostic Monitoring, held as a satellite conference to a recent meeting of the American Epilepsy Society in San Francisco, examined these problems. Specific goals were recognized and are addressed in this volume:

1. To review the clinical indications for intensive neurodiagnostic monitoring and determine the kinds of disturbances of behavior that can be studied.
2. To identify the aims of monitoring and specify the kinds of information that should be obtained.
3. To discuss the setting in which monitoring is performed and list the types of hospitals and clinics that can appropriately do such work. To determine if monitoring can stand alone or if it must be part of an organized diagnostic effort.
4. To determine the appropriate instrumentation for monitoring with special emphasis on combined video/EEG recording, telemetered EEG and 24-hour ambulatory cassette-recorded EEG. The limitations of this instrumentation need to be identified. New directions for future development of instrumentation are pointed out.
5. To study the matter of costs versus benefits because intensive neurodiagnostic monitoring is expensive.
6. To review the roles that monitoring can play in clinical research. It has been suggested that such recordings may help evaluate new anticonvulsant drugs, look at the clinical efficacy of a given drug in a given patient, localize lesions for surgical removal, and deal with patients with infantile spasms.

It is hoped this volume will help clarify the differences that exist within the scientific community and point the way toward new ventures in clinical research. Most important, it should provide guidance about the indications, limitations, techniques, and proper selection of intensive neurodiagnostic monitoring.

Acknowledgments

The preliminary planning for this conference greatly benefited from the advice and participation of the following people: Antonio V. Delgado-Escueta, M.D., Fritz Dreifuss, M.B., F.R.A.C.P., Jean Gotman, Ph.D., John Ives, M.S., Richard Mattson, M.D., and J. Kiffin Penry. Florence Gray and Margaret Jacobs served as staff to the organizers in the early stages. Deborah James McNally from the Minnesota CEP then became the editorial assistant. She worked with the various authors to develop the final manuscript. She and Priscilla Bourgeois of the American Epilepsy Society also organized the International Conference on Intensive Neurodiagnostic Monitoring on which this book is based.

This project was made possible, in part, through funds provided by the National Institutes of Health (grant numbers R13-NS 20816-01 and P50 NS 16308), and with the support of the following sponsors: Biomedical Monitoring Systems, Inc., Del Mar Science Foundation, Oxford Medilog, Inc., and Telefactor Corporation.

Contents

Combined Video and EEG Recording

Ambulatory EEG: Telemetered EEG and Cassette Recorded EEG

Intensive Monitoring in Specific Problem Areas

Data Reduction

Summary

Contributors

Colin D. Binnie, M.D., M.A., B.Chir.
Department of Clinical Neurophysiology
Instituut voor Epilepsiebestrijding
Meer en Bosch
P.O. Box 21
2100 Heemstede, The Netherlands

L. D. Blumhardt, M.D., F.R.A.C.P.
Department of Neurology
Associated Unit of Neuroscience
University of Liverpool, and
Mersey Regional Unit of Medical and Surgical Neurology
Walton Hospital
Rice Lane
Liverpool L91AE, England

Paul H. Crandall
Department of Neurology and Anatomy
University of California at Los Angeles
School of Medicine
Reed Neurological Research Center
Center for the Health Sciences
Los Angeles, California 90024

Antonio Delgado-Escueta, M.D.
Department of Neurology
University of California at Los Angeles School of Medicine, Los Angeles, California 90024; and
Comprehensive Epilepsy Program (UCLA) and Veterans Administration Southwest Regional Epilepsy Center
West Los Angeles Veterans Administration Medical Center (Wadsworth)
Los Angeles, California 90024

Fritz E. Dreifuss, M.B., F.R.C.P., F.R.A.C.P.
Department of Neurology
School of Medicine
University of Virginia
Charlottesville, Virginia 22908; and
Comprehensive Epilepsy Program
University of Virginia Hospital
Charlottesville, Virginia 22901

John S. Ebersole, M.D.
Department of Neurology
Yale University School of Medicine
333 Cedar Street
New Haven, Connecticut 06510, and
Epilepsy Center
Neurology Service
Veterans Administration Medical Center
West Spring Street
West Haven, Connecticut 06516

Jerome Engel, Jr., M.D., Ph.D.
Department of Neurology and Anatomy
University of California at Los Angeles School of Medicine
Reed Neurological Research Center
Center for the Health Sciences
Los Angeles, California 90024

James D. Frost, Jr., M.D.
Department of Neurology
Baylor College of Medicine, and
The Methodist Hospital
6565 Fannin
Houston, Texas 77030

John R. Gates, M.D.
Department of Neurology
University of Minnesota; and
Clinical Neurophysiology Laboratory
Minnesota Comprehensive Epilepsy Program
2701 University Avenue S.E.
Suite 106
Minneapolis, Minnesota 55414

Jean Gotman, Ph.D.
Department of Neurology and Neurosurgery, and
The Montreal Neurological Institute
McGill University
3801 University Street
Montreal, Quebec, Canada H3A 2B4

Robert J. Gumnit, M.D.
Department of Neurology
University of Minnesota; and
Minnesota Comprehensive Epilepsy Program
2701 University Avenue S.E.
Suite 106
Minneapolis, Minnesota 55414

John Ives, M.Sc.
Department of Neuroelectronics
Beth Israel Hospital, and
Department of Neurology
Harvard Medical School
330 Brookline Avenue
Boston, Massachusetts 02215

Peter Kellaway, Ph.D.
Department of Neurology
Section of Neurophysiology
Epilepsy Research Center
Baylor College of Medicine
Texas Medical Center
Houston, Texas 77030

Alfonso G. Lee, M.D.
Comprehensive Epilepsy Program
University of California at Los Angeles School of Medicine
Los Angeles, California 90024

Ilo E. Leppik, M.D.
Department of Neurology
University of Minnesota; and
Antiepileptic Drug Research Laboratory
Comprehensive Epilepsy Program
2701 University Avenue S.E.
Suite 106
Minneapolis, Minnesota 55414

Hector M. Maldonado, M.D. Ph.D
Comprehensive Epilepsy Program
University of California at Los Angeles School of Medicine
Los Angeles, California 90024, and
Veterans Administration Southwest Regional Epilepsy Center
West Los Angeles Veterans Administration Medical Center (Wadsworth)
Los Angeles, California 90073

Richard Mattson, M.D.
Department of Neurology
Yale University School of Medicine
Veterans Administration Medical Center
Neurology Service
West Haven, Connecticut 06516

Venkat Ramani, M.D.
Department of Neurology and Psychiatry
Albany Medical College; and
Section of Epilepsy and Electroencephalography
Albany Medical Center Hospital
Albany, New York 12208

Gregory Stores, M.D., F.R.C.P., F.R.C. Psych.
Department of Neuropsychiatry
National Center for Children with Epilepsy, and
University of Oxford
Department of Psychiatry
Park Hospital for Children
Old Road Headington, Oxford, England

Barbara Swartz, M.D., Ph.D.
Comprehensive Epilepsy Program
University of California at Los Angeles School of Medicine
Los Angeles, California 90024, and
Veterans Administration Southwest Regional Epilepsy Center
West Los Angeles Veterans Administration Medical Center (Wadsworth)
Los Angeles, California 90073

Barry R. Tharp, M.D.
Department of Neurology
Division of Pediatric Neurology
Stanford University School of Medicine
Stanford, California 94305

Gregory O. Walsh, M.D.
Comprehensive Epilepsy Program
University of California at Los Angeles Medical School
Los Angeles, California 90024

Peter D. Williamson, M.D.
Department of Neurology
Yale University School of Medicine, and
Veterans Administration Medical Center
West Haven, Connecticut 06516

ADVANCES IN NEUROLOGY

Volume 46

Advances in Neurology, Vol. 46: Intensive Neurodiagnostic Monitoring, edited by R. J. Gumnit. Raven Press, New York © 1986.

Video Recording During Long-Term EEG Monitoring of Epileptic Patients

J. R. Ives

Department of Neuroelectronics, Beth Israel Hospital, Harvard Medical School, 340 Brookline Avenue, Boston, Massachusetts 02215

The principal goal of long-term video/EEG monitoring in patients with seizures is to provide simultaneous documentation of the clinical manifestations correlated to the EEG changes during the patient's ictal events or seizures. The present day video/EEG investigations stemmed from the use in the early 1930s (5) when Schwab et al. (19) developed and documented elaborate cinefilm techniques using mirrors and lenses to simultaneously record in a "split-screen" format the patient's behavior along with multichannel EEGs obtained from a conventional EEG machine (19). Figures 1A and 1B illustrate an early result taken from Stewart et al. (20). A summary of the variety of methods used was made in the studies of Stewart et al. (20) where the future potential of closed circuit television or video, as we now know it, was mentioned.

The use of cinefilm did produce very high quality pictures (Fig. 1), as demonstrated in the extensive work by Ajmone-Marsan and Abraham (1). Its corresponding drawbacks (tedious, expensive, operational for only short recording periods, lag time in obtaining results) have resulted in the present-day universal use of video for monitoring behavior in conjunction with the EEG.

When the videotape recorder required the hourly change of reel-to-reel videotapes, the use of a time-lapse videotape recorder permitted a single reel to last more than 24 hr, as demonstrated by Ives and Gloor (8) and Jestico et al. (10). This was extremely advantageous when used in conjunction with an automatic EEG recording system, Ives et al. (9). The 3 frames per second presentation created a "Charlie Chaplinish" picture, but it was an acceptable compromise to avoid hourly tape changes and produced relevant diagnostic information over a 24-hr unattended period (17).

With the standardization of the videotape cassette recorders (VCR) using either the VHS or Beta format, 6 or 8 hr can be obtained on one inexpensive cassette. Arrangements can be made to change the cassette when necessary or automatic switching to a second or third VCR can be obtained (4).

The commercialization of the VCR and the related technology now provides inexpensive, reliable, efficient, versatile video equipment that can be used either directly or with minor modification by long-term EEG monitoring labo-

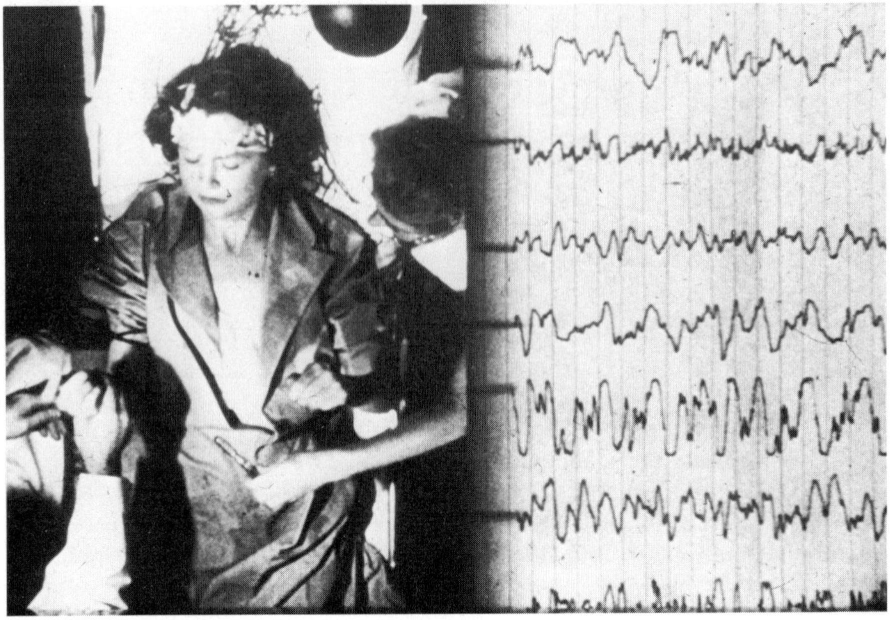

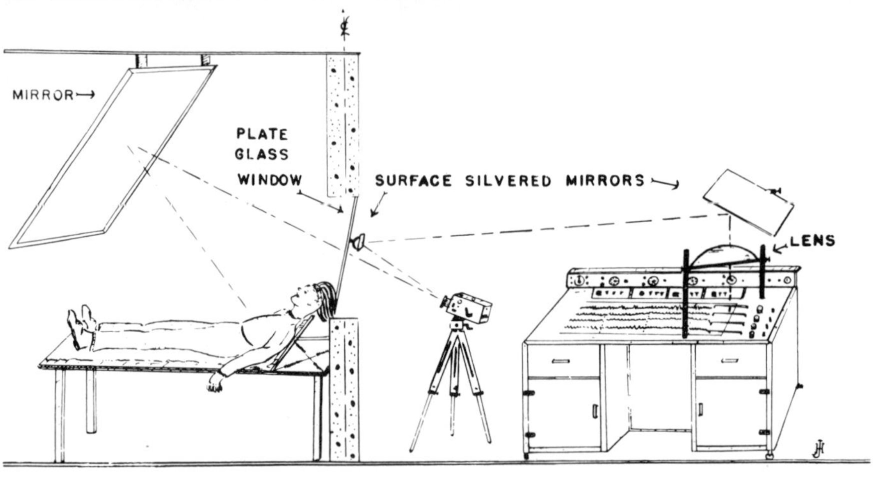

FIG. 1A and B. The "split-screen" image of both the patient and the EEG illustrates the use of cinefilm and its early importance for correlating the behavior with the EEG. (From ref. 20.)

ratories. It is best to obtain industrial grade equipment which ensures high quality as well as high reliability of the equipment. Expensive studio quality, broadcast-grade video equipment is no longer a necessity in order to obtain acceptable results. Thus, for video recording during long-term monitoring, the problems of technical standardization, cost, and reliability have been solved.

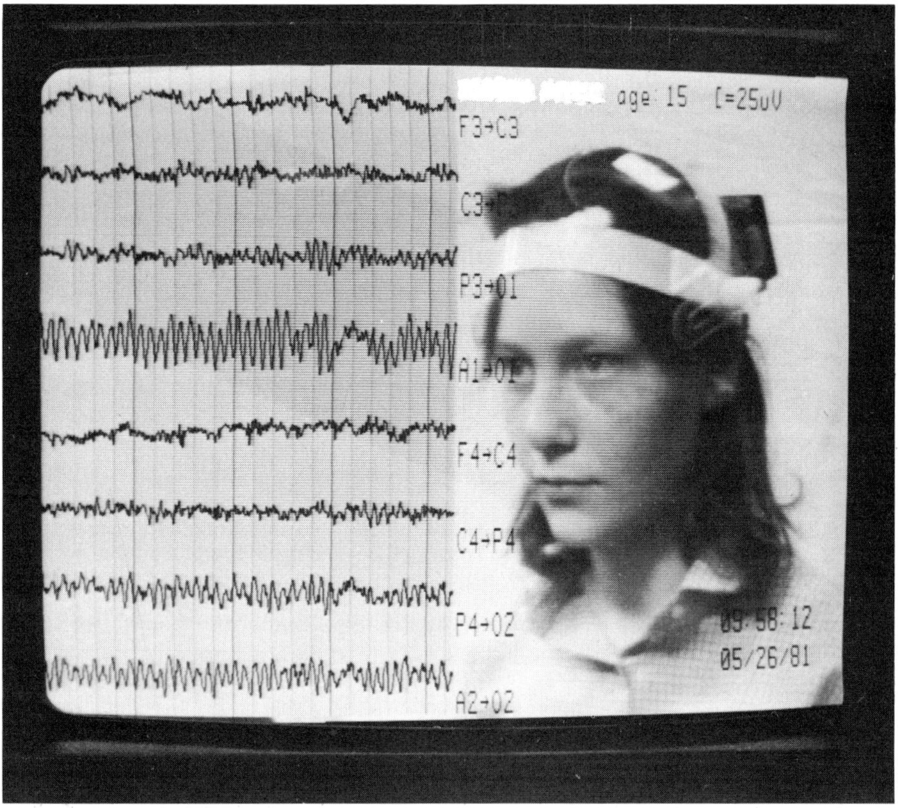

FIG. 2. Demonstrates the reformatting technique which permits viewing of both the patient's behavior and the time-locked EEG. A comparison between Fig. 1A and Fig. 2 illustrates the advancements over nearly a 30-year period. One is struck that, although technology permits one to obtain the above on an efficient, routine basis, the quality of both the EEG and the picture are slightly better in Fig. 1. (Photo courtesy of Telefactor Corporation, Inc.)

GENERAL VIDEO-EEG RECORDING TECHNIQUES

There are a variety of methods used to record both the EEG and the behavioral components of an epileptic patient. Generally, this can be broken down into two basic approaches: (a) EEG and video simultaneously recorded on the same medium, and (b) EEG and video separately recorded on different media but time-locked.

In the technique of simultaneously recording the EEG and the behavior of the patient on the video media, a variety of subtechniques have been used:

1. Two cameras, one for the patient and one for the EEG [Penry et al. (14)].
2. Reformatted (Fig. 2) [Porter et al. (15, 16); Sato et al. (18)].

3. Multiplexed EEG recorded on the audio track.
4. Multiplexed EEG digitally recorded with the video synchronized.

Methods 3 and 4 are available commercially from specialty suppliers.

General Advantages (Simultaneous)

The two separate events (EEG and behavior) are simultaneously recorded and therefore are automatically time-locked.

The recording equipment is the videotape itself and is easy to operate, inexpensive, and reliable.

A continuous recording time of 8 hr can be obtained in the extended mode.

Disadvantages

The replay of the EEG on a video screen may compromise the presentation of the EEG itself due to the video's limitations in frequency and dynamic range.

The replay of the EEG onto other media, e.g., back onto paper, requires a means of synchronization which is a similar problem to separating recordings as discussed below.

The quality of the EEG itself may suffer somewhat in the extended recording mode, especially if reformatting is used (2, 3).

General Advantages (Separate)

In the techniques of recording the multichannel EEG on one medium (e.g., paper, instrumentation tape recorder, cassette tape, digital tape, digital disc, etc.) and the behavior on the usual video media, the main advantage is that the EEG is recorded by an independent, dedicated means, and thus quality can be maintained throughout the recording and playback. An interesting use of this technique has been made by Bio-Medical Systems by using two videotape recorders, one to record the usual clinical activity and the other to record up to 32 channels of digitized EEG (12).

Disadvantages

The main disadvantage is the requirement of a time-locking device such as a common time-of-day (TOD) clock, and the ability to move rapidly and accurately from looking at one medium to another.

An early solution to this problem permitted "blip" time codes to be simultaneously recorded which could be used to time-lock the events. At the practical level, this was difficult to read. A reasonable solution to this was to write out a numerical-like trace which permitted the time of day to be easily read from the paper record (6, 7), or use an ink-jet type of EEG machine that writes out the time directly as readable numbers.

SOME BASIC PROBLEMS

Seizure Frequency

The frequency of the seizures or attacks experienced by the patient can also play an important part in the design of an intensive EEG-video monitoring system and the selection of equipment. The ideal situation, of course, is the one in which the patient's seizure or attack can be obtained on demand, and therefore can be induced at an opportune time. Unfortunately, this type of seizure is rare (particularly with the focal seizure patient group) and can usually be dealt with using conventional EEG and direct observation by the interested parties. The majority of cases have infrequent and unpredictable times for spontaneous seizures or attacks (Fig. 3).

The frequency of attacks or seizures or complaints can be grouped as follows: A, 1 to 2 times per hour; B, 1 to 2 times per day; C, 1 to 2 times per week; D, 1 to 2 times per month; and E, 1 to 2 times per year.

In case A, the high frequency of the attacks is easy to capture using conventional EEG recording methods. In cases D and E, the frequency of attacks is out of range even for long-term monitoring. In cases B and C, the attack frequency is within range of long-term monitoring. It is also the attack frequency experienced by most patients.

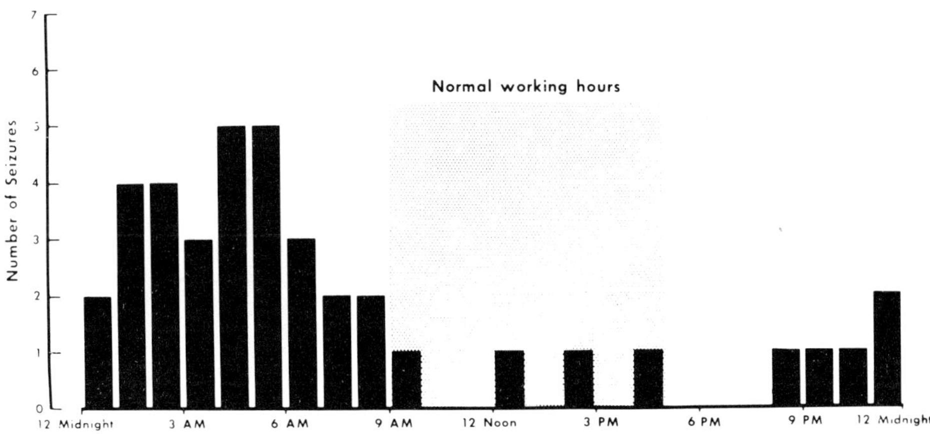

FIG. 3. This graph of the number of seizures occurring over a 20-day in-hospital period plotted on the 24-hr clock demonstrates the difficulty in capturing spontaneous seizures on a 9 A.M. to 5 P.M. Monday to Friday working hour basis. This patient's seizure frequency is very typical of patients with temporal lobe epilepsy (psychomotor, partial complex). Number of observed seizures: 20; average: 2 per day. A.C.: 17 years.

Time of Day of the Attack

In the purely nonepileptic group, the time of the attack is usually during the daytime waking hours, although some patients do indicate that sometimes they are awakened during sleep.

In the true epilepsy group, the majority of seizures statistically occur during the sleep or transient sleep/awake–awake/sleep times. More important, at the practical level, most seizures occur outside of normal working hours as is shown (Fig. 3) in a typical patient with partial complex seizures. In this patient, who was having approximately two seizures per day, if only the hours of 9 a.m. to 5 p.m., Monday to Friday, was available for intensive monitoring, the patient would require approximately 20 days in the hospital to ensure documentation of two or three seizures.

PATIENT'S SEIZURE TYPE AND PURPOSE OF LONG-TERM MONITORING

For organizational simplicity, the classification of the patient's complaint and purpose of performing a long-term EEG-video monitoring on a patient may be expressed as:

1. Nonepileptic versus epilepsy.
2. Documentation of the patient's spontaneous epileptic seizures for (a) classification for diagnosis and treatment; (b) establishing seizure frequency for medication effectiveness; and (c) localization for surgical intervention.

The above have a natural emphasis either for the importance of the EEG over the video or vice versa. In other words, if, in retrospect, a patient has only nonepileptic seizures, the EEG is expected to be negative, while the video documentation of the actual behavior changes during the attack becomes the primary method of making the diagnosis. This is based on the specific activity of the patient during the attack, and whether or not it is consistent with known seizure behavior. It should be emphasized that a negative EEG does not necessarily rule out epilepsy, however, the fact that an EEG demonstrating only muscle and movement artifact mixed with alpha while the patient is clinically involved in a generalized tonic-clonic seizure may significantly contribute to the diagnosis of psychologically induced nonepileptic seizures.

At the other extreme, in a patient being considered for the surgical removal of brain tissue for the treatment of intractable focal epilepsy, the specific details of the EEG are of paramount importance, while the video behavior may only be used to establish that the EEG changes occurred before the clinical changes. Even the most dramatic clinical localization aspect such as head turning cannot be localized or lateralized correctly without the EEG (13). The most significant contribution of the video in this situation is to establish whether the EEG changes or the clinical seizure manifests itself first and the delay before response in the other. If a clinical seizure begins significantly before the change occurs in the EEG (surface or depth), then the seizure focus may be a significant distance from the recording electrodes. Therefore, the type of patients being investigated may influence the emphasis and significance of the two different activities (EEG and behavior) that one is simultaneously monitoring.

SET-UPS: FIXED BASE VERSUS MOBILE

In the establishment of an EEG-video long-term seizure monitoring system, there are basically two physical locations for performing the examination.

The first is to set up a permanent studio or suite where the patient is brought to be monitored in a controlled environment. The second is to develop a mobile monitoring procedure whereby the equipment is brought to and set up in the patient's primary care area.

Suite

In this situation, a dedicated room is established to monitor the patient's behavior and both the clinical activity and the EEG are instrumentated in an elaborate fashion to provide multiple views of the patient as well as multichannel EEG (2, 18). In this controlled environment, the lighting can be specially designed to provide optimum exposure of the subject. The audio can be established to provide input not only from the patient but also the attending staff. With remote pan, tilt and zoom facilities, the patient can be continuously followed and close-ups of important specific behaviors studied. Up to two or three operators may be needed to efficiently operate the systems in order to maintain the high quality of the video and the EEG during normal patient activities. Obviously, if the patient is cooperative or produces seizures at a reasonable frequency, this is probably the best facility to use. If one is dealing mainly with infrequent seizures (as demonstrated by the patient in Fig. 2) which occur outside working hours, then this type of set-up can become very expensive to maintain. Such patients are best handled in very specialized centers.

Mobile

If all the equipment can be mounted on a mobile cart, it can be brought to the patient's bedside and set up within the patient's normal care area (Fig. 4A and B).

PERSONNEL

Usually, three levels of staffing can be used: (a) continuous/dedicated (11); (b) continuous/observation (12); and (c) casual/periodic/normal nursing (4).

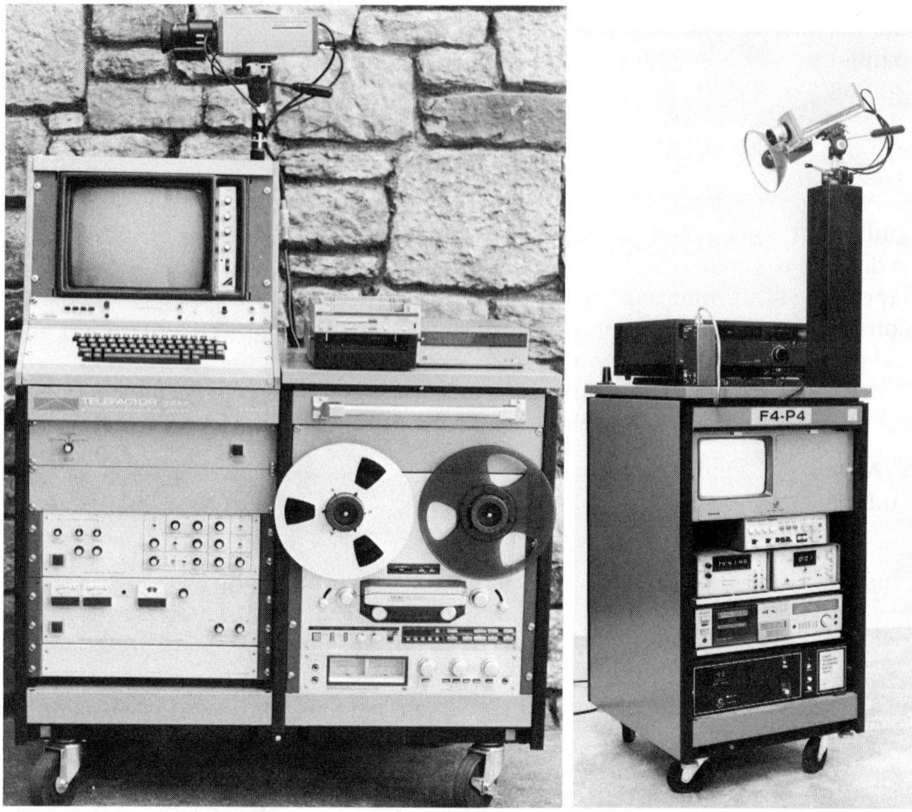

FIG. 4A and B. The configuration of some typical mobile EEG-video monitoring systems which are self-contained units that can be moved easily to the patient's bedside. (Photos courtesy of Telefactor Corporation and Ives Ambulatory Instrumentation, Inc., respectively.)

Obviously, the most efficient level of staffing would be to have one person dealing with the EEG and another one or two people interreacting with the video, e.g., pin, tilt, zoom, and audio, while another interacted with the patient. If a seizure occurred under these conditions, then a great deal of relevant, correlated information would be obtained. At the practical level, this would only work with very frequent or induced seizures. Even if seizures occurred daily, this level of intensive monitoring could not be maintained routinely due to the strain on both patient and staff.

At the next level, one person assigned to the patient/EEG/video with the aid of some automatic devices can very efficiently keep track of the activity of a patient and interreact with him to obtain subjective feelings or states.

At the last level, no one is responsible for the EEG or the video, while the responsibility for the patient rests with the usual nursing staff.

In general, decreasing cost is associated with decreasing effectiveness. At the practical level, the choice of set-up greatly depends on the type of patient, the number of patients being investigated, and the seizure frequency of the patient.

Ambulatory

Although telemetered EEG permits the patient freedom of the nursing unit and ambulatory cassette recorder, and the complete freedom of going home, it is difficult to obtain simultaneous video. It is conceivable that a portable videotape recorder synchronized to the EEG could be operated by the patient's companion to provide simultaneous information during an event (Fig. 5).

Audio

Audio and video are usually recorded together but, in our experience, the audio component has never been found to provide consistent results because of

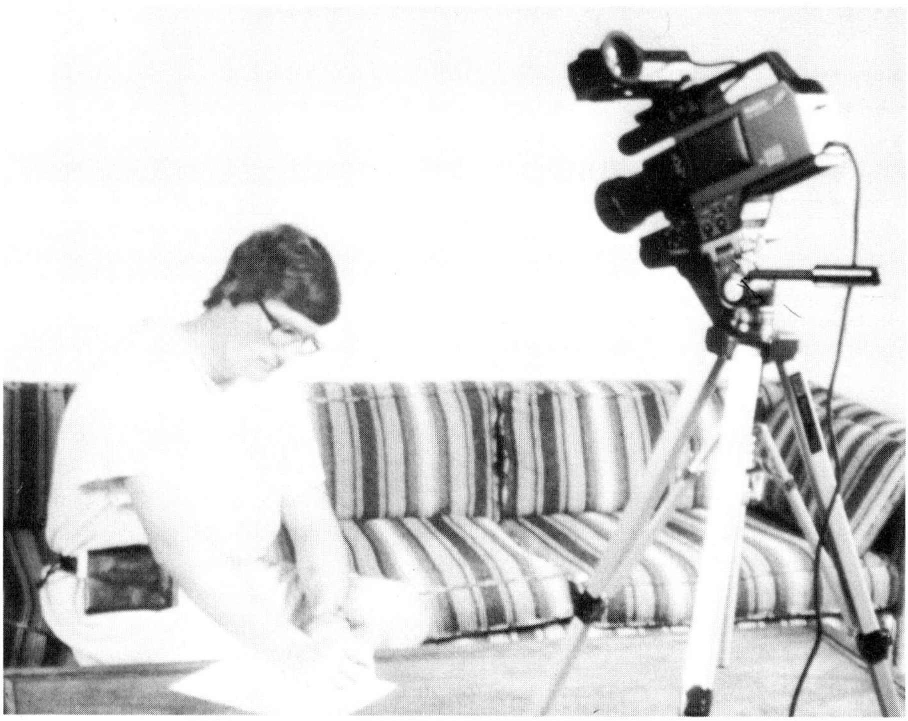

FIG. 5. Even if wearing an ambulatory recorder, the EEG and video can be correlated by recording a synchronizing TOD signal. This illustration demonstrates the practicality of this technique particularly in light of the recent advancements in the video industry of small, lightweight, completely integrated (camera and tape recorder) video systems. (Photo courtesy of Oxford Medilog, Inc.)

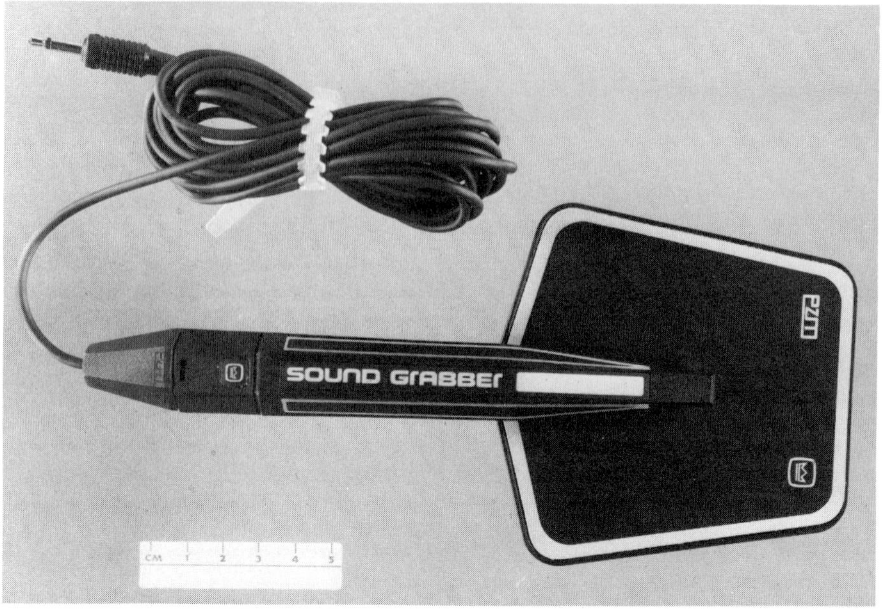

FIG. 6. A new microphone that has unique properties which are advantageous for long-term patient monitoring, particularly when used on the mobile units that are set in the patient's room.

a variety of factors: (a) directionality, (b) dynamic range, (c) sensitivity, (d) distance, and (e) background noise.

Recently, a small compact microphone available from Crown International, Inc. (Model SG-12, called a "sound grabber," "pressure zone microphone," or "flyswatter") has demonstrated unique properties for recording audio from patients' hospital rooms (Fig. 6).

CONCLUSION

The use of video coverage of the patient's behavior changes correlated with the EEG in evaluating epileptic patients has become a well-established routine that can be accomplished simply and inexpensively by most laboratories.

REFERENCES

1. Ajmone-Marsan, C., and Abraham, K. (1960): A seizure atlas. *Electroencephalogr. Clin. Neurophysiol.,* Suppl. 15:215pp.
2. Binnie, C.D., Aarts, J.H.P., van Bentum-De Boer, P.T.E., and Wisman, T. (1985): Monitoring at the Instituut voor Epilepsiebestrijding Meer En Bosch. In: *Long-Term Monitoring in Epilepsy,* edited by J. Gotman, J.R. Ives, and P. Gloor. Elsevier, New York, pp. 341–355.

3. Ebersole, J.S., Mattson, R.H., Williamson, T.D., Spencer, S.S., and Glaser, G.H. (1985): Monitoring at the West Haven VA/Yale University School of Medicine Epilepsy Center. In: *Long-Term Monitoring in Epilepsy,* edited by J. Gotman, J.R. Ives, and P. Gloor. Elsevier, New York, pp. 357–369.
4. Gotman, J., Ives, J.R., Gloor, P., Quesney, L.F., and Bergsma, P. (1985): Monitoring at the Montreal Neurological Institute. In: *Long-Term Monitoring in Epilepsy,* edited by J. Gotman, J.R. Ives, and P. Gloor. Elsevier, New York, pp. 327–340.
5. Hunter, J., and Jasper, H.H. (1949): A method of analysis of seizure pattern and electroencephalogram: a cinematographic technique. *Electroencephalogr. Clin. Neurophysiol.,* 1:113–114.
6. Ives, J.R. (1984): "Time-Scribe": A universal time writer for any EEG/polygraph chart recorder. *Electroencephalogr. Clin. Neurophysiol.,* 57:388–391.
7. Ives, J.R. (1985): Recording the time of day. In: *Long-Term Monitoring In Epilepsy,* edited by J. Gotman, J.R. Ives, and P. Gloor. Elsevier, New York, pp. 83–89.
8. Ives, J.R., and Gloor, P. (1978): A long-term time-lapse video system to document the patient's spontaneous clinical seizure synchronized with the EEG. *Electroencephalogr. Clin. Neurophysiol.,* 45:412–416.
9. Ives, J.R., Thompson, C.G., and Gloor, P. (1976): Seizure monitoring: a new tool in electroencephalography. *Electroencephalogr. Clin. Neurophysiol.,* 45:412–416.
10. Jestico, J., Fitch, P., Gilliatt, R.W., and Willison, R.G. (1977): Automatic and rapid visual analysis of sleep stages and epileptic activity. A preliminary report. *Electroencephalogr. Clin. Neurophysiol.,* 43:438–441.
11. Kellaway, P., and Frost, J.D. (1985): Monitoring at the Baylor College of Medicine, Houston. In: *Long-Term Monitoring In Epilepsy,* edited by J. Gotman, J.R. Ives, and P. Gloor. Elsevier, New York, pp. 403–414.
12. Nuwer, M.R., Engel, J., Sutherling, W.W., and Babb, T.L. (1985): Monitoring at the University of California, Los Angeles. In: *Long-Term Monitoring in Epilepsy,* edited by J. Gotman, J.R. Ives, and P. Gloor. Elsevier, New York, pp. 385–401.
13. Ochs, R., Gloor, P., Quesney, F., Ives, J.R., and Olivier, A. (1984): Does head turning during a seizure have lateralizing or localizing significance? *Neurology,* 34:884–890.
14. Penry, J.K., Porter, R.J., and Dreifuss, F.E. (1975): Simultaneous recording of absence seizures with video tape and electroencephalography. *Brain,* 98:427–440.
15. Porter, R.J., Penry, J.K., and Wolf, A.A., Jr. (1976): Simultaneous documentation of clinical and electrographic manifestations of epileptic seizures. In: *Quantitative Analytic Studies in Epilepsy,* edited by P. Kellaway and I. Petersen, pp. 253–268. Raven Press, New York.
16. Porter, R.J., Sato, S., and Lang, R. (1985): Video recording. In: *Long-Term Monitoring in Epilepsy,* edited by J. Gotman, J.R. Ives, and P. Gloor. Elsevier, New York, pp. 73–82.
17. Quesney, L.F., and Gloor, P. (1985): Localization of epileptic foci. In: *Long-Term Monitoring in Epilepsy,* edited by J. Gotman, J.R. Ives, and P. Gloor. Elsevier, New York, pp. 165–200.
18. Sato, S., Long, R.L., and Porter, R.J. (1985): Monitoring at the National Institute of Neurological and Communicative Disorders and Stroke. In: *Long-Term Monitoring in Epilepsy,* edited by J. Gotman, J.R. Ives, and P. Gloor. Elsevier, New York, pp. 415–422.
19. Schwab, R.S., Schwab, M.W., Wither, D., and Chock, Y.C. (1954): Synchronized moving pictures of patients and EEG. *Electroencephalogr. Clin. Neurophysiol.,* 6:684–686.
20. Stewart, L.F., Jasper, H.H., and Hodge, C. (1956): Another simple method for simultaneous cinematographic recording of the patient and his electroencephalogram during seizures. *Electroencephalogr. Clin. Neurophysiol.,* 8:688–691.

Advances in Neurology, Vol. 46: Intensive Neurodiagnostic Monitoring, edited by R. J. Gumnit. Raven Press, New York © 1986.

Role of Intensive Monitoring in Classification

Fritz E. Dreifuss

Department of Neurology, School of Medicine, University of Virginia, Charlottesville, Virginia 22908

Recent activity in the classification of epileptic seizures and in the classification of the epilepsies has been based on the ability to accurately identify (a) individual seizure types, (b) the progression of one type of seizure into another during the course of a single seizure, and (c) the repertoire of different seizures and other symptoms allowing the identification of epileptic syndromes. Much of this activity has resulted from the technological advances in video recording, long-term electroencephalographic monitoring, and the incorporation of both into the clinical armamentarium.

Throughout history, attempts at classification of seizures and the epilepsies have gone *pari passu* with existing knowledge about these disorders. The ability to discern and describe events in the seizure repertoire has been a limiting factor. It is certain that the recent advances in knowledge, a better inheritance prognosis, and improved therapy of seizures have resulted from the ability to distinguish accurately between different seizure forms, and to objectively identify and measure their effects.

RATIONALE FOR CLASSIFICATION

From the earliest days of attempts at classification, one aim had to do with recognition of the disorder under study. Galen already recognized that seizures might primarily be due to disorders in the brain, or secondarily due to disorders elsewhere in the body, though it would be presumptuous to assume that such words as idiopathic and symptomatic had identical meaning in his day as that ascribed to the second half of the twentieth century. In 1824, Calmeil introduced a classification based on severity. Delasiauve spoke of idiopathic seizures without demonstrable anatomical lesion, symptomatic where there was such a lesion, and sympathetic to describe seizures due to effect on the brain of diseases elsewhere. In the latter part of the 19th century, Hughlings Jackson proposed that classification should include anatomical localization, physiologic disturbance, and pathologic process; and he introduced the concept of generalized and partial seizures, the former called "genuine epilepsy," and the latter "convulsions beginning unilaterally." Jackson ascribed generalized seizures to the "highest level" and partial seizures to a focal cortical discharge.

The concept of relating clinical events to ictal electroencephalographic findings and interictal electroencephalographic correlation was introduced in the international classification of epileptic seizures of 1969. The main feature of the 1969 classification was a distinction between seizures that were generalized from the beginning, and those that were partial or focal at onset and became generalized secondarily. Objective methods for documenting seizures have come into common use in the past decade. Such methods include prolonged EEG recording and the use of videotape, allowing for capture and availability for review of individual seizures. More accurate recognition of individual symptoms during seizures and their elaboration during the course of the seizure has resulted from the application of intensive monitoring technology. In addition, other factors such as anatomical substrate, etiology, and age factors based on other information than intensive monitoring are, at present, being incorporated into a definition of epileptic syndromes.

The 1981 classification of epileptic seizures (3) resulted from the increased information imparted by intensive monitoring capability. Thus, unlike the 1969 version, the current classification schema allows for longitudinal description of evolving seizure manifestations, thereby greatly improving descriptive accuracy. By repetitive replay of videotape, distinctions can be made between simple partial seizures and complex partial seizures because one is able to discern changes in a person's awareness and responsiveness which previously had been sufficiently evanescent to escape observer detection, particularly if the observer was not with the patient at all times. The 1981 classification owes its success to these techniques of better recognition.

Central to the problem of classification of seizures and epileptic syndromes is the recognition of those attacks which are superficially indistinguishable, which with intensive monitoring may be identified as nonepileptic. Not all recurrent episodes of loss of consciousness represent epilepsy, and not all episodes of loss of consciousness in persons with epilepsy are epileptic. Syncope (2), cardiac, vasovagal (11, 18), or reflex may present with loss of consciousness. Many cases of potentially lethal cardiac disease (9, 28), as well as relatively trivial or event-related alterations of the conscious state, may be distinguished by the application of provocative tests while the patient is monitored. Vertigo, periodic syndromes of children including recurrent abdominal pain and/or headache, hyperventilation, breath holding, and various episodic attacks occurring during sleep may be identified if the patient can be appropriately monitored for a prolonged period of time and a relationship established between the seizures, other events, and EEG manifestations (19). A major subgroup of nonepileptic seizures are psychogenic seizures—nonepileptic events associated with a variety of psychological mechanisms. Psychogenic seizures are common both by themselves and in association with epilepsy, and many persons are treated with inappropriate amounts of anticonvulsant medication because of persistence of seizures when, in fact, this persistence is on the basis of attacks other than epilepsy (10, 12, 13).

It is of importance that for purposes of communication there is unanimity of terminology. The common coin of the realm of communication is uniform language, and this has been contributed to by a classification and terminology based on uniform observation. This is particularly true of the classification of epilepsy syndromes which has engaged the Commission on Terminology and Classification of the International League Against Epilepsy (ILAE) for the past 3 years (4). Syndromes are concatenations of symptoms including seizure type, etiology, precipitating factors, age of onset, severity, chronicity, diurnal and circadian cycling, family history, and prognosis. Syndromes are also conditions about which physicians communicate, rather than seizure types, and include such things as infantile spasm syndrome, Lennox-Gastaut syndrome, benign juvenile myoclonus syndrome, etc. These will be further described (*vide infra*).

A further rationale for classification into seizure types and epilepsy syndromes is the use of the most appropriate therapeutic regimen. The development of more and more specific anticonvulsant drugs for individual seizure types has mandated the identification of individual seizure types with great accuracy. In addition, the recognition of the deleterious effects of anticonvulsant medication has emphasized the importance of the judicious use of such medications. The prevention of deleterious consequences of anticonvulsant therapy can be minimized by its most appropriate application and, on occasion, its avoidance and its relatively early discontinuation when the seizure syndrome is such that a benign prognosis may be predicted. Thus, classification has the further rationale of a pragmatic goal, namely, the most appropriate utilization of treatment, the judicious withholding of treatment, and the prediction of prognosis on which may be predicated the decision as to whether and when to attempt the termination of treatment.

USES OF MONITORING

Classification of Epileptic Seizures

In the 1981 classification (3), only clinical seizure type and ictal and interictal electroencephalographic expressions are used. The anatomic substrate, etiology, and age factors were deleted, as these were felt to be relevant more to a classification of the epilepsies than of epileptic seizures; and in a description of seizures rather than epilepsy, the seizures themselves should be the only consideration. The classification was entirely based on visualization of seizures and EEG simultaneously, and no seizure type was included in the classifications which had not been verified by combined video and EEG viewed by members of the Commission of Classification at workshop sessions. The subclassification of absence seizures, the distinction of absence simple and complex partial seizures with impairment of consciousness only (23), and of absence with automatisms and complex partial seizures with automatisms (6) continues to be predicated upon the availability of intensive monitoring techniques (19–26, 30–32).

The classification of epileptic seizures (3) appears in Table 1.

For purposes of classification it is essential that seizures be viewed. This may only require a regular EEG with simultaneous video display or it might require a prolonged recording with attacks precipitated by withdrawal of anticonvulsant drugs and sleep deprivation activation (31, 32).

Between 1975 and the adoption of the present classification of epileptic seizures in 1981, the Commission on Classification and Terminology of the ILAE convened several workshops. One of these concentrated on complex partial seizures, another on generalized seizures, and a third on the variations of absence seizures. Each of these workshops was attended by persons from throughout the world who had made a study of specific seizure types using video techniques and who provided videotape for discussion at the workshops. Each seizure type described in the 1981 classification was viewed by 12 or more persons who replayed each seizure several times until consensus was reached as to what was being observed and where the observed phenomena fit into the proposed classification. In turn, the proposed classification was molded to incorporate the observed phenomena. The conclusions of individual workshop seminars were circulated to all the Chapters of the ILAE and the feedback was provided to the Commission and incorporated into subsequent revisions.

Though unanimity of points of view was not total, disagreements were confined to semantics rather than substantive differences, as the latter had been resolved by repeated viewing of individual seizures and the nuances of their presentation and evolution both clinically and electrographically. The classification thus represents a synthesis of the efforts of many persons examining hundreds of seizures over many years, as was stated by the Commission in its report: "This compilation of knowledge has been brought in line with the state-of-the-art technology without extrapolating to what cannot be observed, but cognizant of the evanescence of any living semantic endeavor which must remain subject to continual revision."

Differential Diagnosis

The differential diagnosis of some seizure types, as previously described, namely, between absence seizures and complex partial seizures, may be difficult on occasion. The monitoring technique here is supplemented by activation techniques such as hyperventilation, and prolonged recording is rarely necessary.

The differential diagnosis of epilepsy from other conditions causing loss of consciousness with or without convulsive activity may, however, require pro-

TABLE 1.

I. PARTIAL (FOCAL, LOCAL) SEIZURES

Partial seizures are those in which, in general, the first clinical and electroencephalographic changes indicate initial activation of a system of neurons limited to part of one cerebral hemisphere. A partial seizure is classified primarily on the basis of whether or not consciousness is impaired during the attack. When consciousness is not impaired, the seizure is classified as a simple partial seizure. When consciousness is impaired, the seizure is classified as a complex partial seizure. Impairment of consciousness may be the first clinical sign, or simple partial seizures may evolve into complex partial seizures. In patients with impaired consciousness, aberrations of behavior (automatisms) may occur. A partial seizure may not terminate, but instead progress to a generalized motor seizure. Impaired consciousness is defined as the inability to respond normally to exogenous stimuli by virtue of altered awareness and/or responsiveness (vide infra: Definition of Terms).

There is considerable evidence that simple partial seizures usually have unilateral hemispheric involvement and only rarely have bilateral hemispheric involvement; complex partial seizures, however, frequently have bilateral hemispheric involvement.

Partial seizures can be classified into one of the following three fundamental groups:

A. Simple partial seizures
B. Complex partial seizures
   1. With impairment of consciousness at onset
   2. Simple partial onset followed by impairment of consciousness
C. Partial seizures evolving to generalized tonic-clonic convulsions (GTC)
   1. Simple evolving to GTC
   2. Complex evolving to GTC (including those with simple partial onset)

Clinical seizure type	EEG seizure type	EEG interictal expression
A. *Simple partial seizures* (consciousness not impaired)	Local contralateral discharge starting over the corresponding area of cortical representation (not always recorded on the scalp)	Local contralateral discharge
1. With motor signs (a) focal motor without march (b) Focal motor with march (Jacksonian) (c) Versive (d) Postural (e) Phonatory (vocalization or arrest of speech)		
2. With somatosensory or special-sensory symptoms (simple hallucinations, e.g., tingling, light flashes, buzzing) (a) Somatosensory (b) Visual (c) Auditory (d) Olfactory (e) Gustatory (f) Vertiginous		
3. With autonomic symptoms or signs (including epigastric sensation, pallor, sweating, flushing, piloerection and pupillary dilatation)		
4. With psychic symptoms (disturbance of higher cerebral function). These symptoms rarely occur without impairment of consciousness and are much more commonly experienced as complex partial seizures (a) Dysphasic (b) Dysmnesic (e.g., déjà-vu) (c) Cognitive (e.g., dreamy states, distortions of time sense) (d) Affective (fear, anger, etc.)		

(contd.)

Clinical seizure type	EEG seizure type	EEG interictal expression
(e) Illusions (e.g., macropsia) (f) Structured hallucinations (e.g., music, scenes)		
B. *Complex partial seizures* (with impairment of consciousness; may sometimes begin with simple symptomatology)	Unilateral or, frequently bilateral discharge, diffuse or focal in temporal or frontotemporal regions	Unilateral or bilateral generally asynchronous focus; usually in the temporal or frontal regions
1. Simple partial onset followed by impairment of consciousness (a) With simple partial features (A.1.–A.4.) followed by impaired consciousness (b) With automatisms 2. With impairment of consciousness at onset (a) With impairment of consciousness only (b) With automatisms		
C. *Partial seizures evolving to secondarily generalized seiures* (This may be generalized tonic-clonic, tonic, or clonic)	Above discharges become secondarily and rapidly generalized	
1. Simple partial seizures (A) evolving to generalized seizures 2. Complex partial seizures (B) evolving to generalized seizures 3. Simple partial seizures evolving to complex partial seizures evolving to generalized seizures		

II. GENERALIZED SEIZURES (CONVULSIVE OR NONCONVULSIVE)

Generalized seizures are those in which the first clinical changes indicate initial involvement of both hemispheres. Consciousness may be impaired and this impairment may be the initial manifestation. Motor manifestations are bilateral. The ictal electroencephalographic patterns initially are bilateral, and presumably reflect neuronal discharge which is widespread in both hemispheres.

Clinical seizure type	EEG seizure type	EEG interictal expression
A. 1. *Absence seizures*	Usually regular and symmetrical 3 Hz but may be 2–4 Hz spike-and-slow-wave complexes and may have multiple spike-and-slow-wave complexes. Abnormalities are bilateral	Background activity usually normal although paroxysmal activity (such as spikes or spike-and-slow-wave complexes) may occur. This activity is usually regular and symmetrical
(a) Impairment of consciousness only (b) With mild clonic components (c) With atonic components		

(*contd.*)

Clinical seizure type	EEG seizure type	EEG interictal expression
(d) With tonic components (e) With automatisms (f) With autonomic components (b through f may be used alone or in combination)		
2. *Atypical absence*	EEG more heterogeneous; may include irregular spike-and-slow-wave complexes, fast activity or other paroxysmal activity. Abnormalities are bilateral but often irregular and asymmetrical	Background usually abnormal; paroxysmal activity (such as spikes or spike-and-slow-wave complexes) frequently irregular and asymmetrical
May have: (a) Changes in tone that are more pronounced than in A.1 (b) Onset and/or cessation that is not abrupt		
B. *Myoclonic seizures* Myoclonic jerks (single or multiple)	Polyspike and wave, or sometimes spike and wave or sharp and slow waves	Same as ictal
C. *Clonic seizures*	Fast activity (10 c/sec or more) and slow waves; occasional spike-and-wave patterns	Spike-and-wave or polyspike-and-wave discharges
D. *Tonic seizures*	Low voltage, fast activity or a fast rhythm of 9–10 c/sec or more decreasing in frequency and increasing in amplitude	More or less rhythmic discharges of sharp and slow waves, sometimes asymmetrical. Background is often abnormal for age
E. *Tonic-clonic seizures*	Rhythm at 10 or more c/sec decreasing in frequency and increasing in amplitude during tonic phase, interrupted by slow waves during clonic phase	Polyspike and waves or spike and wave, or, sometimes, sharp and slow wave discharges
F. *Atonic seizures* (Astatic) (combinations of the above may occur, e.g., B and F, B and D)	Polyspikes and wave or flattening or low-voltage fast activity	Polyspikes and slow wave

III. UNCLASSIFIED EPILEPTIC SEIZURES

Includes all seizures that cannot be classified because of inadequate or incomplete data and some that defy classification in hitherto described categories. This includes some neonatal seizures, e.g., rhythmic eye movements, chewing, and swimming movements.

IV. ADDENDUM

Repeated epileptic seizures occur under a variety of circumstances:

1. as fortuitous attacks, coming unexpectedly and without any apparent provocation; 2. as cyclic attacks, at more or less regular intervals (e.g., in relation to the menstrual cycle, or the sleep-waking cycle); 3. as attacks provoked by: (a) nonsensory factors (fatigue, alcohol, emotion, etc.), or (b) sensory factors, sometimes referred to as "reflex seizures."

Prolonged or repetitive seizures (status epilepticus). The term "status epilepticus" is used whenever a seizure persists for a sufficient length of time or is repeated frequently enough that recovery between attacks does not occur. Status epilepticus may be divided into partial (e.g., Jacksonian), or generalized (e.g., absence status or tonic-clonic status). When very localized motor status occurs, it is referred to as epilepsia partialis continua.

From ref. 3.

longed and repeated monitoring and, on occasion, the application of polygraphic techniques including cardiac monitoring or ambulatory cassette-recording under conditions of exercise, stress, or alterations in the milieu. Polygraphic recording including cardiac monitoring is essential for the delineation of episodes of loss of consciousness on the basis of vasovagal syncope, cardiac syncope, for example, the Ward-Ramano syndrome with prolonged QT interval, and reflex syncope. Different types of breath-holding and hyperventilation and the recurrent syndromes in childhood including headache, abdominal pain, or vomiting may only be definitely identifiable with prolonged polygraphic ambulatory techniques. It is critical to make a distinction between seizures and migraine because, particularly in the childhood age group, inappropriate medication could have side effects which would be too high a price to pay for an inaccurate identification and classification of the child's problem (34).

The various sleep syndromes including narcolepsy, sleep terrors, hypnagogic hallucinations, hypnagogic myoclonus, sleep paralysis, and somnambulism may be distinguishable only by all-night recordings with sleep staging. Without the capability of all-night recording, the accurate identification and classification of recurrent syndromes occurring during sleep is a matter of guesswork and may lead to incorrect management. Polysomnographic monitoring rapidly resolves the problem and results in accurate categorization of the presenting symptom.

Of major differential diagnostic importance are psychogenic seizures which may occur alone in such conditions as malingering, Von Muenchausen syndrome, and under certain medicolegal conditions, or may occur as a hysterical manifestation when it is often seen in persons who are also suffering from epilepsy (10, 12, 13, 33). For accurate management it is essential that combined video/EEG be obtained which may require several monitoring sessions of several hours duration. Prolonged hospital observation may be needed. Here, a patient-triggered device for commencing recordings is frequently useful. On the other hand, some of the seizures occur following prolonged monitoring sessions just as the electrodes are being removed or with the patient out of camera range. Such an event is, however, in itself, sometimes of diagnostic significance.

Some nuances which may have therapeutic implications may be detected. For example, absence with mild clonic components may be distinguished from myoclonic absence. The former usually responds well to either ethosuximide or valproate therapy. The latter may respond only to a combination of ethosuximide and valproate, and much time may be gained by recognition of the seizure types (21, 22, 30, 31).

Communication

The limitation of the classification of epileptic seizures to description of individual seizure types is that the terminology which is used in daily communication between colleagues usually consists of description of syndromes. This is also true of diagnostic entries in hospital records, and communication between collaborators conducting clinical trials (27, 30). An epileptic syndrome is an epileptic disorder characterized by a cluster of signs and symptoms customarily occurring together, and these include such things as type of seizure, etiology, anatomy, precipitating factors, age of onset, severity, chronicity, diurnal and circadian cycling, and sometimes prognosis. Some syndromes are very specific, for example, benign rolandic epilepsy, juvenile myoclonic epilepsy (14, 16), the Lennox-Gastaut syndrome, and the infantile spasm syndrome.

The epilepsies may be classified according to seizure type and EEG findings, e.g., either partial or generalized, or according to etiology, that is, into idiopathic, genetic, or symptomatic. Or they may be anatomically localized, for example, into frontal lobe, rolandic, occipital, or temporal epilepsies; and, finally, they may be classified according to precipitating factors. Age of onset may be of importance, as may certain diurnal influences such as sleep or waking, as well as menstrual cycle. Also, there are specific diseases such as the progressive myoclonus epilepsies.

In tackling the problem of the classification of the epilepsies these factors are taken into account and the proposed classification is outlined in Table 2.

It will be noted that both in the case of localization-related epilepsies and in the case of generalized epilepsies there are subgroups of idiopathic and symptomatic; and this distinction is critical because clinically identical seizures may belong to one or other of these categories depending on factors other than the clinical appearance, such as neurological development, focal or generalized EEG findings, and the presence of a family history. These distinctions have major therapeutic implications both as to the type of treatment employed and the duration of therapy as determined by the prognosis for remission. The distinctions between temporal lobe epilepsies and frontal lobe epilepsies, and between limbic and extralimbic seizures are of critical importance in the design of patient management, both pharmacological and surgical. Such a distinction is predicated on combined video/EEG identification and the resulting classification is the product of workshop sessions with detailed review (4).

It is emphasized that in temporal lobe epilepsies, there is a distinction between hippocampal (or mesial basal limbic) epilepsy and amygdalar (or anterior polar amygdalar) epilepsy. The former is ushered in by motionless stare, oral or alimentary automatisms, and amnesia; the latter is characterized by gradual onset of unconsciousness, staring, automatisms, and amnesia, and autonomic and affective symptoms prevail (1, 7, 8).

Similarly, frontal lobe epilepsies are divided into supplementary motor, characterized by postural changes (e.g., fencing posture), speech arrest, incontinence, cingular seizures with initial sexual features and vegetative signs, orbitofrontal seizures with initial automatisms and olfactory hallucinations, and dorsolateral seizures with version, aphasia, and partial complex seizures with initial automatisms.

TABLE 2. *International classification of epilepsies and epileptic syndromes*

Localization-related (focal, local, partial) epilepsies and syndromes.
- Idiopathic with age-related onset. At present, two syndromes are established, but more may be identified in the future:
  - Benign childhood epilepsy with centro-temporal spike.
  - Childhood epilepsy with occipital paroxysm.
- Symptomatic. This category comprises syndromes of great individual variability, which will mainly be based on anatomical localization, clinical features, seizure types, and etiological factors (if known).

Generalized epilepsies and syndromes.
- Idiopathic, with age-related onset, listed in order of age. Other generalized idiopathic epilepsies, if they do not belong to one of the following syndromes, can still be classified as generalized idiopathic epilepsies:
  - Benign neonatal familial convulsions.
  - Benign neonatal convulsions.
  - Benign myoclonic epilepsy in infancy.
  - Childhood absence epilepsy (pyknolepsy).
  - Juvenile absence epilepsy.
  - Juvenile myoclonic epilepsy (impulsive petit mal).
  - Epilepsy with grand mal seizures (GTCS) on awakening.
- Idiopathic and/or symptomatic, in order of age of appearance:
  - West syndrome (infantile spasms, Blitz-Nick-Salaam Krämpfe).
  - Lennox-Gastaut syndrome.
  - Epilepsy with myoclonic-astatic seizures.
  - Epilepsy with myoclonic absences.
- Symptomatic:
  - Nonspecified etiology.
    - Early myoclonic encephalopathy.
  - Specific syndromes.
    - Epileptic seizures may complicate many disease states. Included under this heading are those diseases in which seizures are a presenting or predominant feature.

Epilepsies and syndromes undetermined as to whether they are focal or generalized.
- With both generalized and focal seizures.
  - Neonatal seizures.
  - Severe myoclonic epilepsy in infancy.
  - Epilepsy with continuous spike-waves during slow wave sleep.
  - Acquired epileptic aphasia (Landau-Kleffner syndrome).
- Without unequivocal generalized or focal features. This heading covers all cases with GTCS where clinical and EEG findings do not permit classification as clearly generalized or localization-related, such as in many cases of sleep grand mal.

Special syndromes.
- Situation-related seizures (Gelegenheitsanfalle).
  - Febrile convulsions.
  - Seizures related to other identifiable situations such as stress, hormonal changes, drugs, alcohol, or sleep deprivation.
- Isolated, apparently unprovoked epileptic events.
- Epilepsies characterized by specific modes of seizure precipitation.
- Chronic progressive epilepsia partialis continua of childhood.

The essence of these distinctions lies in the ability to observe onset and evolution and to evaluate these by reviewing the video-recorded events.

In order to devise the classification of the epilepsies, the Commission on Classification and Terminology again held several meetings and workshop sessions. The childhood epilepsy syndromes formed the basis of a meeting with video workshop participation by an international cadre of pediatric epileptologists, who spent many hours reviewing videotapes and electroencephalographic material to justify the delineation of the individual syndromes (29). A further workshop concentrated on idiopathic or primary epilepsies and symptomatic or secondary epilepsies. The results of this workshop are incorporated into the foregoing scheme proposed for the classification of the epilepsies. This scheme will be further refined and will be modified in accordance with recommendations which will be made after study of the proposal by the individual ILAE Chapters. As in the case of the classification of epileptic seizures, no syndrome has been included which has not received the scrutiny and consensus development made possible by repeated review of the data by the workshop participants, who were chosen for their specialized interest in the syndromes presented.

Implications of Classification for Therapy

All anticonvulsant drug therapies represent a compromise between the therapeutic efficacy and unwanted side effects, and the tempering of therapeutic enthusiasm with an acknowledgment of risks of adverse side effects. This dilemma is faced by everyone in the management of seizure disorders. Anticonvulsant drug therapy should not be entered into lightly, and once entered into, a decision should be made from time to time during the evolution of the treatment process as to the likelihood of future discontinuation of medication. The latter decision may be as important as the institution of treatment. Here the distinction between the two main syndromic subgroups, namely, the primary epilepsies and the secondary (lesional or symptomatic) epilepsies, is of signal importance.

The primary epilepsies are unassociated with underlying pathology, there is frequently a positive family history of similar seizure types, and the child has usually made normal progress up to the time of the development of seizures. Often the seizures are relatively self-limited and respond to medication if appropriately used. The secondary epilepsies have an anatomicopathological substrate; there are frequently neurological abnormalities and, associated with this, there is frequently abnormal neurological development. The seizures are frequent and more difficult to control. There may be a family history of seizures other than those under consideration. These subdivisions can be applied to nearly all the childhood seizure syndromes. Thus, neonatal convulsions may be benign, familial, and require no treatment. On the other hand, they may be secondary or lesional with a very severe prognosis. The infantile spasms may be idiopathic primary epilepsy with normal development prior to the onset of the condition with relatively good prognosis and relatively good response to appropriate therapy. On the other hand, they may be of early onset, on the basis of severe cerebral disease including anoxic encephalopathy, metabolic encephalopathy, etc., with a poor outlook and poor response to therapy, and, yet, seizure type identical to that of the more benign variant. Febrile seizures, again, come in the same two varieties, namely the idiopathic, benign febrile seizure characterized by normal neurological development, a strong family history of similar seizure type, and a seizure with short, nonfocal characteristics; and though it may recur, it is usually not associated with the development of subsequent epilepsy. The converse is true of secondary or lesional febrile seizures. The importance of this distinction is that simple febrile seizures of a benign variety may not require treatment, and the risk benefit analysis may be in favor of withholding therapy because of the side effects of phenobarbital and the potential side effects of valproate which are the drugs of choice in the prevention of febrile seizures. On the other hand, the risk benefit analysis may be in favor of treatment in the secondary variety where the recurrent rate is great, the chance of severe seizures is increased, and the prognosis is less good as regards the development of subsequent epilepsy. Astatic myoclonic seizures, again, consist of two varieties including a relatively benign form described by Kruse (17) and Doose (5), and a severe form, the Lennox-Gastaut syndrome. The former variety responds relatively well to valproate, whereas the latter is relatively intractable to most anticonvulsant drugs and the prognosis with regard to intellectual development is grave. Absence seizures allow themselves to be classified into the same two categories. The primary generalized epilepsy presenting as absence seizures responds well to treatment, where some very similar-appearing secondary or lesional epilepsies are relatively intractable and the prognosis for spontaneous remission is much greater in the first than in the second variety.

The application of video and combined video and EEG recording has contributed to major advances in the identification and management of the epilepsies. Further improvement will occur as we increase our knowledge.

REFERENCES

1. Balafsky, M.A., Carwille, S., Miller, P., Waddell, G., Boxley-Johnson, J., and Delgado-Escueta, A.V. (1979): Prolonged epileptic twilight states: Continuous recordings with nasopharyngeal electrodes and videotape analysis. *Neurology,* 28:239–245.
2. Boudoulas, H., Schaal, S.F., Lewis, R.P., and Robinson, J.L. (1979): Superiority of 24-hour outpatient monitoring over multi-stage exercise testing for the evaluation of syncope. *J. Electrocardiol.,* 12(1):103–108.
3. Commission on Classification and Terminology of the International League Against Epilepsy (1981): Proposal for revised clinical and electroencephalographic classification of epileptic seizures. *Epilepsia,* 22:489–501.
4. Commission on Classification and Terminology of the International League Against Epilepsy (1985): Proposal for classification of the epilepsies. *Epilepsia,* 26:268–278.

5. Doose, H. (1964): Das akinetische petit mal. *Arch. Psychiatr. Nervenkr.,* 205:625–636, 637–654.
6. Dreyer, R., and Wehmeyer, W. (1977): Status mit psychomotorischen Anfallen. Beitrag zur klinischen hirnelektrischen problematik. Eine Video-Band-Analyse von 7 Fallen mit 9 Staten. *Nervenartz,* 48:612–620.
7. Escueta, A.V., Kunze, U., Waddell, G., Boxley, J., and Nadel, A. (1977): Lapse of consciousness and automatisms in temporal lobe epilepsy: A videotape analysis. *Neurology,* 27:144–155.
8. Escueta, A.V., Envile-Bascal, F., and Treiman, D.M. (1982): Complex partial seizures on closed-circuit television and EEG: A study of 691 attacks in 79 patients. *Ann. Neurol.,* 11:292–300.
9. Espinsoa, R.E., Klass, D.W., and Maloney, J.D. (1978): Contribution of the electroencephalogram in monitoring cardiac dysrhythmias. *Mayo Clin. Proc.,* 53:119–122.
10. Finlayson, R.E., and Lucas, A.R. (1979): Pseudoepileptic seizures in children and adolescents. *Mayo Clin. Proc.,* 54:83–87.
11. Gastaut, H. (1958): Syncope and seizure. *Electroencephalogr. Clin. Neurophysiol.,* 10:571–572.
12. Gross, M. (1979): Pseudoepilepsy: A study in adolescent hysteria. *Am. J. Psychiatry,* 136:210–213.
13. Herpin, T. (1867): *Des Acces Incomplets d'Epilepsie.* Bailliere, Paris.
14. Holmes, G.L., Sackellares, J.C., Ragland, M., and Dreifuss, F.E., (1980): Pseudoseizures in childhood: A clinical appraisal using prolonged EEG telemetry and videotape monitoring. *J. Pediatr.,* 97:554–558.
15. Jackson, J.H. (1931): On epilepsy and epileptiform convulsions. In: *Selected Writings of J. Hughlings Jackson,* Vol. 1, edited by J. Taylor. Hodder & Staughton, London.
16. Janz, D. (1969): *Die Epilepsien. Spezielle Pathologie and Therapie.* Georg Thieme Verlag, Stuttgart.
17. Kruse, R. (1968): *Das myoklinisch-astatisches Petit Mal.* Springer-Verlag, Berlin.
18. Lai, C.-W., and Ziegler, D.K. (1981): Syncope problem solved by continuous ambulatory simultaneous EEG/ECG recording. *Neurology,* 31:1152–1154.
19. Niedermeyer, E., and Lopes Da Silva, F. (1982): *Electroencephalography. Basic Principles, Clinical Applications and Related Fields.* Urban and Schwarzenberg, Baltimore.
20. Penin, H. (1968): Neuartige Diagnostik und Forschungsanlagen in der Universitats-Nervenklinik Bonn. *Acta Medicotechn.,* 16:76–78.
21. Penry, J.K., Porter, R.J., and Dreifuss, F.E. (1971): Patterns of paroxysmal discharge in 12-hour telemetered EEGs of untreated children with absence (petit mal) seizures. *Neurology,* 21:392.
22. Penry, J.K., Porter, R.J., and Dreifuss, F.E. (1975): Simultaneous recording of absence seizures with video-tape and electroencephalography: A study of 374 seizures in 48 patients. *Brain,* 98:427–440.
23. Porter, R.J., Penry, J.K., and Dreifuss, F.E. (1973): Responsiveness at the onset of spike-wave bursts. *Electroencephalogr. Clin. Neurophysiol.,* 34:239–245.
24. Porter, R.J., Penry, J.K., and Lacy, J.R. (1977): Diagnostic and therapeutic re-evaluation of patients with intractable epilepsy. *Neurology,* 27:1006–1011.
25. Porter, R.J., Penry, J.K., and Wolf, A.A., Jr. (1976): Simultaneous documentation of clinical and electroencephalographic manifestations of epileptic seizures. In: *Quantitative Analytic Studies in Epilepsy,* edited by P. Kellaway and I. Petersen, pp. 253–268. Raven Press, New York.
26. Porter, R.J., Wolf, A.A., and Penry, J.K. (1971): Human electroencephalographic telemetry: A review of systems and their applications and a new receiving system. *Am. J. EEG Technol.,* 11:145–159.
27. Redenbaugh, J.R., Sato, S., Dreifuss, F.E., Penry, J.K., and Kupferberg, H.J. (1977): Sodium valproate: A pilot study of pharmacokinetics and adverse reactions in patients with intractable seizures. *Neurology,* 27:376.
28. Regis, H., Toga, M., and Righini, C. (1961): Clinical, electroencephalographic and pathological study in a case of Adams-Stokes syndrome. In: *Cerebral Anoxia and the Electroencephalogram,* edited by H. Gastaut and J.S. Meyer. Thomas, Springfield, Illinois.
29. Roger, J., Dravet, C., Bureau, M., Dreifuss, F.E., and Wolf, P. (1985): *Epileptic Syndromes in Infancy, Childhood and Adolescence.* Libby, Paris.

30. Sato, S., Penry, J.K., Dreifuss, F.E., and Dyken, P.R. (1977): Clonazepam in the treatment of absence seizures; a double-blind clinical trial. *Neurology,* 27:371.
31. Sato, S., Penry, J.K., and Dreifuss, F.E. (1976): Electroencephalographic monitoring of generalised spike-wave paroxysms in the hospital and at home. In: *Quantitative Analytic Studies in Epilepsy,* edited by P. Kellaway and I. Petersen, pp. 237–251. Raven Press, New York.
32. Stefan, H., and Penin, H. (1980): Standardized methods of video-documentation in intensive monitoring. In: *Advances in Epileptology: Xth Epilepsy International Symposium,* edited by J.A. Wada and J.K. Penry, p. 130. Raven Press, New York.
33. Stores, G. (1981): Differential diagnosis of seizures (psychiatric aspects). In: *Advances in Epileptology: The XIIth Epilepsy International Symposium,* edited by M. Dam, L. Gram, and J.K. Penry, pp. 259–263. Raven Press, New York.
34. Sutula, T.P., Sackellares, J.C., Miller, J.Q., and Dreifuss, F.E. (1981): Intensive monitoring in refractory epilepsy. *Neurology,* 31:243–247.

Advances in Neurology, Vol. 46: Intensive Neurodiagnostic Monitoring, edited by R. J. Gumnit. Raven Press, New York © 1986.

Closed-Circuit Television Videotaping and Electroencephalography Biotelemetry (Video/EEG) in Primary Generalized Epilepsies

*Alfonso G. Lee, *,**Antonio V. Delgado-Escueta, *,**Hector M. Maldonado, *,**Barbara Swartz, and *Gregory O. Walsh

**Comprehensive Epilepsy Program, University of California at Los Angeles School of Medicine, Los Angeles, California 90024; and **Veterans Administration Southwest Regional Epilepsy Center, West Los Angeles Veterans Administration Medical Center (Wadsworth), Los Angeles, California 90073*

HISTORICAL DEVELOPMENT OF THE CONCEPT OF PRIMARY GENERALIZED EPILEPSIES

> Three lines of inquiry should be pursued . . . It is an anatomical inquiry to seek the organ or part damaged . . . It is a physiological inquiry to search into defective working of the nervous tissue of the organ damaged, the functional affection. It is a pathological inquiry to trace the processes by which nutrition of nervous tissue is altered [J. Hughlings Jackson, 1863, (56)].

It is said that the modern era of research in the epilepsies had its beginnings with the pioneer work on electroencephalography by Hans Berger half a century ago. Through the electroencephalograph (EEG), Berger (7, 8), Lennox (62–66), Penfield (81–89), and Jasper (86) confirmed the nature of epileptic seizures as abnormal paroxysmal neuronal discharges. However, the concept of the epilepsies as recurrent disorders produced by abnormal neuronal discharges within the central nervous system, symptomatic of a variety of diseases affecting the brain, began over 120 years ago when Reynolds (101), Jackson (56), Gowers (43), and Turner (120) observed and studied the detailed signs and symptoms of epileptic attacks. In 1861, J. Russell Reynolds published a book entitled *Epilepsy: Its Symptoms, Treatment and Relation to Other Convulsive Disorders* (101); in so doing, he inspired Sir William Gowers to write his classic detailed clinical descriptions of epilepsies 20 years later (43). But it was J. Hughlings Jackson who further completed our knowledge of the clinical epilepsies through his careful classical observations in the last two decades of the 19th century. And in 1907, W. Aldren Turner published a volume entitled *Epilepsy: A Study of the Idiopathic Disease* (120) following the principles of inquiry espoused by Jackson.

By 1863, Jackson distinguished between "symptomatic" and "genuine" or "idiopathic" forms of the epilepsies (56). In dividing chronic convulsions into two groups or classes, Jackson recognized the concept of (a) primary generalized epilepsies, e.g., "those in which the spasm affects both sides of the body almost contemporaneously—usually called epileptic and sometimes cases of 'genuine' or 'idiopathic' epilepsy," and (b) partial epilepsies: "those in which the fit begins by deliberate spasm on one side of the body and in which parts of the body are affected one after the other." Jackson sought the anatomical, physiological, and pathological bases of seizures (56). His three lines of inquiry also remain cornerstones in modern diagnostic approaches to epileptic seizures, and are followed by the International League Against Epilepsy (ILAE), and by Dreifuss in the revised 1980 and 1984 Classification of Seizures (17). This ILAE classification distinguishes between seizures that are generalized from the beginning (generalized seizures), and those that are partial at onset (partial seizures) and become generalized secondarily. It is interesting that the ILAE, in recognizing the etiologic implications of its classification of the epilepsies, also incorporated Gower's principles (43). Gower had maintained a clear distinction between "convulsions which are the result of organic disease such as can be recognized after death and those which are the expression of a condition of the brain which is not evidenced by any visible alteration." The ILAE classification, following Gower's distinction, also recognizes that generalized epileptic seizures consist of two subgroups: (a) primarily generalized seizures without any signs of organic brain disorder [e.g., Calmeil's epileptic absence of 1824 (13) or Esquirol's petit mal of 1838 (29)], and Gower's grand mal clonic-tonic-clonic seizures of 1885 (43), and (b) secondarily generalized seizures caused by a presumed or demonstrable organic brain disease.

The ILAE classification of epileptic seizures, as it has evolved since 1970, serves well as a taxonomic scheme for analysis of individual attacks. It is clear, however, that if defects in the structural gene or molecule or neurotransmitter systems of the brain are to be defined, if an accurate prognosis for specific epilepsies are to be determined, if we are to know which epilepsies spontaneously remit, which epilepsies undergo cure or remission after antiepileptic drug treatment, which epilepsies stay symptomatic for a lifetime, and which epilepsies are cured by corticectomy or lobectomy, clinicians must understand and apply in their practice a classification of epilepsies or epilepsy syndromes and not a classification of individual seizures. Such a classification of the epilepsies should follow the clinical pathologic principles espoused by Reynolds (101), Jackson (56), Gower (43), and Turner (120), but refined by the modern experiences of Penfield and Jasper (86), Talairach and Bancaud (116), and Gastaut et al. (31–33).

Descriptions of the clinical attack recorded on closed-circuit television videotape and EEG biotelemetry (video/EEG), the age at onset and remission of epileptic seizures, the interictal neurological status, the etiology and trigger mechanisms of epileptic attacks, the interictal and ictal EEG, different responses to antiepileptic medication, remission rates after drug treatment and, if pertinent and available, patterns of hereditary transmission should all be considered in describing specific epilepsies (Table 1). Although no truly satisfactory unitary classification of the epilepsies exists at present, the general scheme of the classification in Table 1 is currently being considered by the ILAE Commission on Classification as the new classification of the epilepsies. It distinguishes primary generalized and primary partial or focal epilepsies (those in

TABLE 1. *Classification of the epilepsies*[a]

Idiopathic or primary epilepsies
Idiopathic or primary generalized epilepsies: Genetically determined and specific age penetrance
Absence epilepsies
Childhood absence with diffuse 3-Hz spike-and-wave complexes
Juvenile absence with diffuse 8-Hz to 12-Hz rhythms and/or 3-Hz spike-and-wave complexes and 3- to 6-Hz multispike-and-wave complexes
Myoclonic absence with diffuse 3-Hz to 6-Hz multispike-and-wave complexes
Myclonus absence: staring, fragmentary myoclonus, automatisms, and diffuse 12-Hz rhythms
Myoclonic epilepsies
Benign myoclonic epilepsy of infancy
Benign familial epilepsies of West syndrome
Benign myoclonic seizures of early childhood, with 3-Hz to 6-Hz multispike-and-wave complexes without mental retardation (idiopathic and familial forms of Lennox-Gastaut syndrome)
Benign juvenile myoclonic seizures or "impulsiv petit mal" of Janz
Grand mal epilepsies
Clonic-tonic-clonic epilepsy (commonly awakening)
Tonic-clonic epilepsy
Idiopathic or primary partial epilepsies: Genetically determined with specific age penetrance
Benign childhood epilepsy with centrotemporal spikes or benign Rolandic epilepsy
Benign childhood epilepsy with versine seizures and occipital spike-and-wave complexes or sharp waves
Childhood epilepsy hemicorporeal (unilateral) seizures
Neonatal seizures
Symptomatic or secondary epilepsies
Symptomatic or secondary partial epilepsies: Caused by a structural lesion(s)
Epilepsies not involving the limbic system or partial epilepsies without loss or impairment of consciousness
Sensorimotor
Partial or focal motor epilepsies
Kojewnikow's syndrome
Occipital epilepsies
Epilepsies involving the limbic system or partial epilepsies with loss or impairment of consciousness
Temporal lobe epilepsies
Hippocampal-amygdalar epilepsy or medial basal limbic epilepsy
Amygdalar or anterior temporal polar-amygdalar epilepsy
Lateral posterior temporoparietal epilepsy
Opercular-insular or Island of Reil epilepsy
Lateral temporal neocortical epilepsy

TABLE 1. *Continued*

Frontal lobe epilepsies
- Cingulate or cingular epilepsies
- Supplementary motor epilepsies
- Orbitofrontal and prefrontal epilepsies
- Dorsolateral frontal epilepsies

Medial Occipital-hippocampal epilepsies

Symptomatic or secondary generalized epilepsies: caused by a structural lesion(s)
- Symptomatic or secondary tonic clonic epilepsies
- Simple partial evolving to tonic-clonic seizures
- Symptomatic neonatal seizures
- Infantile spasms (propulsive petit mal, infantile myoclonic encephalopathy with dysrhythmia or West syndrome)
- Myoclonic astatic or atonic epilepsies of early childhood (epileptic drop attacks, atypical absence, tonic seizures of Lennox-Gastaut in children with mental retardation)
- Progressive myoclonic epilepsies in adolescent and adults with dementia (myoclonic epilepsies of Unverricht, Lafora, Lundborg-Hartung, Ramsay-Hunt, Kuf, and Zeman)

Unclassified epilepsies
- Undetermined whether focal or generalized, or epilepsies with both focal and generalized features

Special epilepsy syndromes
- e.g., "stress convulsions," isolated convulsive tonic-clonic seizure, reflex epilepsies

[a] Modified from classification of A. V. Delgado-Escueta and from a simplified version of the classification proposed by the Commission of Classification and Terminology, ILAE.

which the etiology is unknown and major genetic contributions with specific age penetrance are accepted) from secondary partial or focal epilepsies (those in which the etiology is clinically identifiable and structural lesions presumably cause epileptic seizures). This classification also recognizes undetermined and unclassifiable epilepsies and special epilepsy syndromes (17).

In classifying epilepsies as primary and generalized with specific age penetrance, modern clinicians generally have assumed a monogenic or polygenic basis. After classifying epileptic attacks as secondary, clinicians compulsively look for the presence of a structural lesion using modern methods of brain imaging. Gower's and Jackson's concepts that some forms of epilepsies do not have demonstrable structural lesions and could have an hereditary basis was first espoused by Hippocrates. Such concept found support in the 1950 studies of Lennox and colleagues (62–66), who found a high degree of concordance (74%) of primary generalized epilepsy in uniovular twins. Lennox also found five times as great incidence of epileptic seizures (2.7%) in near relatives of epileptics compared to the incidence of epilepsy in the general population.

In the 1960s, the Metrakos' (75) showed a high occurrence of epileptiform discharges in the EEGs of relatives of patients with generalized *or* partial epilepsies, and provided further convincing evidence of the importance of heredity not only in generalized epilepsies, but also in some partial epilepsies. Noebels (76), in showing that a single gene defect can cause focal epilepsy and absence attacks in experimental animals, has provided even stronger arguments that some of these so-called idiopathic epilepsies can be due to a single gene defect. In stark contrast, some of the partial epilepsies appear to be due solely to environmental insults, such as are caused by the meningococcal and pneumococcal bacteria, or the herpes simplex, and slow measle viruses.

Thus, today, clinicians recognize primary generalized epilepsies and primary partial epilepsies (see classification in Table 1). There is new information delineating partial epilepsies that are purely environmental from partial epilepsies that are purely genetic. In the future we hope to advance to the point that we can differentiate between the contributions of genetic lesions and environmental insults in the multifactorial forms of secondary partial epilepsies.

Our purpose in this chapter is to show how video/EEG (1, 2, 9–11, 20–23, 28, 34–38, 49–53, 55, 59, 72, 77) can help the practitioner manage patients with primary or idiopathic epilepsies. Stalberg (111), Sindrup (110), Penry and Porter et al. (90, 91, 94, 98), Sutula (115), Binnie and co-workers (9–11), and Aarts et al. (1, 2) all emphasized how video/EEG monitoring has led to reclassification of seizure types (in as much as 43% of patients), answered questions of referring physicians in 67% to 81% of instances, e.g., cognitive impairment, sensory perception, pseudoseizures, and in 35% of cases led to changes in therapy. They further argue that 50% of patients referred involve the differentiation of pseudoepileptic seizures from epileptic attacks. "Unsuccessful, inconsistent treatment extended over years with repeated hospitalizations characterized such patients. The potential savings in hospitalization and outpatient medical care, achieved by an unequivocal diagnosis should readily cover the costs of epilepsy monitoring," according to Binnie (9).

In this chapter, the concept of primary epilepsies is as that proposed by Reynolds, Gowers, Jackson, and Turner. Specifically, we show how video/EEG has refined the diagnostic approach to subvarieties of primary generalized epilepsies; how video/EEG differentiates pseudoepileptic seizures from primary generalized and secondary generalized epileptic seizures; and how video/EEG can be used as a practical tool for assessing drug or surgical treatment results. Video/EEG can now be used to detect early recurrence of seizures after antiepileptic drug withdrawal. Video/EEG can also be used to follow patients who are in remission and/or are cured. These practical uses of video/EEG and the clinical decisions made with their help are best appreciated and illustrated by case studies. These case studies were obtained from 644 cases whose epilepsies were studied in three different units (the Duke-Durham Veterans Administration Epilepsy Unit, the Reed Unit at University of California at Los Angeles, and the Epilepsy Inpatient Unit at Wadsworth Veterans Administration Medical Center) (20–23).

METHODS

Patient Data Base and Recording Epilepsy Attacks

Six hundred and forty-four patients, suffering from different types of epilepsies (Fig. 1), underwent video/EEG monitoring for various periods of time ranging from 3 hr to 35 days. More than 5,000 seizures were recorded on video/EEG, but the major concern of our present report is the description of seizures that occur in (a) childhood absence epilepsies, (b) juvenile absence epilepsies, (c) benign juvenile myoclonic epilepsy, (d) the rare forms of absence epilepsies (myoclonus epilepsy and myoclonic epilepsy), and (e) the grand mal tonic-clonic, clonic-tonic-clonic epilepsies.

At the epilepsy unit, three to ten attacks of the patient's habitual seizures are recorded on video/EEG (20–24, 54, 55). Both split-screen analysis and a digital clock superimposed on videoimages and transcribed in code on the EEG are used for ascertaining time relations between the clinical attack and electrographic patterns. A close view of the patient's face on video/EEG, and bedside examinations by a nurse specialist in epilepsy, helps determine the exact onset of alterations of consciousness. In our experience, the clinical signs of impaired consciousness are best demonstrated on video/EEG by examining the patients' responses and reaction times to varying command stimuli.

Most patients were followed regularly and were familiar with the routine tests performed during prolonged EEG and videotape-monitoring sessions. They were familiar with methods of responding to the auditory monotone stimuli, such as pushing a response button immediately, delaying response by 3 sec, or pushing the response button five times on command. They were also familiar with tests instructing them to turn off flashing lights of various colors, using an off-switch for each color, or reading instructions printed with large letters.

During periods of prolonged cloudiness, all patients were tested for apraxia, written and spoken language, identifying and naming objects, and right and left orientation. Responses to pinprick, corneal stimulation, and deep pain were tested every 1.5 to 3 min. Muscle tone, muscle stretch reflexes, and plantar responses were examined. In some cases amnesia during the attacks was verified when patients were shown the tape-recorded attacks after they had recovered. The duration of attacks was timed from the historically verified onset of altered consciousness to the total disappearance of amnesia.

A 16-channel Grass Model 6 or 8 EEG apparatus was used to record brain waves through 22 scalp electrodes (10–20 system); in cases where EEG patterns suggested secondary bilateral synchrony two nasopharyngeal or sphenoidal electrodes were also used (54). Videotape recordings were obtained by mounting multiple cameras directed to the patient and the EEG. In some patients, black-and-white reproductions of eight to twelve EEG channels and of the patient's entire body were displayed split-screen on a television monitor for on-line viewing (20, 23, 24, 27).

Data Analysis

During the past 15 years, all the videotaped attacks were independently analyzed second-by-second by two or three associates (most recently Maldonado, Lee, and Swartz) in addition to the two senior epileptologists (Walsh and Delgado-Escueta). In the most recent patients, a computerized program for data analysis was also used. Split-screen video/EEG analysis of seizures was performed independently by viewing videotaped recordings of seizures at least ten times independently and without knowledge of the clinical history. Automatisms were described according to conventional classifications (3, 6, 19, 23, 26, 93). To help analyze the clinical and EEG data second-for-second, the behavioral state of the patient recorded by the television camera and displayed on the television monitor (sometimes by split-screen with telemetered EEG) was imprinted by a rapid-sequence camera (3, 34, 38, 41, 52). Polygraphic recordings of telemetered EEG were also reproduced by camera, and the digital time code, recorded on both the videotape and telemetered EEG, was used to line up the clinical and EEG data second-for-second. Final decisions on clinical diagnosis were made with confidence using the second-for-second analysis.

RESULTS

In general, our experience has taught us that the video/EEG can be used in most epilepsies (73–75, 78, 79, 81, 90–94, 96–99, 102–105, 108–112, 121) for (a) electroclinical analysis of epileptic attacks, aided by second-for-second correlation of electrographic and behavioral manifestations; and (b) for quantitation of epileptic attacks before, during, and after trials with conventional and experimental drugs, and also, before and after surgical intervention.

In primarily generalized epilepsies, we have found video/EEG useful in both diagnosis and treatment. In the group of patients in whom it is difficult to determine whether attacks are epileptic in origin, video/EEG recording of attacks can be especially useful in differentiating pseudoepileptic seizures (24, 49, 51, 61, 70) from true epileptic attacks. Simultaneous EEG and electrocardiography during video/EEG monitoring can also sieve out attacks of unconsciousness caused by disorders other than epilepsy such as cardiac dysrhythmias, carcinoid syndromes, and basilar insufficiency (12, 44).

Most recently, we have also found video/EEG useful in differentiating the various forms of epileptic convulsive syndromes, in classifying nonconvulsive epilepsies, and in providing a guide to specific pharmacotherapy. Whereas in the past, we had found the chief application of intensive monitoring in patients being evaluated for neurosurgical treatment, we are now also convinced of its practical use in uncontrolled primary generalized epilepsies (21, 23). It differentiates primary or genetically determined generalized clonic-tonic-clonic or tonic-clonic epilepsies from symptomatic or secondary generalized seizures. It also helps differentiate classic absences from atypical absences and complex partial seizures, pure absence from juvenile absence, juvenile myoclonic epilepsy (JME), myoclonus absence, and myoclonic absence.

Of the patients with primary generalized epilepsies, 27 had classical absence only (Fig. 1). The diagnosis of absence only was documented on the basis of the scalp EEG and absence attacks captured on the videotape. The number of attacks varied from 20 to approximately 100 episodes per day. Duration of the attacks most commonly ranged from 3 to 10 sec, but 20- to 60-sec or 30-min attacks were rarely recorded. In these patients, tonic-clonic convulsions or myoclonic jerks were not present.

Thirteen patients had myoclonic absence, six patients suffered from myoclonus absence, and 25 patients had juvenile absence with 8- to 12-Hz rhythms. All of these patients also had tonic-clonic convulsions.

We appreciated even further the usefulness of video/EEG in 152 patients with JME or "impulsiv petit mal" of Janz. Over half of these patients were referred because of uncontrolled grand mal convulsions. The nature of the syndrome had not been appreciated and video/EEG was required in over 60% of these patients to document the character of the grand mal attacks and the presence of mild myoclonic seizures. Out of these 152 patients, 20 cases required admission as inpatients. The other 132 patients underwent video/EEG monitoring for 3 to 12 hr as outpatients.

We found video/EEG particularly valuable in determining the primary nature of convulsive attacks classically called grand mal (23). Thirty-seven patients, diagnosed as grand mal epilepsy only, were studied and the diagnosis documented on the basis of video/EEG. Nineteen of these patients suffered clonic-tonic-clonic seizures and the other 18 had tonic-clonic attacks. Absence and myoclonic seizures were not present in these pure cases of grand mal. video/EEG documented clonic-tonic-clonic manifestations of grand mal attacks in 16 patients and pure tonic-clonic attacks in 11 patients. In our experience, clonic-tonic-clonic seizures are almost always primary and idiopathic in nature, and do not result from a partial or focal disorder. Rarely do clonic-tonic-clonic convulsions result from heredodegenerative or degenerative disorders, like Kuf, Lafora, and Lundborg diseases. Clonic-tonic-clonic convulsions can also appear in uremia or anoxic encephalopathy. Both patient groups had convulsive seizure breakthroughs with phenytoin, carbamazepine, and primidone; and valproate or benzodiazepines were required to stop convulsions.

Video/EEG was also important in determining why and what forms of seizures persisted in cases of Lennox-Gastaut syndrome (14, 15). Atypical absences, complex partial seizures, and generalized tonic seizure commonly underlie the complaints of uncontrolled convulsive disorders in symptomatic forms of Lennox-Gastaut syndrome. These seizures, especially tonic attacks, occur frequently during sleep.

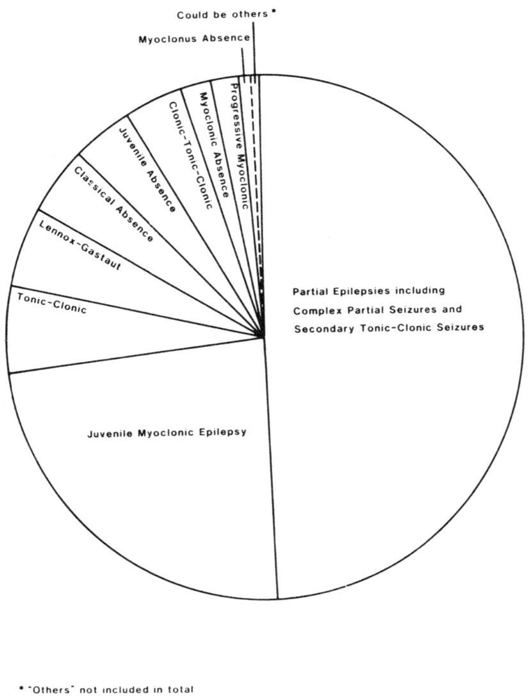

	Number of Patients
Partial Epilepsies including Complex Partial Seizures and Secondary Tonic-Clonic Seizures	319
Juvenile Myoclonic Epilepsy	152
Tonic-Clonic	34
Clonic-Tonic-Clonic	24
Classical Absence	27
Juvenile Absence	25
Myoclonic Absence	13
Myoclonus Absence	6
Progressive Myoclonic Epilepsies (Kufs, Lafora, Lundborg-Hartung; Mitochondrial Encephalopathy)	11
Lennox-Gastaut	33
TOTAL	644

FIG. 1. Patient data base.

We now also use video/EEG to follow up patients with uncontrolled primary generalized epilepsies who are under drug trials or who have been successfully treated with drugs. Remission or recurrence of seizures are best documented by 1 to 3 days of video/EEG done at 1- to 3-month intervals as antiepileptic drugs are withdrawn.

Partial epilepsies were the most common type of seizure disorder diagnosed in our series. Of 319 patients with partial seizures 1,535 attacks were documented on video/EEG. Most of these patients were being evaluated for uncontrolled seizures and some were candidates to receive surgical treatment. One hundred and six simple partial seizures and five secondary tonic-clonic attacks were recorded in five patients. The rest of the patients (314) showed 74 secondary generalized tonic-clonic seizures and 1,350 complex partial attacks. Because many of the characteristics of the secondary generalized epilepsy are similar to those of the pure generalized seizures, the role of the video/EEG in identifying the initial behavioral and electrographic signs was crucial in making the differential diagnosis. Thirty-three patients were diagnosed as Lennox-Gastaut syndrome and admitted to the telemetry unit. One hundred and forty-seven other patients with Lennox-Gastaut were managed as outpatients and did not need inpatient video/EEG monitoring.

During the past 15 years, 11 patients, suffering from progressive myoclonic epilepsy (Lafora, Lundburg-Hartung, Kuf, and Ramsey Hunt syndromes), were admitted into the telemetry units for diagnostic purposes. An additional 26 cases of progressive myoclonic epilepsy were admitted to the regular neurology service for diagnostic workup. Of patients with juvenile myoclonic epilepsy 152 underwent video/EEG monitoring as outpatients or inpatients from 3 to 6 hr to 15 days.

CASE ILLUSTRATIONS

Case 1: Pure Absence Without Tonic-Clonic Seizures: Documentation and Quantitation

A 5-year-old girl developed absence attacks with blinking of eyelids, upward stare, and loss of contact with the environment, lasting less than 10 sec. She had no tonic-clonic convulsions or myoclonic seizures, but several hundred seizures occurred each day and a variety of antiepileptic drugs (ethosuximide, valproate, phenytoin, and clonazepam) failed to suppress seizures. Moreover, the mother was concerned that many were now characterized by "rearrangements of items on the table, recurring postural changes and a hesitation." The patient claimed these were not seizures since she was conscious during these events. The EEG biotelemetry showed bilaterally synchronous and symmetrical 3/sec spike-and-wave complexes only when staring episodes and unconsciousness were identified on the television monitor. She has a maternal uncle with a history of posttraumatic seizures. The patient was also placed on video/EEG in order to document the nature and frequency of absence attacks that were resistant to ethosuximide. During the first 3 days of hospitalization, ethosuximide measured 95 μg/ml in the plasma while 13 attacks of absence with spike-and-slow-wave complexes lasting 6 to 10 sec to as long as 18 sec were recorded every 3 hr. Valproate, clonazepam, and trimethalione as single entry drugs did not reduce seizure frequency. With ethosuximide and tridione, 1 to 2 absences were recorded every week (Fig. 2).

Comments

In primary generalized epilepsies, video/EEG monitoring is most useful in identifying frequently occurring attacks that are easily overlooked by the patient's family (9–11) or observers (46, 49). Video/EEG is also useful in differentiating the clinical manifestations of absence from normal behavior, e.g., thinking, meditating, a posture or hesitation, and mouth movements which may be mistaken for arrest, and staring with lip-smacking (1, 2). When first-line drugs fail, it is necessary to establish a baseline count of absence attacks before new drugs are entered into the treatment plan. When therapeutic plasma levels of a new drug are achieved, a second count of absence attacks is then obtained.

Case 2: Absence in Clusters; and Assessment of Remission After Drug Withdrawal

An 11-year-old boy failed the fifth grade twice. He was scheduled to repeat the same year for the third time and the mother had been told by his teachers that he might be mentally retarded. Several EEGs including 3 and 6 hr EEG biotelemetry were reported to be normal. At 3 years of age he had one tonic-clonic seizure. Family history was negative for seizures. During our evaluation, physical examination was normal including intelligence quotient. During his hospital stay, video/EEG biotelemetry showed normal results except for clusters of classic absence attacks with 3-Hz spike-and-wave complexes all occurring within 30- to 60-min epochs. Characteristically, the rest of the day and night recordings did not record absence attacks on videotape (Fig. 3).

After 2 years of valproate plasma levels at 60 to 68 mcg/ml and suppression of seizures, valproate was gradually discontinued. Video/EEG monitoring, 3 months after valproate was discontinued, detected 2 to 3 absence attacks per day. The mother was advised to restart valproate but she did not comply. Two tonic-clonic attacks appeared in the next 2 weeks. Valproate was resumed for another year. Valproate was discontinued again at 14 years of age and annual video/EEG recordings have failed to show absence attacks for the past 2 years.

Comments

We do not know how many cases of childhood absence attacks cluster within short periods of the day (80). It would seem that in these infrequent cases, radiotelemetry or even portable cassette recorders that can monitor the freely

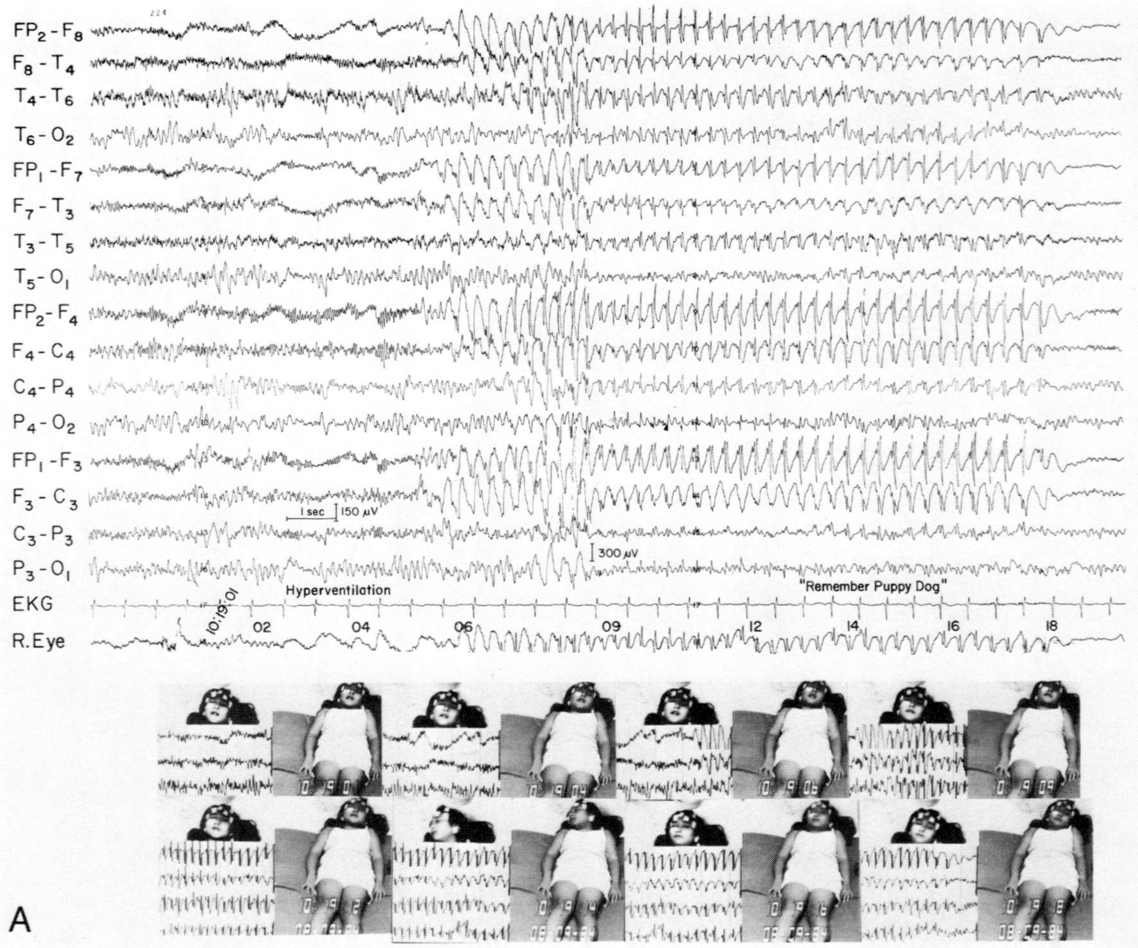

FP2 - F8
F8 - T4
T4 - T6
T6 - O2
FP1 - F7
F7 - T3
T3 - T5
T5 - O1
FP2 - F4
F4 - C4
C4 - P4
P4 - O2
FP1 - F3
F3 - C3
C3 - P3
P3 - O1
EKG
R.Eye
1 sec
150 µV
300 µV
10:19:01
Hyperventilation
"Remember Puppy Dog"
02
04
06
09
12
14
16
18
A

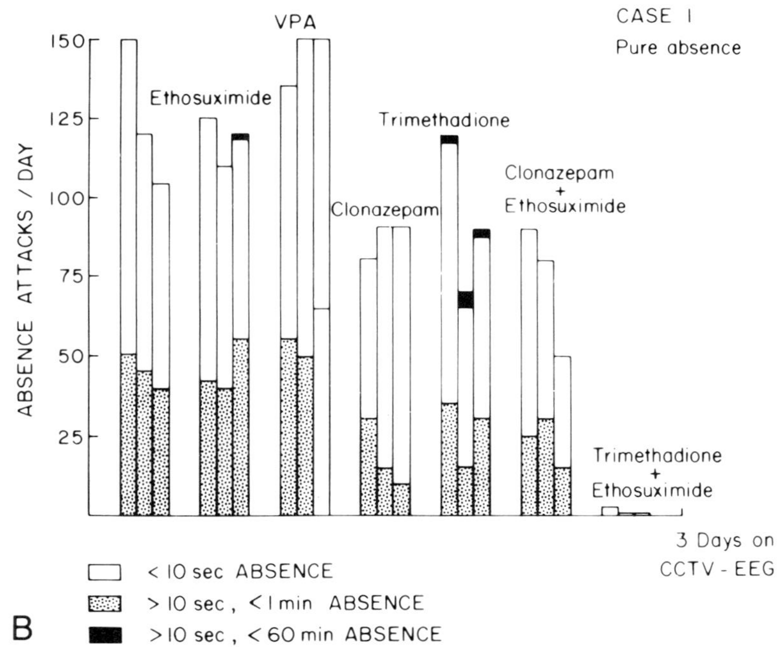

FIG. 2. Absence of childhood: Classical absence attack induced by hyperventilation: **(A)** occurred spontaneously from 100 to 150 instances in a day. They were counted on 3 consecutive days; **(B)** as antiepileptic drugs were varied. Trimethadione in combination with ethosuximide suppressed the seizures significantly. There were no tonic-clonic convulsions.

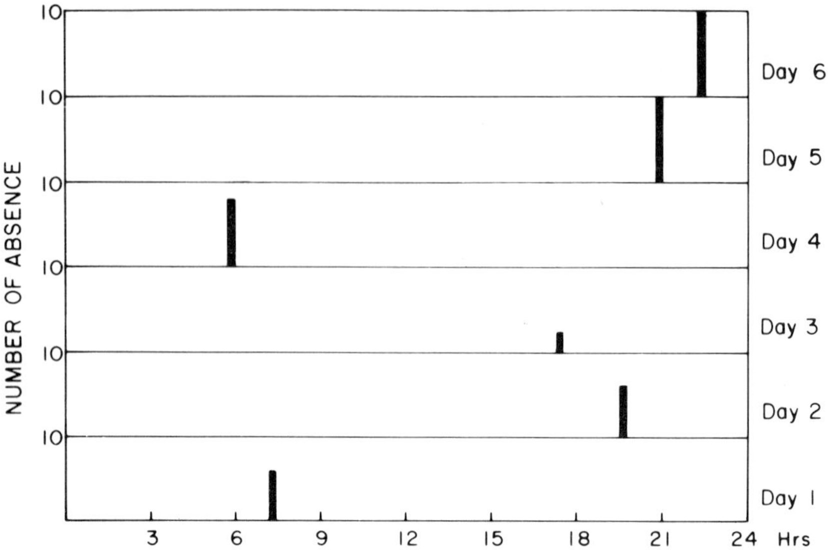

FIG. 3. Absence of childhood with infrequent tonic-clonic convulsions. Attacks occurred in clusters of 6 to 10 consecutive or repeated seizures. Twenty-four-hour monitoring was necessary to document the attacks.

moving patient for 24 hr would be the ideal technology (28, 30, 53, 104, 105). Had either of these systems been used, this patient's diagnosis would have been made earlier. It is difficult to predict when therapy should be discontinued when absence occurs with tonic-clonic convulsions. Fifty-eight to 65% of these cases relapse when successful treatment for 2 to 5 years is stopped.

Case 3: Myoclonic Absence: Differentiation from Classic Absence

A 15-year-old female was referred with the diagnosis of classic absence without tonic-clonic seizures; the referring physician and the family claimed that absence had been completely controlled by ethosuximide for 4 years. The patient and her family, however, were distraught with the presence of awakening momentary leg and arm jerks, sometimes symmetrical and less often asymmetrical and migratory, left more than right. These occurred once or twice a day, lasting 2 to 10 sec, usually without loss of consciousness. Video/EEG revealed rhythmic 3/sec bilaterally symmetrical truncal and appendicular jerks and unconsciousness during diffuse 3-Hz multispike-wave complexes, lasting 2 to 10 sec. The family was informed that the patient had myoclonic absence and cross-over to valproate was instituted.

Comments

In this particular patient, we do not know whether absence of childhood developed into myoclonic absence or whether the patient had myoclonic absence from the onset of illness. In retrospect, the family admitted that truncal and arm jerks were frequently present during attacks of unconsciousness when they were first noticed at 11 years of age. According to Penry et al., 17% of absence attacks have mild clonic components as the sole accompaniment of unconsciousness, and another 19% have mild clonic components together with automatisms. The most common clonic components consisted of eye-blinks; less commonly facial muscle twitches were observed (90, 92–94). Wolf and Inoue reported in 1984 that 8.2% of patients with childhood absence also have asymmetrical, mild myoclonic jerks in the shoulders and hands similar to those of "impulsive petit mal" (123). These clonic movements are milder, asymmetrical, arrhythmic, and clearly different from the more pronounced rhythmic, bilaterally symmetrical truncal and appendicular jerks of myoclonic absence. In myoclonic absence flexor muscles and trunk muscles usually predominate and jerk against a background of arrest of movement. The arms increasingly flex with the 3-Hz multispike-wave bursts and may rise above the head. The legs also jerk rhythmically. Myoclonic absence can develop in early or middle childhood, and is almost always associated with 3-Hz multispike-and-wave complexes. Frequently they are associated with diffuse 12-Hz rhythms. They are incompletely suppressed by ethosuximide, diones, or benzodiazepines. Lugaresi et al. (68, 69) and Tassinari et al. (117) claim that myoclonic absence can evolve towards a Lennox-Gastaut syndrome. Our experience shows that they occur mainly in intellectually normal patients as shown by cases 3 and 4.

Case 4: Myoclonic Absence, Grand Mal, and Photosensitivity: Differentiation from Juvenile Myoclonic Epilepsy

Attacks of impaired consciousness, lip-smacking, and ambulatory automatisms started at 9 years of age and occurred frequently until 12 years of age. Turning the room light on at night, opening the refrigerator door, or sudden exposure to sunlight triggered seizures. At 12 years of age, she had a single tonic-clonic seizure. The patient is now 29 years old, has been married for 5 years, and has 3 children. Because of ambulatory automatisms, she had a working diagnosis of complex partial seizures and secondary tonic-clonic convulsions. In every pregnancy, she had one to two convulsive seizures in the first and last trimester. During the last pregnancy, she had two convulsive seizures in the third trimester, and labor had to be induced. Now she complains of awakening nervousness, convulsions at 4 to 6 a.m., and frequent momentary blackouts in the middle of sleep as well as during the daytime in spite of phenytoin, primidone, and phenobarbital. Two absence attacks with 3- to 6-Hz multispike-wave complexes (Fig. 4) occurred during hyperventilation and photic stimulation. Closer analysis of the attacks on video/EEG records showed mild rhythmic clonic jerks of the extremities and trunk during absence attacks. These rhythmic clonic jerks were contrasted from the isolated muscular jerks of shoulder and extremities which cause items to be dropped. The latter are present in juvenile myoclonic epilepsy. Cross-over to valproate was instituted and phenytoin, primidone, and phenobarbital was discontinued. Because of continuing myoclonic absence attacks early in the morning, higher doses of valproate were used to raise plasma levels to 96 μg/ml. Family history was negative for clinical epileptic attacks and febrile convulsions.

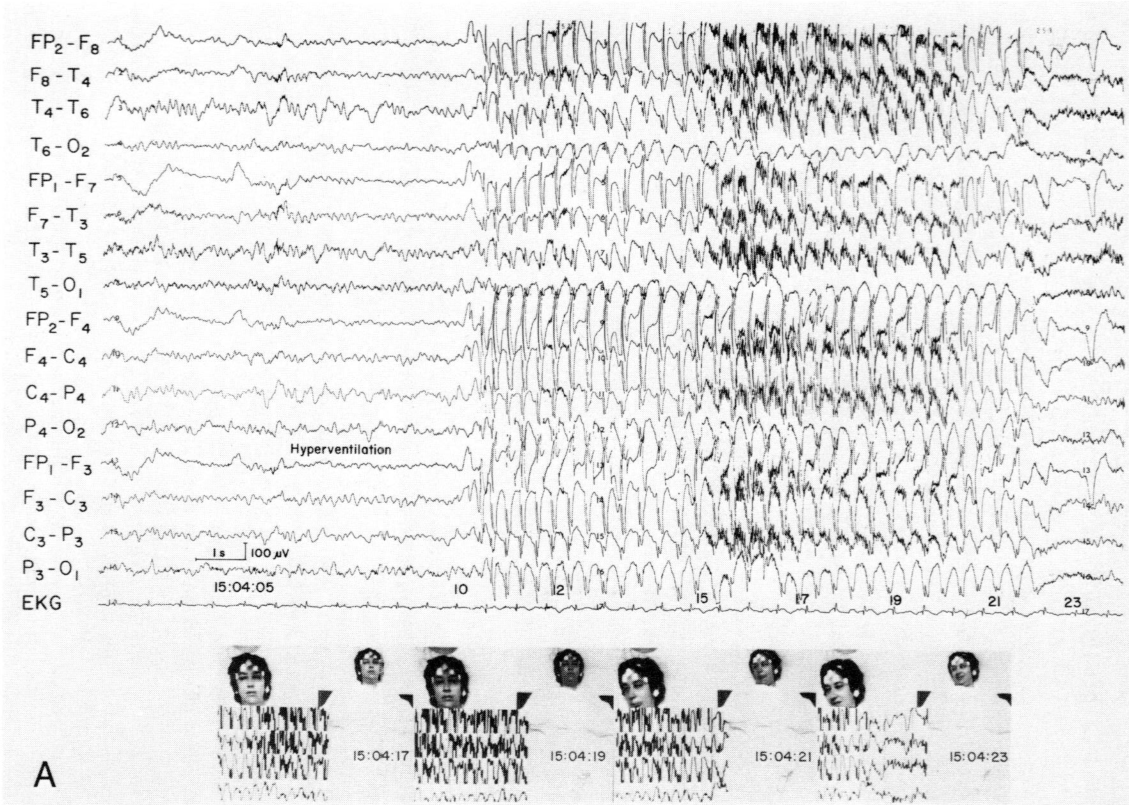
FP2 - F8
F8 - T4
T4 - T6
T6 - O2
FP1 - F7
F7 - T3
T3 - T5
T5 - O1
FP2 - F4
F4 - C4
C4 - P4
P4 - O2
FP1 - F3
F3 - C3
C3 - P3
P3 - O1
EKG
Hyperventilation
1 s
100 μV
15:04:05
10
12
15
17
19
21
23
15:04:17
15:04:19
15:04:21
15:04:23
A

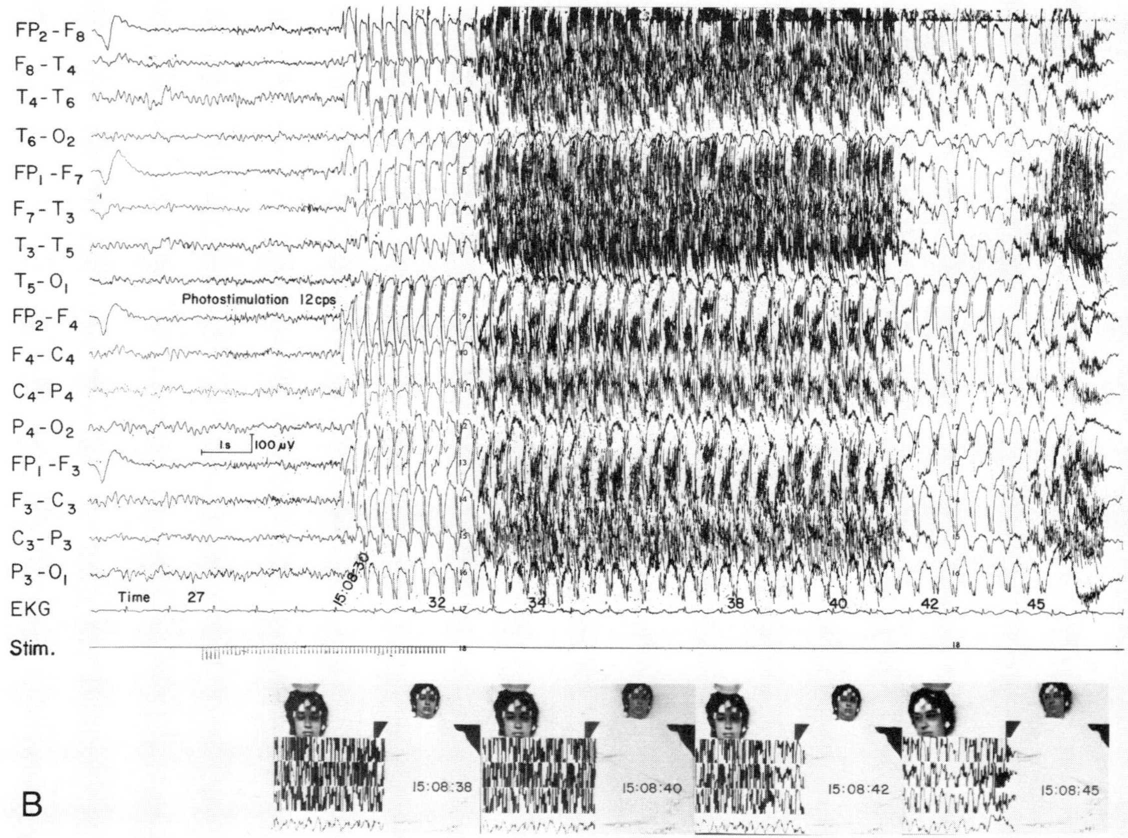

FIG. 4. Absence in a 29-year-old woman whose chief complaint was uncontrolled convulsions. Attacks were induced by hyperventilation (**A**) and photic stimulation (**B**) and were associated with mild rhythmic clonic jerks of extremities and trunk.

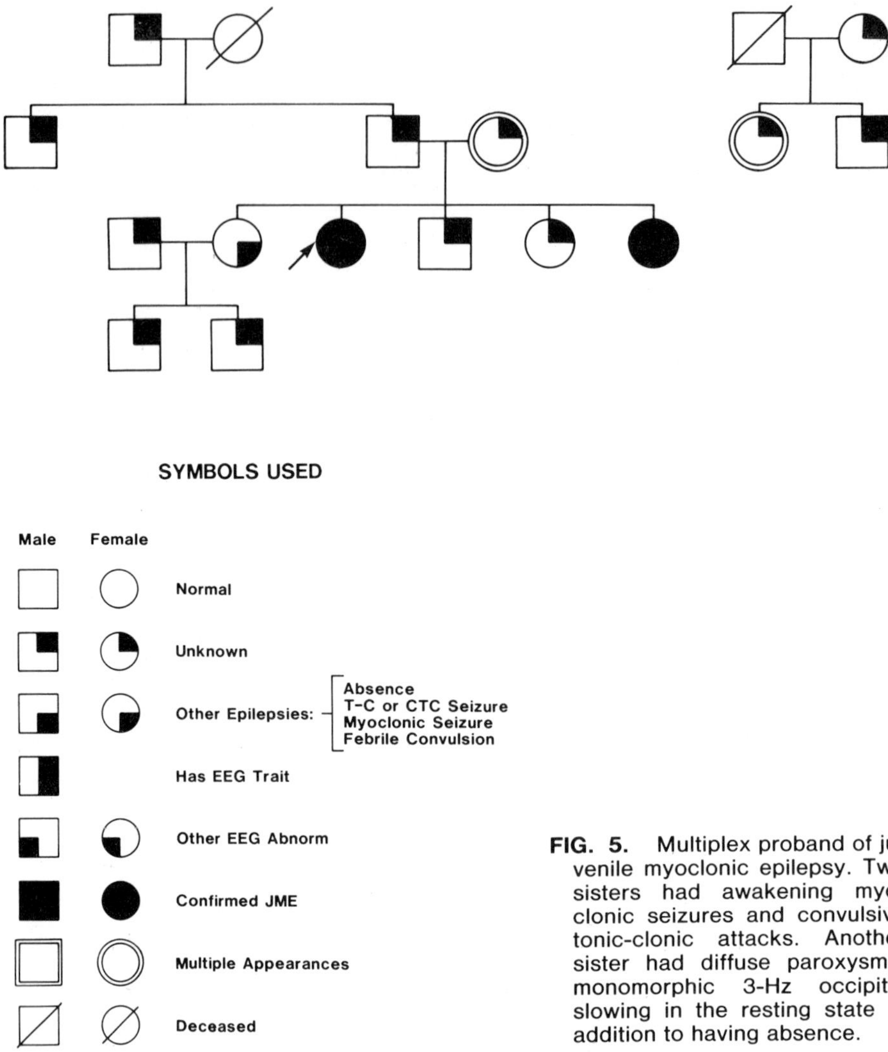

FIG. 5. Multiplex proband of juvenile myoclonic epilepsy. Two sisters had awakening myoclonic seizures and convulsive tonic-clonic attacks. Another sister had diffuse paroxysmal monomorphic 3-Hz occipital slowing in the resting state in addition to having absence.

Comments

This was a difficult diagnostic problem and only after CCTV-EEG did the presence of myoclonic absence become clear. We had originally suspected juvenile myoclonic epilepsy. Photosensitivity, however, should have made the referring physicians realize that the diagnosis of partial seizures was unlikely (60, 74). Thirty percent of patients with juvenile myoclonic epilepsy are reported by Janz to be photosensitive (57, 58). Our figures for photosensitivity in juvenile myoclonic epilepsy are not as high (20%). Most agree that 13 to 15% of pure awakening grand mal, 8% of juvenile absence, and 20% of childhood absence are sensitive to photic stimulation (57). But atypical absences, parietooccipital epilepsy, and drop attacks can also be triggered by light stimuli (60).

Case 5: Multiplex Probands of Juvenile Myoclonic Epilepsy

Two sisters, aged 29 and 22 years, were referred because of uncontrolled convulsions. The older sister described awakening clonic-tonic-clonic convulsions and denied any myoclonic jerks until she heard her younger sister describe disabling shoulder and hand jerks during a medical interview. The younger sister described dropping a coffee mug or a pen while her hand jerked. Sometimes a single jerk would appear when she would be applying makeup to her eyebrows with an eyebrow pencil; the pencil would strike straight up to her forehead. The younger sister also admitted to awakening clonic-tonic-clonic convulsions. Both sisters described onset of mild shoulder and hand jerks at 13 years of age, but the older sister had ascribed it to nervousness and lack of sleep. At 16 years of age, convulsions (clonic-tonic-clonic) appeared. A maternal aunt and a maternal grandmother had tonic-clonic convulsions (Fig. 5). The interictal EEGs in both sisters showed 4- to 6-Hz multispike-wave complexes diffusely. Valproate stopped seizures in both sisters.

Comments

In Janz's and our experience, more than three-fourths of cases with juvenile myoclonic epilepsy begin between the ages of 12 and 18 years (21, 22, 57, 58). The mean age at onset of seizures is 13.5 years. Only rarely is the correct diagnosis made before the first tonic-clonic or clonic-tonic-clonic convulsion. The latter term has been used because a series of jerks leads to the tonic-clonic convulsions; Jasper and Kershman referred to this as "myoclonic grand mal" in 1949, and Janz and Christian called this "impulsive grand mal" in 1957. A positive family history is obtained in 38% of patients with juvenile myoclonic epilepsy.

Case 6: Self-Induced Absence Attacks and Uncontrolled Grand Mal Tonic-Clonic Convulsions in Juvenile Myoclonic Epilepsy

Grand mal tonic-clonic seizures persisted in a 29-year-old nursing student in spite of ethosuximide, phenytoin, carbamazepine, and phenobarbital. As a 9-year-old child, he had black-out spells that were precipitated by watching black and white television or by opening and closing eyes against a bright sunlight. His father, a physician, worried about self-induction of seizures. He looked at the sun and waved one hand in front of the eyes to induce attacks. Sometimes he would slowly open and close his eyes in front of sunlight. At 14 years of age, tonic-clonic convulsions started. Work-up then included an EEG which was reported to have shown a left parietal 3- to 5-Hz spike-slow-wave focus. The patient had a normal skull X-ray, CSF analysis, and lumbar puncture, computerized brain scan tomography, bilateral carotid angiogram, and pneumoencephalography. He continued to have grand mal tonic-clonic seizures from 24 attacks a month to as little as 4 to

8 seizures a year. There was no family history for epilepsy. An early morning seizure was recorded during video/EEG monitoring. Loss of consciousness with clonic jerks were followed by tonic and then clonic movements of all extremities. No focality was noted and he bit his tongue, had urinary incontinence, and was amnesic for the event. Video/EEG also showed bilateral diffuse and symmetrical 4- to 6-Hz multispike-and-wave complexes during photostimulation at 12 to 16 flashes/sec. Myoclonic jerks involving all the limbs were recorded on CCTV during the photostimulation. Juvenile myoclonic epilepsy was suspected and prompted valproate treatment. To explore the familial nature of this disorder in this family, an EEG was performed in the nuclear family members. A half-brother (26-years-old, of the same father) had the 3- to 6-Hz multispike-wave complexes, but no clinical attacks were recorded on the video/EEG (Fig. 6).

Comments

Tsuboi and Christian (119) and Janz (57, 58) reported 21% of patients with juvenile myoclonic epilepsy induced polyspike-wave discharges and absence or jerks by slowly closing the eyes, or staring at a light and waving a hand in front of the eyes to produce flicker. Janz reports that 30.5% of patients with JME have photic-induced absence and myoclonic seizures (57, 58). Our experience agrees with these figures. In case 6, light could induce absence or jerks. Self-induction of seizures has long been associated with mentally retarded patients, but our recent experience has shown the same phenomenon in juvenile myoclonic epilepsy, in juvenile absence, and rarely in childhood absence, where normal or superior intelligence is the rule. Self-induced seizures are notoriously resistant to treatment (8, 18, 45).

In our experience, 2% of childhood absence and 8% of juvenile absence can be induced solely by repeated eye closure (22). In some of these patients flicker production by hand movements during eye closure are used to induce attacks. Video/EEG is extremely useful in these cases because the frequency of spontaneous absence are commonly less than the self-induced attacks. In these instances, behavior modification with the help of psychiatrists and psychologists are more important than drug treatment. In planning behavior modification, it is well to remember that some patients can induce seizures by eye closure alone, while some patients need both eye closure and light. Gooses studied this phenomenon well and showed that 16% of childhood absence, 7.5% of juvenile absence, and 16.5% of juvenile myoclonic epilepsies are both light- and eye-closure-sensitive (40).

Case 7: Pure Grand Mal: Diagnosis and Treatment of Clonic-Tonic-Clonic Grand Mal Without Myoclonic Seizures

The patient was a term product of a normal delivery but was described to be a "blue baby." He is a 37-year-old white male, a successful professional in the movie industry who reported normal developmental milestones as a child. At the age of

16 years, he sustained head trauma, hitting a goalpost with the top of his head, with loss of consciousness but no other sequela. At 18 years of age, the patient was at work at 6 a.m. setting the props for a stage, when he lost consciousness and had a generalized tonic-clonic seizure. On 600 mg/day Dilantin, he was free of seizures for 1½ years. Deprivation of sleep during periods of film production induced a second episode of convulsions where he was noted to be jerking all of his extremities, turned blue, and foamed at the mouth. There is no epilepsy in the family. Interictal EEG was normal; photic stimulation and hyperventilation did not induce abnormalities. Video/EEG monitoring and EEG telemetry, showed clonic-tonic-clonic sequences during grand mal convulsions. Generalized 4- to 6-Hz slow waves and clonic jerks preceded fast 8- to 16-Hz frequencies and a tonic state, which evolved to polyspike-wave sequences and clonic convulsions. Video/EEG did not record any morning shoulder or truncal or extremity jerks or absence attacks. Convulsions persisted with 130 μg/ml valproate plasma levels and 10 μg/ml tegretol blood concentrations. Eighteen μg/ml of phenytoin in combination with valproate and tegretol stopped all convulsions.

Comments

The average age at onset for pure awakening grand mal is between 16 and 18 years. Like juvenile myoclonic epilepsy, sleep deprivation is a very effective method of provoking awakening grand mal seizures. Fifteen to 20% of those patients show 3.5- to 5-Hz polyspike-wave complexes in their interictal EEG (21, 31). Epilepsy with pure grand mal tonic-clonic seizures and without myoclonic seizures or absence is a rare clinical activity.

Case 8: Differentiation of Tonic from Tonic-Clonic Seizures in Lennox-Gastaut Syndrome

At the age of 3½ years, the patient was noted to drop whatever she had in her left hand, lean to her left side frequently, and laugh in a funny way. This usually progressed to tonic-clonic seizures. She frequently had falls, where both arms shook and her legs got rigid, pointing down. This shaking lasted a few seconds to 45 sec, worse on the left side on her face and her trunk, the left facial muscles, eyes and mouth twitching considerably. For a few years, her seizure frequency ranged from 18 to 35 attacks a day. She had been treated in several medical centers with poor results. The patient's age is now 16 years and the mother claimed her developmental milestones were normal. At the present time the mother claims her main seizures consist of left arm clonic jerks, which progress to a sudden fall to the floor, impairment of consciousness, and tonic-clonic convulsions. These complaints persist in spite of 37 mcg/ml of phenobarbital and 67 mcg/ml of valproic in plasma. There is no history of epilepsy or neurological disorder in her family. Physical and neurological examinations were normal except for intelligence quotient of 85 and slow intellectual functions. Video/EEG telemetry recorded eight generalized seizures lasting 20 to 30 sec consisting mainly of a tonic posture when the EEG showed generalized flattening and low-voltage 18- to 22-Hz rhythms. Another eight seizures were preceded by postural movements of the left hand, with adversive movements of the head to the left. The EEG showed generalized 1½- to 3-Hz irregularly formed bilateral and diffuse spike-and-sharp-wave formations (14, 15,

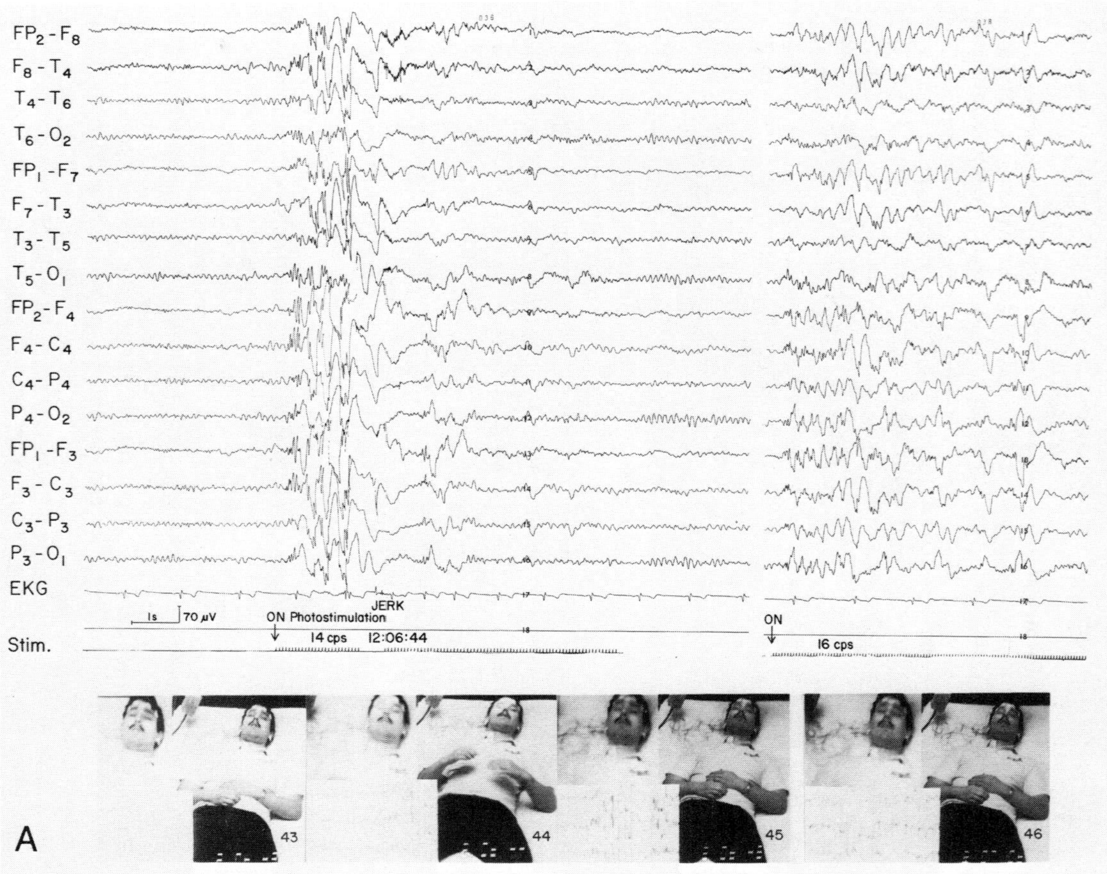
FP2 - F8
F8 - T4
T4 - T6
T6 - O2
FP1 - F7
F7 - T3
T3 - T5
T5 - O1
FP2 - F4
F4 - C4
C4 - P4
P4 - O2
FP1 - F3
F3 - C3
C3 - P3
P3 - O1
EKG
Stim.
1s
70 μV
ON Photostimulation
JERK
14 cps
12:06:44
ON
16 cps
43
44
45
46

A

B

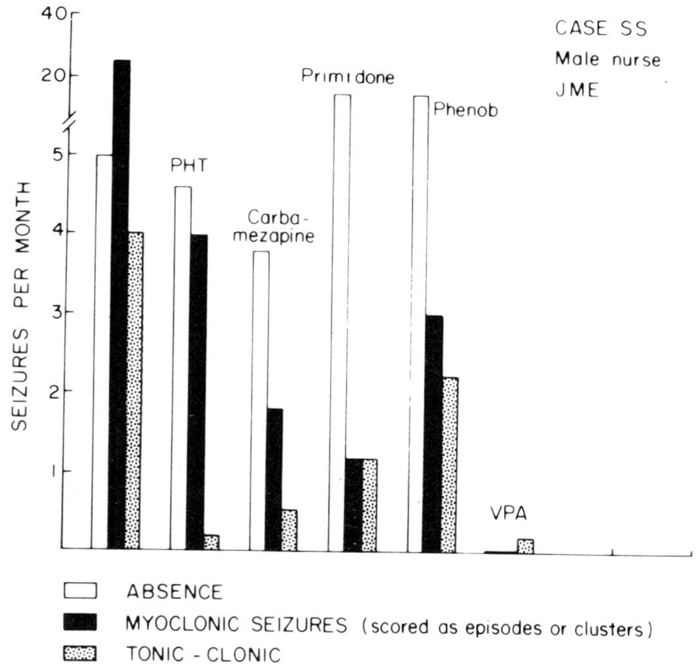

FIG. 6. Juvenile myoclonic epilepsy. A 29-year-old nursing student had uncontrolled tonic-clonic convulsions and light sensitive myoclonic jerks **(A)**. At 9 years of age, he had self-induced absence attacks which disappeared in adolescence. Seizures were suppressed by valproate **(B)**.

31, 33). Nine μg/ml of carbamazepine significantly decreased the tonic and postural seizures.

Comments

Drug suppression of seizures in Lennox-Gastaut syndrome remains difficult. Video/EEG, however, can frequently decipher the main seizure types that persist. Valproate in combination with carbamazepine is the best drug combination for this syndrome where incomplete control of seizures occurs in two-thirds of the cases.

Case 9: Secondary Tonic-Clonic Seizures, Primary Tonic-Clonic Seizures and Pseudoepileptic Seizures in the Same Patient

A 42-year-old Spanish Basque male has had convulsions since 5 years of age consisting of short absence attacks, myoclonic jerks, generalized tonic-clonic seizures, and olfactory hallucinations. The patient has a first cousin with "drop attacks." Physical examination, ancillary studies including CAT scan and bilateral cerebral angiography were normal. Two years ago, he was in a vehicle accident, lacerated his left forehead and lost consciousness for 20 min. Since then, the patient has described a typical seizure as follows: "the onset is with flashing lights, red and white, which increase in number with time." An EEG was performed and showed high-amplitude left occipital spikes. The patient's other seizure included myoclonic twitches of the left eye or left arm; occasionally, he experienced malodorous smells. Video/EEG recorded four secondary tonic-clonic seizures preceded by flashing lights and rapid 16-Hz spikes in the left occipital area. At high plasma levels of phenytoin, carbamazepine, and valproate, seizures persisted as an outpatient. He was readmitted and video/EEG telemetry recorded three attacks with clinical manifestations, similar to habitual seizures described by the patient, and a leading left occipital spike focus. Twelve behavioral changes consisting of body jerks and arm, pelvis, and leg contortions without associated EEG correlates were also recorded. A psychiatric consult followed.

Comments

Practitioners are commonly surprised to hear their patients have both epileptic seizures and pseudoepileptic attacks. Video/EEG can demonstrate effectiveness of drug treatment, partial or total suppression of epileptic seizures, persistence of pseudoepileptic attacks, and emphasize the need for refocusing psychiatric management goals.

Case 10: Diagnosis of Spike-Wave Stupor or Petit Mal Status

The patient started to have tonic-clonic seizures at age 27 (6). Four years later, generalized tonic-clonic seizures occurred once a year despite anticonvulsant therapy (phenytoin, primidone, carbamazepine). At age 41 years, seizures persisted and he became ataxic, lethargic, and dysarthric. Blood levels of phenytoin and phenobarbital were in the toxic range. He was being studied to determine why seizures were intractable. Pneumoencephalography showed mild cortical and cerebellar atrophy. One day after the pneumoencephalograph, generalized tonic-clonic seizures were followed by a prolonged state of impaired consciousness and confusion. He appeared to stare, there were brief periods of eye blinking and lip-smacking. He did not respond properly to the auditory monotone stimuli and could not identify colors or objects, but he responded when the Achilles tendon was pinched. Video/EEG monitoring showed frequent bursts of irregular diffuse 2- to 4-Hz multiple spike-and-slow-wave complexes which appeared most prominently in the frontal and central regions. The posterior temporal, parietal, and occipital regions showed irregular low-voltage 7- to 8-Hz waves. Phenytoin (1,100 mg) and phenobarbital (1,000 mg) were administered intravenously with no immediate effects on the clinical or EEG features. Six milligrams of intravenous diazepam decreased the spike-and-wave complexes and abolished the stereotyped eye blinking and lip smacking. Six hours after the onset of confusion, he was awake and alert.

Comments

Spike-wave stupor (synonyms: prolonged twilight state with spike-and-waves or petit mal status) can develop in adult patients who have never had absence in childhood or who have never had epilepsy (6). Most commonly, however, petit mal status occurs in patients who are known to suffer from absence epilepsy, absence with tonic-clonic seizures, juvenile myoclonic epilepsy, or the Lennox-Gastaut syndrome. Marked clouding of confusion, immobility, and speech arrest most commonly characterize spike-wave stupor. Infrequently, slight clouding of consciousness, or impairment of attention, memory, lethargy, somnolence, or psychosis can be presenting symptoms. In half of the cases, associated convulsive signs appear, e.g., myoclonic jerks of limbs, or chin muscles.

DISCUSSION

Evaluation and Preparation for Video/EEG Monitoring

When generalized seizures are inadequately controlled, factors other than pharmacological intractability are usually considered: (a) noncompliance, (b) inadequate drug dosage, (c) improper drug or combination of drugs, (d) precipitating or aggravating factors, e.g., stressful home or work situations, alcohol, sleep deprivation, or menstrual period, (e) drug interactions that influence plasma drug levels, (f) drug toxicity, and (g) not infrequently, a slowly progressive neurological disorder such as a slowly progressive myoclonic encephalopathy, or a deep-lying neoplasma in midline structures (22).

If generalized seizures continue to interfere seriously with the individual's life, treatment with first-line and adjunctive drugs fail, and none of the previously listed factors appear to be significant, the practitioner should consider prolonged video/EEG monitoring. To prepare the patient, the practitioner should carefully review the patient's life history and neurological examination, the description of the patient's attacks by the spouse, parents, or friends, and the results of radiologic and brain-imaging examinations. The results of neuropsychological tests must also be assessed looking for signs of diffuse or focal brain damage or evidence of a psychiatric disorder. Do seizures continue because there is more than one type of epileptic attack or are some attacks pseudoepileptic in nature? Once the practitioner is assured of a generalized process, it is important to relook for clues of a progressive process in the EEG, e.g., slow background process, evidence of secondary bilateral synchronies, a focal polymorphic delta slow-wave focus. When the practitioner is convinced that an underlying progressive lesion is not responsible for inadequate control of seizures, video/EEG monitoring should now proceed.

When diffuse spike-wave complexes are present, the interictal EEG must be studied closely for evidences and differential points of primary or secondary bilateral synchronies (Tables 2 and 3). The random occurrence of interictal epileptiform paroxysms in the EEG and of clinical seizures should explain why a

TABLE 2. *Bilaterally synchronous spike-and-wave complexes on the electroencephalograph*

EEG	Secondary bilateral synchrony	Primary bilateral synchrony
Frequency	Usually 1.5 to 2.5 Hz	2.5- to 3.5-Hz diffuse spike-slow complexes at ages 3–15 years 4- to 6-Hz diffuse multispike-wave complexes during adolescence but frequently 13–15 years
Form	Differs in form, amplitude, and wave components from complex to complex	Regularity in repetition from complex to complex
	May consistently be asymmetrical	Usually symmetrical
	A single phase reversal over the sagittal plane is the rule	Phase reversals over both hemispheres are common
Background rhythms	May have disorganized background	Normal background activity in EEG
	Usually does not have posterior rhythmic 1- to 3-Hz bursts	May have posterior rhythmic 1- to 3-Hz bursts
	Reduction of background activity may be evident on one side of the midline; potentialized by IV pentothal	None
Focal signs	Usually has a cortical or subcortical focus on ECOG and depth recordings	Do not usually have a focus
	Focal cortical discharges may precede spike-and-wave complexes	Sudden appearance without premonitory EEG changes
	May have postparoxysmal focal extinction and recovery signs	None

single routine 30- to 45-min EEG fails more often than not in providing evidence for the diagnosis of epilepsy (4). Fortunately, in generalized epilepsies, the interictal EEG yields useful information. The interictal EEG activated by hyperventilation and/or photic stimulation or sleep deprivation commonly provides evidence for the presence of a seizure disorder in most patients with generalized epilepsies. Routine 30-min EEGs show spike-slow-wave or multispike-slow complexes in 15 to 20% of patients with generalized tonic-clonic (GTC) seizures (21, 31). Half of all patients with isolated myoclonus or GTC seizures with myoclonus show epileptiform paroxysms, and 80 to 90% of patients with absences or petit mal attacks show diffuse 2.5- to 3.5-Hz spike-wave complexes during hyperventilation (21, 31). When the practitioner is convinced that an underlying, progressive lesion is not responsible for inadequate control of seizures, video/EEG monitoring should now proceed.

Some Clinical Concepts Useful in Video/EEG Monitoring of Primary Generalized Epilepsies

In 1969, Gloor modified the concept of the centrencephalic epilepsies and introduced the term "corticoreticular" epilepsies. He abandoned the concept of a focal subcortical pacemaker and proposed that diffuse oscillatory mechanisms between corticoreticular pathways mediate diffuse spike-wave complexes. Corticoreticular seizures have since been subdivided into four groups: (a) The genetically determined primary generalized epilepsies, such as absence or petit mal of childhood, juvenile myoclonic epilepsy, grand mal epilepsy, and the rare forms of absence epilepsies; (b) seizure disorders, associated with renal failure, hypoglycemia, or hypocalcemia; (c) generalized convulsive and nonconvulsive seizures in diffuse progressive encephalopathies, such as lipid storage disorders, affecting the cortical and subcortical gray matter; and (d) focal cortical seizures originating in the orbital frontal, dorsolateral frontal, frontopolar, and medial frontal lobe, with secondary bilateral synchrony.

This clinical subdivision conforms to Gastaut's EEG classification of diffuse spike-wave complexes. (a) Three-Hz spike-wave complexes correspond to childhood absence of petit mal seizures. (b) The slower 1.5- to 2-Hz spike-wave discharges almost always indicate diffuse brain damage, as in symptomatic Lennox-Gastaut syndrome or lipid storage diseases. (c) Faster 4- to 6-Hz spike-wave and multispike-wave complexes are observed in benign myoclonic epilepsies of early childhood, juvenile myoclonic epilepsy of Janz, myoclonic and tonic-clonic seizures in renal and metabolic failure, and in progressive myoclonic encephalopathies, such as Lafora, Kuf, or Lundborg-Hartung syndromes (Table 4).

Our experience is in agreement with Gloor's concept and Gastaut's EEG classification of spike-wave complexes. As noted above, we observed several forms of absence epilepsies in over 200 patients with generalized epilepsies (see

TABLE 3. *Clinical correlates of bilaterally synchronous spike-and-wave complexes*

Correlates	1.5–2.5 Hz S-W Complexes[a]	2.5–3.5 Hz S-W Complexes		4–6 Hz Multi-S-W Complexes	
Etiology	Diffuse cortical and subcortical lesions, i.e., Lennox-Gastaut syndrome, anoxia, birth injury neuronal storage diseases, severe encephalopathies from trauma	Idiopathic but genetic (petit mal) in 5–10-year-old children	Orbital/medial, frontal, or cingulate focus associated usually with static structural lesions, rarely with neoplasms, usually in adults	Idiopathic but genetic, 8–20 years old with juvenile myoclonic epilepsy	Biochemical brain lesion, i.e., Lafora, Lundborg, Hartung, Kuf, gangliosidosis, or ceroid lipofuchsinosis
Clinical accompaniments	Infants and children usually with mental retardation				
Response to anticonvulsants	Poor; 33% achieve partial control with valproate and carbamazepine	Excellent response to ethosuximide or valproate	Partial or complete control with carbamazepine or phenytoin	Excellent response to valproate	Partial response to diazepam, carbamazepine, or valproate

CCTV-EEG					
Clinical attacks during EEG S-W bursts	Episodes of impaired consciousness or even transitory changes in cognition are usually not evident during S-W bursts	Impaired consciousness or transient alterations in cognition almost always appear during S-W bursts	Pseudo-absence attacks: short periods of impaired consciousness with or without postural arm or leg movements may appear with S-W bursts	Absence attacks of impaired consciousness or transient diminution of cognitive powers can appear during 3 Hz or 4–6 Hz S-W bursts	Impaired consciousness or cognition rarely appear with S-W bursts
Drop attacks during EEG desynchrony or low voltage slowing or S-W bursts	Frequently appear as patient collapses to the floor	Collapse to the floor during absence should make the clinician consider another form of epilepsy other than petit mal	Collapse to the floor during S-W bursts can appear	Rarely collapse to the floor appears during massive myoclonic seizures	Collapse to the floor usually does not appear with S-W bursts

[a]S-W = Spike-and-wave.

TABLE 4. *Progressive familial myoclonic epilepsies*

Epilepsies	Age of onset (decade)	Inheritance	Sequence of clinical signs and symptoms	Pyramidal tract signs	Duration of disease (years until death)	Pathology
Unverricht (1891)	1–2	Autosomal Recessive	Epilepsy→dementia→cerebellar signs→myoclonic seizures myoclonus	May be present	5–6	Unknown
Lafora (1911)	2	Autosomal Recessive	Epilepsy→dementia→cerebellar signs→myoclonic seizures myoclonus	In 12 to 24 months	5–10	Lafora inclusion bodies
Lundborg-Hartung (1903)	2	Autosomal Dominant	Myoclonus, myoclonic seizures and no or minimal organic mental dysfunction	None	20–40	Unknown
Ramsay-Hunt (1903), Gilbert (1963)	1–2	Autosomal Dominant	Cerebellar signs and/or myoclonic jerks→with or without Freidreich's or Marie's ataxia	None	20–30	Degeneration of neuronal systems
Kuf's disease	2–3[a]	Autosomal Recessive	Myoclonus, myoclonic seizures→ tonic-clonic seizures→cerebellar signs→dementia	Middle or terminal stages	7–12	Ganglioside storage
Zeman's disease	3–4[a]	Autosomal Dominant	Myoclonus, myoclonic seizures→tonic-clonic seizures→cerebellar signs→dementia	Middle or terminal stages	5–10	Ceroid lipofuchsinosis

[a] Rarely during the first 5 years of life.

TABLE 5. *Myoclonic jerks on video/EEG*[a]

Common symptoms or complaints used to explain myoclonic jerks	No. of patients
Nervousness of hands or legs	9
Ataxia (impaired gait)	3
Tics (nervous habits)	1
Slurred speech (jerks of mouth and tongue muscles)	2
Unilateral jerks as focal seizures (especially during antiepileptic drug treatment)	4
Frequent sighs and deep breathing	3
Early morning nervousness (need the first morning hours to get steady and stabilize)	5
Step backwards	2
Difficulty eating, chewing, and swallowing	2

[a] Some common interpretations by patients and/or referring physicians as elicited by historical account.

Table 5 for the subvarieties of absence epilepsies and their differential points). The first and most well-known type consisted of the classical absence of childhood, associated with diffuse 3-Hz spike-wave complexes (synonyms: simple petit mal, pure petit mal, pykno-epilepsy). Absence accounts for 3 to 4% of all epilepsies and for 10% of all childhood seizure disorders. Penry and co-workers prospectively studied childhood absence on video/EEG (90–94, 96–99). They found automatisms accompanied at least one attack in 88% of patients with absence, and automatisms were exhibited in 63% of all absence seizures. They differentiated absence from complex partial seizures by the following criteria (90–94, 96–99, 107): (a) In absence, an aura does not precede the abrupt onset; (b) the duration of absence is generally 10 sec, much briefer than that of complex partial seizures; (c) the prolonged third phase of confusion and quasipurposeful behavior of psychomotor attacks is absent; and (d) mental clarity returns instantly at the end of the absence attacks. We have noted, in addition, that bizarre complex bilateral motor automatisms, such as running away, bicycle pedaling, and swimming motions, are not found as automatisms in absence seizures, whereas they appear as part of complex partial seizures of extratemporal origin, e.g., parietal or frontal lobe origin (22, 23, 36).

It is these brief absences that can go unnoticed by the patients' families and those relatives and friends who report on seizure frequency that can cause difficulty at school or work. In childhood absence, the associations of impaired consciousness or cognition with 3-Hz spike-wave bursts are so close that it is more practical sometimes to count the spike-wave bursts than spend hours analyzing the videotaped attacks. If the sequences of spike-wave bursts are longer than 1.5 sec, arrest of movements and loss of consciousness can be detected on the videotape. Diffuse 3-Hz spike-wave complexes that last seconds can be detected as a staring attack without the aid of a videotape. Ninety-five percent of patients with diffuse 3-Hz spike-wave complexes have clinical epilepsy. Interseizure discharges probably do not occur in absence seizures. Even 3-Hz spike-wave sequences of less than 1.5 sec duration are associated with problems in responsiveness and cognition. Goode et al. (39) explored latency and accuracy of responses during spike-wave bursts in absence and showed that impairment in responses were noted more during continuous performance tasks where the stimuli were randomly delivered. Such impairment of cognitive powers during EEG paroxysms had been reported by Schwab in 1939 (107), and more recently by Binnie in 1980 (9). Prolonged performance testing should therefore be done during video/EEG monitoring in forms of random command auditory stimuli, the use of cards for memory testing, and even television games. In absence of childhood, performance testing is done during the first monitoring sessions. If transitory impaired cognition or unconsciousness always occur with the 3-Hz spike-wave sequences, subsequent monitoring sessions may not require such rigorous performance testing. The frequency of absence attacks can be more conveniently determined by counting the spike-wave bursts and these practical applications can be very important as the frequency of seizures is determined during trials with antiepileptic drugs.

In contrast to the above observations, alterations in consciousness or cognition are not necessarily present when the generalized patterns of Lennox-Gastaut syndrome (1.5- to 2-Hz spike-wave complexes), the rare forms of absence epilepsies (myoclonic absence, juvenile absence) and progressive myoclonic encephalopathies (4- to 6-Hz spike-wave complexes) appear. These are important facts to consider in video/EEG monitoring. If a child has drug-resistant absence with 3-Hz spike-wave complexes, almost all of the hundreds of seizures recorded on video/EEG will be associated with problems in responsiveness and/or cognition. As mentioned above, it is important to document the latter during the first monitoring sessions. When treatment with a single drug or new drug combinations are then tried, the frequency of electroclinical attacks can be more conveniently done by counting the number of spike-wave sequences, since one can presume behavioral or cognitive changes with every diffuse 3-Hz spike-wave sequence. This important baseline also becomes useful when one or two drugs successfully stop absence attacks for 2 to 3 years and the patient enters the phase of antiepileptic drug withdrawal. Counts of electroclinical attacks after drug withdrawal can be compared to the count obtained on the initial video/EEG monitoring.

Attempts at computerized detection and quantitation of diffuse spike-waves during long-term video/EEG monitoring have been reported by DeVries et al. (19), Quy et al. (100), Gergely and Paul (37), and Gotman (41, 42). The goal is to consume less time in analyzing data acquired during the prolonged monitoring sessions. When these systems are used to identify epochs at which clinical seizures may have occurred (so-called buffering), they can successfully reduce the data for naked eye or visual analysis.

More studies, however, are necessary to develop systems of spike-wave detection and quantification which have a low incidence of false positive and false negative detections (16, 109). The above reported quantifiers for spike-wave paroxysms all suffer from these shortcomings and cannot be used alone. All require some validation by the naked eye to guard against false positive and false negative results. Worse uncertainties about the reliability of on-line spike detection exist with the sole exception of the studies of Gotman et al. (41, 42) who have used a spike detector to trigger the recognition of ictal activity.

Video/EEG monitoring unaided by buffering systems that can reduce data collected from 24 hr of recording can be even more time consuming for the nurse clinicians or psychologists when absence epilepsies other than childhood petit mal are present, e.g., myoclonus absence, myoclonic absence, juvenile absence (Table 5). Prolonged performance testing for documentation of impaired consciousness and decreased cognitive powers during bursts of 3- to 5-Hz or 4- to 6-Hz multispike or single-spike-wave sequences or diffuse 12-Hz rhythms will need to be done more often. Rare forms of juvenile absence seizures may be associated with high-voltage, bilaterally synchronous, diffuse 8- to 12-Hz rhythms rather than spike-wave sequences. Monitoring personnel must be trained to distinguish these attacks from childhood absence seizures with spike-wave complexes (Table 5). Another rare form of absence in childhood, described in cases 3 and 4, is myoclonic absence where staring is associated with symmetric myoclonic jerking of the limbs and trunk during diffuse 8- to 12-Hz rhythms or diffuse 3- to 6-Hz multispike-wave complexes; here, the myoclonic activity is more prominent than in classical absence, but the patients are not propelled to the floor, as in Lennox-Gastaut syndrome (see cases 3 and 4 in patient illustrations). Like classical absence, these two subvarieties of absence seizures respond to valproic acid. Another rare form of absence starts in adolescence and consists of short attacks of unconsciousness (8–10 sec), automatisms, and asymmetric myoclonic activity with diffuse 8- to 12-Hz rhythms (myoclonus absence).

The importance of video/EEG in prospective studies of absence seizures was shown by Sato et al. (103), who quantitated attacks on videotape and by radiotelemetry. Seventy-eight percent of patients who initially suffered from absence seizures alone were attack-free after 16 years. In contrast, only 31% of patients who initially had both absence and GTC seizures were attack-free. Lack of generalized tonic-clonic seizures, an IQ of at least 90, and no family history of seizures were favorable factors for the future cessation of all types of seizures. For the cessation of absence seizures, however, normal EEG background activity and an IQ of 90 or more were significant. Similar prospective studies are now being applied to other types of absence epilepsies.

Perhaps the most common form of generalized epilepsies consists of impulsive petit mal or juvenile myoclonic epilepsy of Janz (synonyms: benign myoclonic and clonic-tonic-clonic seizures of adolescence). They account for 10 to 22% of all epilepsies and are probably responsible for old incidence figures which claim absence accounting for 10 to 12% of seizures in adults and adolescents. Ten to 37% of patients with juvenile myoclonic epilepsy of Janz also have absence attacks in addition to grand mal tonic-clonic and myoclonic seizures. As a rule, absence attacks are simple, relatively infrequent, and appear a few years before the myoclonic jerks do. According to Janz, 4.6% of childhood absence develop into juvenile myoclonic epilepsy when patients have reached the peak age onset of impulsiv petit mal. Janz also reports that impulsiv petit-mal-type jerks are found in 8.2% of patients with childhood absence and 15.9% of juvenile absence.

Over 50% of patients with juvenile myoclonic epilepsy have both grand mal convulsions and myoclonic jerks. Most often, patients with juvenile myoclonic epilepsy come for referral because of uncontrolled grand mal convulsions. Only when their histories are carefully reviewed are the presence of small, single, or repeated shoulder and arm jerks recognized. Some patients report that only one arm or leg jerks, and most frequently they pay no attention to the jerks until something is thrown or dropped from their hand. Table 5 lists explanations given by patients, family members, and practitioners as to why they mistook myoclonic seizures for nonepileptic events, and why they disregarded the myoclonic jerks. Rarely is a correct diagnosis of impulsiv petit mal or juvenile myoclonic epilepsy made before the first grand mal convulsion occurs. In this regard, it is of interest to note that 8 to 17% of impulsiv petit mal are manifested by myoclonic seizures alone without tonic-clonic convulsions or absences.

Juvenile myoclonic epilepsy affects children and adolescents who are otherwise normal neurologically and have normal to high intelligence. What is characteristic is the appearance of mild myoclonic jerks of neck and shoulder flexor muscles and by clonic-tonic-clonic seizures shortly after awakening. Most commonly the interictal EEG trait consists of the fast or 4- to 6-Hz variety of diffuse spike-and-wave sequences or multispike-and-wave complexes. In 30% of patients, 3-Hz multispike-wave complexes are present during absence seizures. During actual myoclonic seizures, diffuse high-amplitude rapid spikes fire in both hemispheres at 16 to 24 Hz. The age at onset peaks at 13 years, but electroclinical traits persist into the later decades of life. Forty-one percent of relatives of probands have myoclonias with the highest incidence among females; 15% of family members of probands have the EEG trait without clinical attacks.

Pure grand mal occurs as the only type of attack in 4 to 10% of all patients with epilepsy. In these patients, there are no associated myoclonic or petit mal absence attacks. True primary grand mal epilepsy should be differentiated from "lesional" or secondary tonic-clonic convulsions which result from structural lesions. Two forms of primary grand mal epilepsy are now recognized. The first consists of awakening clonic-tonic-clonic seizures and is usually triggered by sleep deprivation, excessive fatigue, and alcohol intake. Consciousness is still preserved during myoclonic jerks and it is lost when the head, face, neck, and trunk extend with tonic contraction. This tonic phase lasts 10 to 20 sec and leads to a final phase of clonic trunk and limb jerks. These seizures have an interictal EEG trait of diffuse 4- to 6-Hz multispike-and-wave complexes. During ictus, diffuse 14- to 24-Hz multispikes fire during brief and violent flexor spasms of the entire body (initial clonic phase). The second subvariety of grand mal epilepsy consists of tonic-clonic seizures with an interictal EEG trait of well formed diffuse 3-Hz spike-and-wave complexes. During ictus, epileptic recruiting patterns of 9- to 12-Hz diffuse rhythms herald the tonic phase. Tonic-clonic seizures frequently occur during both diurnal and nocturnal hours.

The practitioner should differentiate these treatable primary generalized epilepsies from the difficult-to-treat infantile spasms of West syndrome, the symptomatic myoclonic astatic seizures of Lennox-Gastaut, and the difficult-to-treat to untreatable progressive heredofamilial myoclonic epilepsies with dementia. Although symptomatic relief can occur in some infantile spasms and myoclonic astatic epilepsies during treatment with antiepileptic drugs and ACTH, diffuse brain damage with mental subnormality is frequently present, and continued freedom from seizures after withdrawal of antiepileptic drugs does not occur. In the progressive heredofamilial myoclonic epilepsies with dementia, not only can seizures be resistant but the relentless progress of the disease usually results in severe neurologic disability and death.

Outpatient Versus Inpatient Video/EEG Monitoring

As is evidenced in the above discussion, the diagnosis of a seizure disorder and the presence of a primary generalized epilepsy can commonly be made with the clinical history and the interictal EEG. When seizures persist in spite of antiepileptic drugs, prolonged video/EEG monitoring can provide evidence for the presence of one or more seizure types, as well as provide clues as to the type of epilepsy present.

The epilepsy monitoring service should, at the time of referral, decide whether prolonged video/EEG can be done as an outpatient (diurnal 3–12 hr) or as an inpatient (24-hr monitoring). Generalized absence seizures usually occur so frequently that 3 or 6 hr of video/EEG monitoring as an outpatient may suffice and answer the following diagnostic issues[1]:

1. Is there more than one type of electroclinical seizure, e.g., impaired consciousness associated with 3-Hz diffuse spike-wave complexes, impaired consciousness with diffuse 12-Hz rhythms, and impaired consciousness with low-voltage slowing. Can all be present in the same patient with varying sensitivity or resistance to valproate or ethosuximide?
2. Is consciousness impaired with every diffuse burst of spike-wave complexes?

[1] This is in contrast to partial seizures which usually do not occur in such frequencies as to encourage shorter monitoring sessions in the outpatient. Moreover, sleep increases the likelihood of capturing complex partial seizures; hence, we recommend round-the-clock inpatient video/EEG monitoring for most partial seizures which require documentation.

3. If consciousness is not impaired with every diffuse burst of spike-wave sequences, are cognitive functions disabled, e.g., latency of response, rapidity of information processing?
4. How frequent were the electroclinical attacks? Do seizures occur in clusters or are they spread evenly over the period of intensive video/EEG monitoring? Frequency and duration of attacks should be noted, e.g., 15 classic absence with 3-Hz spike-wave sequences lasting 3 to 8 sec/hr and 1 prolonged absence attack with 3-Hz spike-wave sequences lasting 30 min/6 hr can occur in the same patient. In this latter example, it is ideal to do 24-hr recordings to accurately quantitate the frequency of prolonged absence attacks.

Once the type(s) of epileptic seizures are documented on video/EEG, the combination of epileptic seizures and the clinical setting in which it occurs, the age at onset, the frequency and temporal distribution of seizures and their precipitants should give more clues as to the type of epilepsy present and the presumed etiology responsible. It is well for the practitioner to appreciate that pure forms of generalized epilepsy are very rare on the video/EEG. A single form of generalized epileptic seizures can occur alone, but they are more frequently observed in combination with clonic-tonic-clonic or tonic-clonic seizures. Pure absence without tonic-clonic seizures is also rare; it is more frequent to record the many absence attacks mixed with prolonged (10–30 min) absence, or tonic-clonic seizures or occasional myoclonic jerks. As we have learned from our 15 years experience in intensive monitoring, apparently pure tonic-clonic seizures are often associated with or preceded immediately by an absence attack or bilateral myoclonic jerks.

At the conclusion of outpatient video/EEG monitoring, it is our custom to ask ourselves if there is any information we may have missed. We compare the patient's historical account of his/her habitual seizures with what we see on the videotape. When the seizures recorded on outpatient monitoring do not conform to the habitual seizures; when seizures occur only at night during induction of sleep; when seizures are provoked during transfer from night-time sleep to wakefulness, e.g., awakening grand mal, awakening myoclonic seizures; when seizures are not frequent enough to be recorded in a 3- to 12-hr session; when there is the possibility of tonic-clonic status epilepticus; or when there are medical reasons to have the patient admitted to the inpatient unit, we elect to perform video/EEG recordings as an inpatient. The latter instances are especially true when the practitioner decides to cross-over to another antiepileptic drug or when a decision to switch from polypharmacy to monotherapy is made.

Follow-up

After a new drug trial is instituted, cross-over is successful and steady-state kinetics are achieved, it is clinically prudent to quantitate the electroclinical seizures again. Particular attention is given to whether a specific electroclinical seizure persists or disappears, e.g., after ethosuximide, classic absence seizures may disappear; but rhythmic myoclonic jerks or assymetrical myoclonus may persist with minimal impairment of consciousness if myoclonic absence is present and ethosuximide is used. Similarly, valproate may suppress absence and 3-Hz spike-wave sequences but absence with diffuse low-voltage slowing persists in the same patient.

When two drugs are required and cross-overs to different drugs have to be done to find a successful drug combination, quantitation and documentation of electroclinical states often help in deciding if a given drug combination is working. When successful treatment controls seizures for a few years, a decision should be made on (a) whether the patient is cured of his/her epilepsy, (b) whether the epilepsy has run its natural course and spontaneously remitted, or (c) whether antiepileptic drug treatment has only suppressed the clinical expression of seizures but the epilepsy genotype persists. In making these decisions, it is well to consider available information on remissions and cure of generalized epilepsies, realizing that no prospective study has accurately delineated the natural course and behavior of each of the subvarieties of generalized epilepsies. In this decision, there is no substitute to good and prudent clinical judgment and the results of prolonged video/EEG monitoring are of great help.

REFERENCES

1. Aarts, J.H.P., Binnie, C.D., Smit, A., and Wilkins, A.J. (1982): Performance testing during epileptiform EEG activity. In: *Mobile Long-term EEG Monitoring: Proceedings of the MLE Symposium,* edited by H. Stephan and W. Burr, pp. 161–168. Fischer, Stuttgart.
2. Aarts, J.H.P., Binnie, C., Van Bentum-de Boer, P.T.E., et al. (1982): The value of telemetric EEG-monitoring in epilepsy. *Br. J. Clin. Pract. (Suppl.),* 18:5–9.
3. Ajmone-Marsan, C., and Abraham, K. (1960): A seizure atlas. *Electroencephalogr. Clin. Neurophysiol. (Suppl),* 15:215.
4. Ajmone-Marsan, C., and Zivin, L.S. (1970): Factors related to the occurrence of typical paroxysmal abnormalities in the EEG records of epileptic patients. *Epilepsia,* 11:361–381.
5. Beaumanoir, A., Nahory, A., and Potoliccio, S. (1982): Indication of tele-electroencephalography coupled to videoscopy in the study of higher functions in the epileptic child. *Rev. Electroencephalogr. Neurophysiol. Clin.,* 12:315–318.
6. Belafsky, M.A., Rosman, N.P., Miller, P., Waddell, G., Boxley-Johnson, J., and Delgado-Escueta, A.V. (1978): Prolonged epileptic twilight states: continuous recordings with nasopharyngeal electrodes and videotape analysis. *Neurology,* 28:239–245.
7. Berger, H. (1929): Uber das elektrendephalogram des meuschen. I mitteilung arch psychiat. *J. Nervenkr.,* 87:527.
8. Berger, H. (1935): Uber die entstehung der erscheinungen des grossen epileptischen anfalls. *J. Klin. Wochenschr.,* 14:217.
9. Binnie, C.D. (1980): Detection of transitory cognitive impairment during epileptiform EEG discharges: Problems in clinical practice. In: *Epilepsy and Behavior '79,* edited by B.M. Kulig, H. Meinardi, and G. Stores, pp. 91–97. Swets and Zeitlinger, Lisse.
10. Binnie, C.D. (1983): Telemetric EEG monitoring in epilepsy, In: *Recent Advances in Epilepsy,* edited by T.A. Pedley and B.S. Meldrum, pp. 155–178. Churchill Livingston, New York.
11. Binnie, C.D., Rowan, A.J., Overweg, L., Meinardi, H., Wisman, T., Kamp, A., and

Lopes da Silva, F. (1981): Telemetric EEG and video monitoring in epilepsy. *Neurology,* 31:298–303.

12. Boudoulas, H., Schaal, S.F., Lewis, R.P., and Robinson, J.L. (1979): Superiority of 24-hour outpatient monitoring over multistage exercise testing for the evaluation of syncope. *J. Electrocardiol.,* 12:103–108.
13. Calmeil, L.F. (1824): De l'epilepsie, étudiée sous le rapport de son siege et de son influence sur la production de l'alienation mentale. *Thesis,* Paris.
14. Chevrie, J.J., and Aicardi, J. (1972): Childhood epileptic encephalopathy with slow spike waves. *Epilepsia (Amst.),* 13:259–271.
15. Chevrie, J.J., and Aicardi, J. (1972): Childhood epileptic encephalography with slow spike-wave. A statistical study of 80 cases. *Epilepsia (Amst.),* 13:259–271.
16. Comley, R.A., and Brignell, J.E. (1981): Real time detection of the epileptic precursor. *J. Phys. (E.),* 14:963–967.
17. Commission on Classification and Terminology of the International League Against Epilepsy (1984): Closed workshop for revised clinical and electroencephalographic classification of epilepsies. Bethesda, Maryland.
18. Darby, C.E., de Korte, R.A., Binnie, C.D., and Wilkins, A.J. (1980): The self-induction of epileptic seizures by eye-closure. *Epilepsia,* 21:31–42.
19. De Vries, J., Wisman, T., and Binnie, C.D. (1981): Evaluation of a simple spike-wave recognition system. *Electroencephalogr. Clin. Neurophysiol.,* 51:328–330.
20. Delgado-Escueta, A.V. (1979): Epileptogenic paroxysms: Modern approaches and clinical correlations. *Neurology,* 29:1014–1022.
21. Delgado-Escueta, A.V., Kunze, U., Waddell, G., Boxley, J., Nadel, A. (1977): Lapse of consciousness and automatisms in temporal lobe epilepsy: A videotape analysis. *Neurology,* 27:144–155.
22. Delgado-Escueta, A.V., Lee, A.G., Maldonado, H.M., Swartz, B., Enrile-Bacsal, F., and Walsh, G.O. (1986): Electroclinical studies in pedigrees of juvenile myoclonic epilepsy. *Ann. Neurol. (Submitted).*
23. Delgado-Escueta, A.V., Treiman, D.M., and Walsh, G.O. (1983): The treatable epilepsies, *N. Engl. J. Med.,* 308:1508–1514; 1576–1584.
24. Delgado-Escueta, A.V., and Walsh, G.O. (1985): Type I complex partial seizures of hippocampal origin: excellent results of anterior lobectomy. *Neurology,* 35:143–154.
25. Desai, B.T., Porter, R.J., and Penry, J.K. (1982): Psychogenic seizures: a study of 42 attacks in six patients, with intensive monitoring. *Arch. Neurol.,* 39:202–209.
26. Dreyer, R., and Wehmeyer, W. (1978): Laughing in complex partial seizure epilepsy: a video tape analysis of 32 patients with laughing as symptom of an attack. *Fortschr. Neurol. Psychiatr.,* 46:61–75.
27. Dreyer, R., and Wehmeyer, W. (1978): The symptom of EEG-flattening accompanying psychomotor attacks, their frequency, duration, form and significance. A video-band analysis of 78 patients with 187 attacks. *Arch. Psychiatr. Nervenkr.,* 225:263–274.
28. Ebersole, J.S., and Leroy, R.F. (1983): Evaluation of ambulatory cassette EEG monitoring: III. Diagnostic accuracy compared to intensive inpatient EEG monitoring. *Neurology,* 33:853–860.
29. Esquirol, J.E.D. (1838): Des maladies mentales considerées sous les rapports médical, hygienique at médico-legal. Paris.
30. Finnegan, T., Abraham, P., and Docherty, T. (1982): Ambulatory monitoring in the Himalayas. *Electroencephalogr. Clin. Neurophysiol.,* 54:21.
31. Gastaut, H. (1970): Clinical and electroencephalographic classification of epileptic seizures. *Epilepsia,* 11:102–113.
32. Gastaut, H., Roger, J., and Lob, H. (1967): *Les États de Mal Épileptiques,* p. 379. Masson, Paris.
33. Gastaut, H., Roger, J., Soulayrol, R., Tassinari, C.A., Regis, H., Dravet, C., Bernard, R., Pinsard, N., and Saint-Jean, M. (1966): Childhood epileptic encephalopathy with diffuse slow spike-waves (otherwise known as 'petit mal variant') or Lennox's syndrome. *Epilepsia,* 7:139–179.
34. Gastaut, H., and Bert, J. (1954): EEG changes during cinematographic presentation, *Electroencephalogr. Clin. Pres.,* 6:433–444.
35. Geier, S. (1971): A comparative tele-EEG study of adolescent and adult epileptics. *Epilepsia,* 12:215–223.

36. Geier, S., Bancaud, J., and Talairach, J., et al. (1977): Ictal tonic postural changes and automatisms of the upper limb during epileptic partial lobe discharges. *Epilepsia,* 18:517–524.
37. Gergely, S., and Paul, R. (1975): Delayed signal EEG trigger. *Biomed. Eng. (Lond.),* 10:105–107.
38. Goldensohn, E.S. (1966): Simultaneous recording of EEG and clinical seizure using the kineoscope. *Electroencephalogr. Clin. Neurophysiol.,* 21:623.
39. Goode, D.J., Penry, K., and Dreifuss, F.E. (1970): Effects of paroxysmal spike-wave on continuous visual motor performance. *Epilepsia (Amst.),* 11:241–254.
40. Gooses, D. (1985): Photosensitivity in age related generalized idiopathic epilepsies (*submitted*).
41. Gotman, J. (1981): Automatic recognition of epileptic seizures in the EEG. *Electroencephalogr. Clin. Neurophysiol.,* 54:530–540.
42. Gotman, J. (1982): A computer system to assist in the evaluation of the EEGs of epileptic patients. *Behav. Res. Meth.,* 13:525–531.
43. Gowers, W.R. (1901): *Epilepsy and Other Chronic Convulsive Diseases: Their Causes, Symptoms and Treatment (2nd ed.).* Church, London.
44. Graf, M., Brunner, G., Weber, H., Auinger, C., and Joskowicz, G. (1982): Simultaneous long-term recording of EEG and ECG in 'syncope' patients. In: *Mobile Long-term EEG Monitoring: Proceedings of the MLE Symposium in Bonn 1982,* edited by H. Stefan and W. Burr, pp. 67–75. Fischer, Stuttgart.
45. Green, J.B. (1966): Self-induced seizures: clinical and electroencephalographic studies. *Arch. Neurol.,* 15:579–586.
46. Guey, J., Bureau, M., Dravet, C., and Roger, J. (1969): A study of the rhythm of petit mal absences in children in relation of prevailing situations: the use of EEG telemetry during psychological examinations, school exercises and periods of inactivity. *Epilepsia,* 10:441–451.
47. Gulick, T.A., Spinks, I.P., and King, D.W. (1982): Pseudoseizures: ictal phenomena. *Neurology,* 32:24–30.
48. Herpin, T. (1852): *Du Pronostic et du Traitement Curatif de l'Épilepsie.* Ouvrage couronne par l'Institut, Paris.
49. Holmes, G.L. (1984): Partial complex seizures in children: an analysis of 69 seizures in 24 patients using EEG FM radiotelemetry and videotape recording. *Electroencephalogr. Clin. Neurophysiol.,* 57:13–20.
50. Holmes, G.L., Sackellares, J.C., McKievnan, L., Ragland, M., and Dreifuss, F.E. (1980): Evaluation of childhood pseudoseizures using EEG telemetry and video tape monitoring. *J. Pediatr.,* 97:(4):554–558.
51. Holmes, G.L., Sackellares, J.C., McKiernan, J., Ragland, M., and Dreifuss, F.E. (1980): Evaluation of childhood pseudoseizures using EEG telemetry and video tape monitoring. *J. Pediatr.,* 97:554–558.
52. Hunter, J., and Jasper, H.H. (1949): A method of analysis of seizure patterns. *EEG Clin. Neurophysiol.,* 1:113–114.
53. Ives, J.R. (1982): A completely ambulatory 16-channel cassette recording system. In: *Mobile Long-term EEG Monitoring: Proceedings of the MLE Symposium, Bonn 1982,* edited by H. Stefan and W. Burr, pp. 205–217. Fischer, Stuttgart.
54. Ives, J.R., and Gloor, P. (1977): New sphenoidal electrode assembly to permit long-term monitoring of the patient's ictal or interictal EEG. *Electroencephalogr. Clin. Neurophysiol.,* 42:575–580.
55. Ives, J.R., and Gloor, P. (1978): A long-term time-lapse video system to document the patient's spontaneous clinical seizure synchronized with the EEG. *EEG Clin. Neurophysiol.,* 45:412–416.
56. Jackson, J.H. (1931): Selected writings of John Hughlings Jackson. In: *On Epilepsy and Epileptiform Convulsions, Vol. 1,* edited by J. Taylor. Hodder and Stoughton, London.
57. Janz, D. (1969): *Die Epilepsien.* Thieme, Stuttgart.
58. Janz, D., and Christian, W. (1957): Impulsiv-Petit Mal. In: *Dtsch. Z. Nervenheilk.,* 176:346–386.
59. Kamp, A., Mars, N.J.I., and Wisman, T. (1979): Longterm monitoring of the electroencephalogram in epileptic patients. In: *A Handbook on Biotelemetry and Radio Tracking,* edited by C.J. Amlaner and D.W. Macdonald, pp. 499–503. Pergamon Press, Oxford.

60. Kasteliejn-Nolst Trenite, D.G.A., Binnie C.D., de Korte, R.A., et al. (1982): Correlative electrophysiological and clinical studies in photosensitive epilepsy. *Br. J. Clin. Prac. (Suppl.)*, 18:81–83.
61. King, D.W., Gallagher, B.B., Murvin, A.L., Smith, D.B., Marcus, D.J., Hartlage, L.C., and Ward, L.C. (1982): Pseudoseizures: Diagnostic evaluation. *Neurology,* 32:18–23.
62. Lennox, W.G. (1936): The physiological pathogenesis of epilepsy. *Brain,* 59:113.
63. Lennox, W.G. (1945): The petit mal epilepsies; their treatment with tridione, *JAMA,* 129:1069.
64. Lennox, W.G. (1951): Phenomena and correlates of the psychomotor triad. *Neurology,* (Minneapolis), 1:357.
65. Lennox, W.G. (1960): *Epilepsy and Related Disorders, Vol. 1 and 2,* p. 1168. Little, Brown, Boston.
66. Lennox, W.G., Gibbs, F.A., and Gibbs, E.L. (1936): Effect on the electroencephalogram of drugs and conditions which influence seizures. *Arch. Neurol. Psychiatry,* 36:1236.
67. Lloyd, D.S.L., Binnie, C.D., Stenfors, S.G.B., and Roberts, J.R. (1972): Character generation on a moving chart recorder. *Biomed. Eng. (Lond.)*, 7:274–277.
68. Lugaresi, E., Pazzaglia, P., Bureau, M., Ambrosetto, G., Roger, J., and Tassinari, C.A. (1973): Prognosis and evolution of petit mal absences. In *Prognosis and Evolution of Epilepsy,* edited by E. Lugaresi, P. Pazzaglia, and C.A. Tassinari. Aulo Gaggi, Bologna.
69. Lugaresi, E., and Tassinari, C.A. (1967): Brèves considérations sur l'état de petit mal. In: *Les États de Mal Epileptiques,* pp. 119–128. Masson, Paris.
70. Luther, L.S., McNamara, L.O., Carwile, S., Miller, P., and Hope, V. (1982): Pseudoepileptic seizures: Methods and video analysis to aid diagnosis. *Ann. Neurol.,* 12:458–462.
71. Manson, G. (1974): EEG radio telemetry. *Electroencephalogr. Clin. Neurophysiol.,* 37:441–413.
72. Mattson, R.H. (1983): Closed-circuit-televised video tape recording and electroencephalography (CCTV/EEG) in convulsive status epilepticus. In: *Advances in Neurology, Vol 34: Status Epilepticus,* edited by A.V. Delgado-Escueta, C.G. Wasterlain, D.M. Treiman, and R.L. Porter. Raven Press, New York.
73. McGrath, D.M. (1983): Video recording seizure activity in children. *MCN,* 8:218–220.
74. Meier-Ewert, K., and Broughton, R.J. (1967): Photomyoclonic response of epileptic and non-epileptic subjects during wakefulness, sleep and arousal. *Electroencephalogr. Clin. Neurophysiol.,* 23:142–151.
75. Metrakos, K., and Metrakos, J.D. (1961): Genetics of convulsive disorders. II. Genetic and electroencephalographic studies in centrencephalic epilepsy, *Neurology, (Minneapolis)*, 11:474–483.
76. Noebels, J. (1979): Analysis of inherited epilepsy using single locus mutations in mice. *Fed. Proc.,* 38:2405–2410.
77. O'Kane, M.L., and Santer, R. (1977): Long-term intensive monitoring of epileptic patients. In: *Epilepsy: the Eighth International Symposium,* edited by J.K. Penry, pp. 125–129. Raven Press, New York.
78. O'Kane, M., O'Kane, F., and Mothersill, I. (1982): On the telemetric monitoring of ictal events. In: *Mobile Long-term EEG Monitoring: Proceedings of the MLE Symposium, Bonn 1982,* edited by H. Stefan and W. Burr, pp. 137–147. Fischer, Stuttgart.
79. Oller-Daurella, A.L. (1967): Contribucion al Estudio de las Absencias Epilepticas. *Arch. Pediatr. (Barcelona)*, 18:239–260.
80. Overweg, J., Binnie, C.D., van der Geest, P., Meinardi, H., and van Parys, J.A. (1981): Clinical evaluation of EEG telemetry and videomonitoring in 212 patients with epilepsy. *Ned. Tijdschr. Geneeskd.,* 125:1600–1604.
81. Penfield, W. (1958): *The Excitable Cortex in Conscious Man.* Liverpool University Press, Liverpool, England.
82. Penfield, W. (1968): Engrams in the human brain. *Proc. Rev. Soc. Med.,* 61:831.
83. Penfield, W., and Bridges W.H (1942): Progressive tissue destruction in epileptogenic lesions of the brain. *Trans. Am. Neurol. Assoc.,* 67:158–163.
84. Penfield, W., and Cage, L. (1933): Cerebral localization of epileptic manifestations, *AMA Arch Neurol. Psychiatr.,* 30:709.
85. Penfield, W., and Humphreys, S. (1942): Epileptogenic lesions of the brain. *Arch. Neurol. Psychiatry,* 43:240–261.

86. Penfield, W., and Jasper, H.H. (1954): *Epilepsy and the Functional Anatomy of the Human Brain,* p. 20. Little, Brown, Boston.
87. Penfield, W., and Kristiansen, K. (1951): *Epileptic Seizure Patterns,* Thomas, Springfield, Illinois.
88. Penfield, W., and Perot, P. (1963): The brain's record of auditory and visual experience, *Brain,* 86:595.
89. Penfield, W., and Roberts, L. (1959): *Speech and Brain-Mechanisms,* Princeton University Press, Princeton, New Jersey.
90. Penry, J.K., Porter, R.L., and Dreifuss, F.E. (1975): Simultaneous recording of absence seizures with video tape and electroencephalography. *Brain,* 98:427–440.
91. Penry, J.K., and Porter, R.J. (1977): Intensive monitoring of patients with intractable seizures. In: *Epilepsy: the Eighth International Symposium,* edited by J.K. Penry, pp. 96–101. Raven Press, New York.
92. Penry, J.K., and Dreifuss, F.E. (1969): Automatisms associated with the absence of petit mal epilepsy. *Arch. Neurol.,* 21:142–149.
93. Penry, J.K., and Dreifuss, F.E. (1969): A study of automatisms associated with the absence of petit mal. *Epilepsia, (Amst.),* 10:417.
94. Penry, J.K., Porter, R.J., and Dreifuss, F.E. (1971): Quantification of paroxysmal abnormal discharge in the EEGs of patients with absence (petit mal) seizures for evaluation of antiepileptic drugs. *Epilepsia,* 12:278–279.
95. Perry, T.R., Gumnit, R.J., Gates, J.R., and Leppik, I.E. (1983): Routine EEG vs. intensive monitoring in the evaluation of intractable epilepsy. *Public Health Rep.,* 98:384–389.
96. Porter, R.J., Penry, J.K., and Dreifuss, F.E. (1973): Responsiveness at the onset of spike-wave bursts. *Electroencephalogr. Clin. Neurophysiol.,* 34:239–245.
97. Porter, R.J., Penry, J.K., and Lacy, J.R. (1977): Diagnostic and therapeutic reevaluation of patients with intractable epilepsy. *Neurology, (Minneapolis),* 27:1006–1011.
98. Porter, R.J., Theodore, W.H., and Schulman, E.A. (1981): Intensive monitoring of intractable epilepsy: a two-year follow-up. In: *Advances in Epileptology: XIIth Epilepsy International Symposium,* edited by M. Dam, L. Gram, and J.K. Penry, pp. 265–268. Raven Press, New York.
99. Porter, R.J., Wolf, A.A., and Penry, J.K. (1971): Human electroencephalographic telemetry. *Am. J. Med. Technol.,* 11:145–159.
100. Quy, R.J., Fitch, P., and Willison, R.G. (1980): High-speed automatic analysis of EEG spike and wave activity using an analogue detection and microcomputer plotting system. *Electroencephalogr. Clin. Neurophysiol.,* 49:187–189.
101. Reynolds, R.J. (1861): *Epilepsy: Its Symptoms, Treatment, and Relation to Other Convulsive Diseases.* Churchill, London.
102. Rohrbaugh, J.W., Fischer, A.Q., Bennett, D.R., and Ellingson, R.J. (1983): Intensive monitoring of epileptic patients. *Nebr. Med. J.,* 68:132–136.
103. Sato, S., Dreifuss, F.E., and Penry, J.K. (1976): Prognostic factors in absence seizures. *Neurology (Minneapolis),* 26:788–796.
104. Sato, S., Penry, J.K., and Burch, J.D. (1978): Eight-channel EEG digital cassette recorder for monitoring partial and generalized seizures. In: *ISAM 1977, Proceedings of the 2nd International Symposium on Ambulatory Monitoring, London,* edited by F.D. Scott, E.B. Raftery, P. Slight, and L. Goulding, pp. 93–103. Academic Press, London.
105. Schmidt, D., Machus, B., Porter, R.J., and Penry, J.K. (1982): The variability of ictal signs in complex-partial seizures: a videotape analysis. In: *Mobile Long-term EEG Monitoring: Proceedings of the MLE Symposium, Bonn,* edited by H. Stefan and W. Burr, pp. 149–159. Fischer, Stuttgart.
106. Schwab, R.S. (1939): A method of measuring consciousness in petit mal epilepsy. *J. Nerv. Ment. Dis.,* 89:690–691.
107. Schwab, R.S. (1939): Method of measuring consciousness in petit mal epilepsy. *Arch. Neurol. Psychiatry,* 41:215–217.
108. Schwab, R.S., Schwab, M.W., Withec, D., and Cock, Y.C. (1954): Synchronized moving pictures of patients and EEG. *Electroencephalogr. Clin. Neurophysiol.,* 6:684–686.
109. Seino, M., Yagi, K., and Takeuchi, I. (1981): A self-tracking system for intensive monitoring of epileptic seizures. *Abstracts Epilepsy International Congress, Kyoto,* p. 191.

110. Sindrup, E. (1980): Technical contributions to the differential diagnosis in epilepsy. *Acta Neurol. Scand. (Suppl)*, 79:47–48.
111. Stalberg, E. (1976): Experiences with long term telemetry in routine diagnostic work. In: *Quantitative Analytic Studies in Epilepsy,* edited by P. Kellaway and I. Petersen, pp. 269–278. Raven Press, New York.
112. Stevens, J.R., Milstein, V.M., and Dodds, S. (1969): Prolonged recording of EEG by radiotelemetry: an aid to localization and treatment of epilepsy. *Electroencephalogr. Clin. Neurophysiol.,* 27:544.
113. Stores, G., and Brankin, P. (1982): Recent development in ambulatory EEG monitoring. *Br. J. Clin. Pract. (Suppl.)*, 18:10–15.
114. Stores, G., Brankin, P., and Crawford, C. (1982): Aspects of differential diagnosis using ambulatory monitoring. In: *Mobile Long-term EEG Monitoring: Proceedings of the MLE Symposium, Bonn,* edited by H. Stefan and W. Burr, pp. 55–60. Fischer, Stuttgart.
115. Sutula, T.P., Sackellares, J.C., Miller, J.Q., and Dreifuss, F.E. (1981): Intensive monitoring in refractory epilepsy. *Neurology,* (NY), 31:243–247.
116. Talairach, J., and Bancaud, J. (1974): Stereotaxic exploration and therapy in epilepsy. In: *The Epilepsies (Handbook of Clinical Neurology)*, edited by O. Magnus and A.M. Lorentz DeHaas, pp. 758–782. American Elsevier, New York.
117. Tassinari, C.A., Lyagoubi, S., Santos, V., Gamborelli, F., Roger, J., Dravet, C., and Gastaut, H. (1969): Étude des décharges de pointe-onde chez l'homme. Les aspects cliniques et electroencephalographiques des absences myocloniques. *Rev. Neurol.,* 3:379–383.
118. Tissot, T. (1790): *Traite de l'Épilepsie.* Lausanne.
119. Tsuboi, T., and Christian, W. (1973): On the genetics of primary generalized epilepsy with sporadic myoclonias of the impulsive petit mal type: and clinical electroencephalographic study of 399 probands. *Humangenetik,* 19:155–12.
120. Turner, W.A. (1907): *Epilepsy: A Study of the Idiopathic Disease.* New Burlington, London.
121. Vignaendra, V., Walsh, J., and Burrows, S. (1979): The application of prolonged EEG telemetry and videotape recording to the study of seizures and related disorders. *Clin. Exp. Neurol.,* 16:81–94.
122. Walsh, G.O., and Delgado-Escueta, A.V. (1984): Type II complex partial seizures: Poor results of anterior temporal lobectomy. *Neurology,* 34:1–13.
123. Wolf, P., and Inoue, Y. (1984): Therapeutic response of absence seizures in patients of an epilepsy clinic for adolescents and adults. *J. Neurol.,* 231(4):225–229.
124. Zetterlund, B. (1982): Quantification of spike-and-wave episodes in 24-hr tape recordings of EEG. In: *Mobile Long-term EEG Monitoring: Proceedings of the MLE Symposium, Bonn,* edited by H. Stefan and W. Burr, pp. 237–244. Fischer, Stuttgart.

Advances in Neurology, Vol. 46: Intensive Neurodiagnostic Monitoring, edited by R. J. Gumnit. Raven Press, New York © 1986.

Intensive Monitoring of Complex Partial Seizures: Diagnosis and Subclassification

Peter D. Williamson

Department of Neurology, Yale University School of Medicine, New Haven, Connecticut 06510; and West Haven Veterans Administration Medical Center, West Haven, Connecticut 06516

Over 100 years have passed since Jackson originally described the epileptic "dreamy state" and related it to lesions in the medial temporal lobe (23, 24). Since then there have been numerous detailed but diverse descriptions of complex partial seizures (CPSs). Although there are certain distinctive features, it is now recognized that these seizures can present with an almost endless variety of clinical manifestations. Furthermore, CPSs may resemble nonepileptic medical or psychiatric conditions and diagnostic errors can occur in either direction (7, 32, 50, 56, 57).

Since CPSs usually do not occur frequently enough to allow direct observation by a trained observer, except by chance, the initial diagnosis often depends on an accurate history. Signs and symptoms are often vague or peculiar and additional studies are needed to confirm the diagnosis. However, routine diagnostic studies may not be helpful. Outpatient EEGs may reveal paroxysmal features, but frequently they are normal or nonspecific (29). Computerized tomography (CT) may reveal an unsuspected lesion, but much more often it is normal. When all tests are normal or nondiagnostic, the treating physician must decide whether the historical evidence is strong enough to justify empirical anticonvulsant therapy. A favorable response to anticonvulsant medication helps confirm the diagnosis. Lack of response can have several explanations, such as incorrect diagnosis or inappropriate medication. When an anticonvulsant drug fails in a patient with suspected seizures, there is a tendency to add more medications. Polypharmacy can compound the problem with drug interactions and toxicity.

The introduction of closed circuit television monitoring and simultaneous EEG recording (video/EEG) has greatly expanded our ability to diagnose, evaluate, and manage patients with convulsive disorders (32, 40, 54, 55). The study of video/EEG records has furthered our understanding of CPSs and is beginning to supply evidence for their subclassification related to region of seizure origin. Although video/EEG monitoring has certain limitations, they are far outweighed by the advantages. The discussion that follows first examines the advantages and limitations of video/EEG monitoring of patients with complex partial seizures, and then reviews the progress in better characterizing and subclassifying these seizures.

VIDEO/EEG MONITORING

Advantages

Establishing the correct diagnosis is the most obvious advantage of video/EEG monitoring. Continuous recording throughout the day and night increases the probability of detecting EEG abnormalities and capturing habitual seizures (32, 40). Seizure frequency can be increased by gradual or partial anticonvulsant drug withdrawal in the safety of a hospital environment. This does not result in misleading or atypical withdrawal seizures (45) and precipitation of convulsive status epilepticus has not been a problem in patients with CPSs. Secondary generalized convulsive seizures, however, can occur during or after drug withdrawal and the patients and their families should be warned of this.

Recorded seizures can be examined repeatedly. When review of the videotape demonstrates automatisms, altered responsiveness, and confusion, and simultaneous EEG recording reveals paroxysmal changes over one or both temporal regions, the diagnosis of CPSs is established (Fig. 1). However, all patients monitored with video/EEG do not have such obvious results. In a previous analysis of patients referred for intractable epilepsy, 20% had nonepileptic attacks (32). Alternative diagnosis included transient cerebral ischemia, movement disorders, anticonvulsant drug toxicity, and, most often, psychogenic seizures. Although the correct diagnosis can be made after observing and recording attacks in the majority of patients, an occasional patient will prove very difficult. The problem usually involves determining whether attacks are epileptic seizures or psychogenic seizures in patients with or without documented epilepsy. Even after extensive evaluations during which numerous episodes have been recorded, the diagnosis can still be in doubt. The following case is an example of this problem.

A 28-year-old man with a 16-year history of medically refractory seizures was referred for surgical evaluation. The referring physician, who had never witnessed an attack, described typical CPSs consisting of a warning of an epigastric sensation and fear followed by confusion and automatisms. Seizures occurred up to ten times per day and lasted several seconds to 1 min. Previous EEGs were interpreted as normal. Neurological examination was normal. Psychiatric evaluation revealed no significant psychopathology and neuropsychological assessment provided no evidence for focal disease. Minnesota Multiphasic Personality Inventory (MMPI) profile was consistent with an hysterical personality disorder. CT scan and baseline EEG were normal. Interictal EEG recording was consistently normal during continuous wake and sleep monitoring. Numerous episodes were recorded. In some, he would signal the nurse and stated he was having a seizure. Although fully responsive to testing, he claimed to be confused, but exhibited no objective evidence of seizures. Other attacks also began with the patient signaling the nurse, then he exhibited bizarre behavior such as rapidly shaking the bed side-rail, vio-

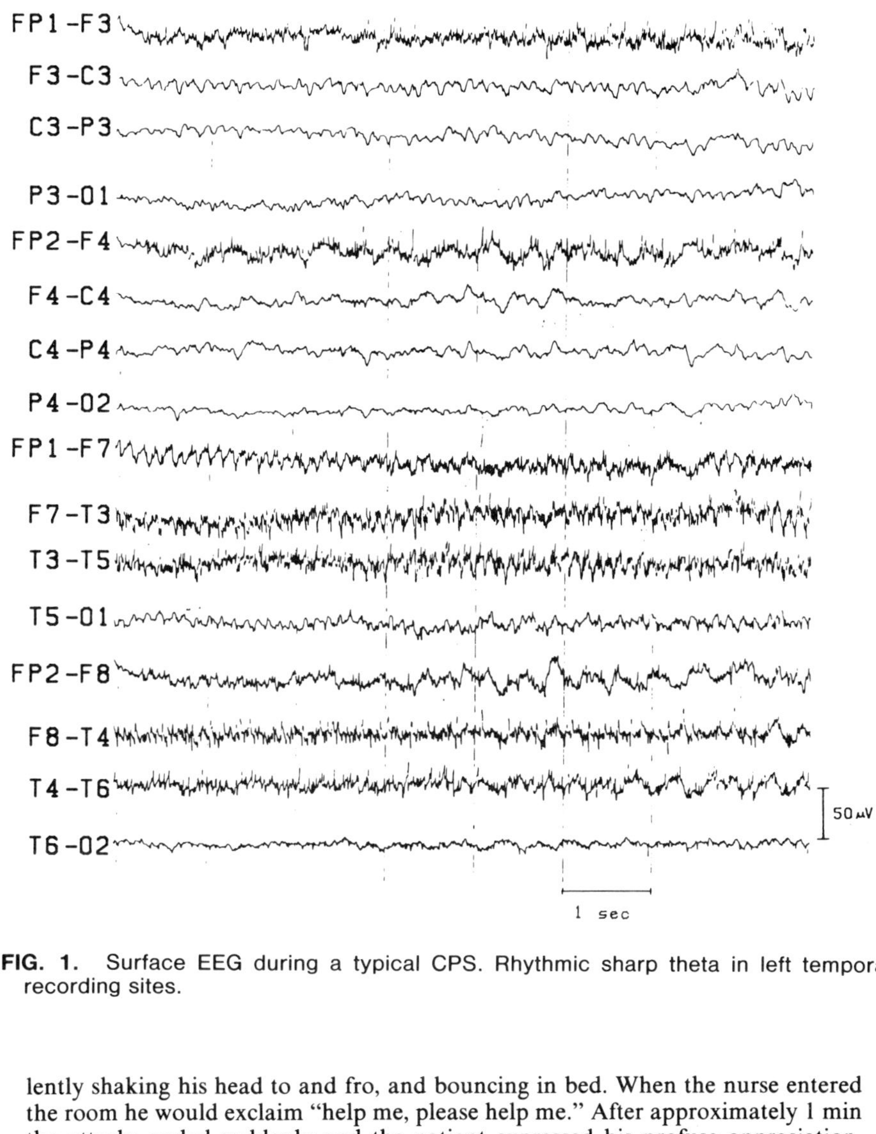

FIG. 1. Surface EEG during a typical CPS. Rhythmic sharp theta in left temporal recording sites.

lently shaking his head to and fro, and bouncing in bed. When the nurse entered the room he would exclaim "help me, please help me." After approximately 1 min the attacks ended suddenly and the patient expressed his profuse appreciation. There were no EEG changes during the brief attacks. There were no obvious paroxysmal EEG changes during the more prolonged attacks but the records contained considerable movement and muscle artifact. There was no postictal slowing.

At the conclusion of the evaluation, opinions differed whether this patient had pseudoseizures or real seizures. Favoring seizures was the 16-year history of typical CPSs. Favoring pseudoseizures were very atypical appearing attacks, normal interictal and inconclusive ictal EEGs, and a hysterical MMPI profile. Since the patient was incapacitated by his attacks, he was readmitted for a

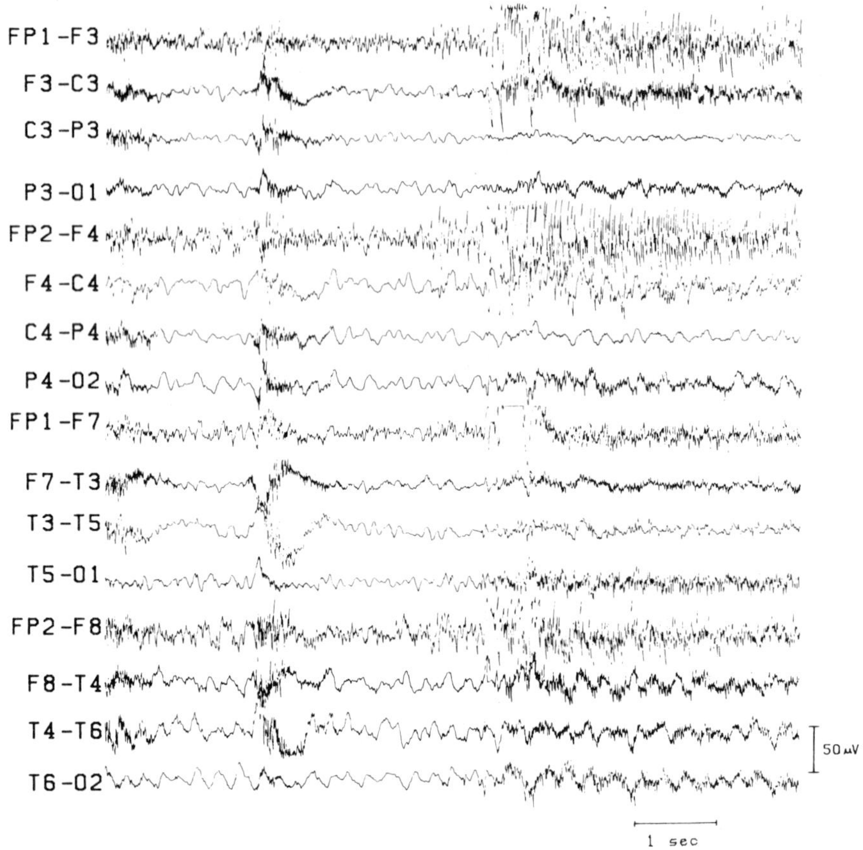

FIG. 2. Surface EEG during a bizarre, atypical seizure. Semi-rhythmic slowing maximal over right side.

"second look" 3 months after the initial evaluation. Interictal recording remained normal but EEGs during some attacks were unequivocally abnormal with rhythmic changes over the right frontal and temporal regions (Fig. 2). Exactly the same recording techniques were used during both admissions, however, ictal records were not as obscured by artifact during the second evaluation. The temptation to label all atypical attacks hysterical should be resisted. We have repeatedly documented epilepsy in patients with very bizarre seizures (56).

Limitations

Passive video/EEG monitoring will document many of the important features of seizures but much can be missed. Whenever possible, a trained observer should examine patients during seizures and report findings as they are detected (13). Pupillary size and reactivity, skin color, salivation, and other autonomic functions are usually not apparent in video recordings. Degree of responsiveness, language function, ability to read and recognize simple objects, motor function, visual fields, and orientation should be tested. Repeated examinations should continue until the patient has completely recovered from the seizure. The form and timing of examination must correspond to the situation. The importance of examination at seizure onset has been stressed (8), but this cannot be consistently done unless seizures are occurring very frequently.

Ambulatory activity often occurs during CPS and in some patients it can be the most prominent feature of the seizure. Although it is technically possible to document ambulatory behavior using telemetry and mobile cameras, this is not practical except in special circumstances in specialized centers. Indeed, when such behavior is anticipated, it may be best to place the patient in light restraints to prevent injury during monitoring. Ambulatory activity is best documented by history.

Severely disturbed, aggressive, or violent patients are sometimes referred for video/EEG monitoring to determine if some of their unacceptable behavior is due to CPSs. These patients are difficult to manage in the best of circumstances and an epilepsy intensive monitoring unit is usually ill-suited to handle their demands. They should be carefully screened to determine if there is any realistic possibility of epilepsy. The referring physicians should be reminded that directed aggression is extremely rare during seizures (10).

CHARACTERIZATION OF COMPLEX PARTIAL SEIZURES

Video/EEG monitoring makes it possible to critically examine clinical events and compare them with other episodes from the same and different patients. Evaluations of this type have resulted in better definition of certain seizure types. Penry and colleagues (38, 39) have shown that typical absence epilepsy is much more complicated than originally described. The myoclonic epilepsies have been better defined and subclassified into several fairly homogeneous types (A.G. Lee et al. *this volume*).

Although studies of CPSs using video/EEG have not been entirely consistent, there has been some progress. Delgado-Escueta and his colleagues analyzed videotaped seizures and concluded there were two types of CPSs (8, 12). Type I seizures began with a motionless stare, followed by total unresponsiveness and stereotyped automatisms, and ended with a period of semipurposeful or reactive automatisms. Type II seizures lacked a motionless stare but began suddenly with stereotyped motor automatisms and/or reactive automatisms. Theodore et al. (50) subsequently analyzed a series of videotaped CPSs and could not verify the type I and II differences. They emphasized the ictal and postictal features of CPSs. Simple, stereotyped automatisms occurred during the ictal phase, whereas partially responsive, semipurposeful behavior characterized the postictal phase. The postictal phase was defined as beginning when the patient first began to respond. We have observed ictal and postictal behavioral differences in some patients during depth electrode evaluations, but responsiveness is often delayed well beyond the ictus. They also proposed a method of differential diagnosis dependent on their observations of the clinical manifestations and duration of CPSs. Their table listing characteristics of psychogenic seizures includes features we use to define a specific CPS syndrome (*vide infra*) (56).

The analyses of video/EEG records cited above have focused our attention on some of the fine details of CPSs, but a consistent definition of these seizures was not documented. It may be the clinical manifestations of CPSs are so diverse that a unified concept cannot be established. It is also possible that the problem is being approached the wrong way due to insufficient data. The previous reports relied heavily on evaluation of videotapes. EEGs were limited to extracranial recording. Depth electrode recording of patients with CPS combined with CCTV has the advantage of better defining seizure origin, spread, and duration and comparing them with clinical characteristics. There is converging evidence from studies using depth electrode recording that not only can CPSs be better defined but also they can be subclassified depending on region of seizure origin (16–19, 31, 35, 49, 55, 56).

SUBCLASSIFICATION

Since Jackson's initial observation of the localizing value of olfactory hallucinations (23, 24), there have been numerous reports of the potential localizing and/or lateralizing value of seizure signs and symptoms. Some of these reports have greatly expanded our knowledge and understanding of epilepsy (1, 2, 37), but consistent complexes of findings were not described for CPSs. Recent studies using video/EEG during depth electrode investigations have first determined the region of seizure origin and then examined the clinical features. Wieser (53) reported his findings from 51 patients with CPSs being evaluated for surgery. He described five clinical syndromes related to regions of seizure origin: four temporal and one frontal. Walsh and Delgado-Escueta studied a series of patients with depth electrodes and concluded patients with type II seizures had extratemporal, probable frontal seizure onset (51). We have reported our findings from patients with CPSs of occipital and frontal lobe origin (55, 56). Finally, reports of limited numbers of patients with CPSs originating extratemporally as determined by intracranial recording have helped verify the findings of larger series (5, 16–19, 31, 35, 49).

The following discussion of CPS subclassification is intended as a first approximation. It includes observations from our series of 95 patients studied with depth electrodes. We have previously reported the superior localizing capability of depth EEG in the first 32 patients from this series (46) and opinions have not changed after evaluating 63 additional patients. We recognize, however, that even when numerous multicontact electrodes are used, sampling errors will persist (20, 34). Specific discussions of scalp and depth EEG results are beyond the scope of this report. The emphasis will be on clinical manifestations with the assumption that intracranial localization of seizure origin has been reasonably accurate.

Temporal Lobe CPSs

Temporal lobe seizures were designated complex partial in part, because it was realized that some of these attacks began extratemporally (15). The fact remains, however, that most CPSs begin in temporal lobe structures. The proportion of CPSs that originate in the temporal lobes has not been specifically reported. An anlysis based on scalp interictal data reported 80 to 85% temporal foci (26). In our series, 87 patients had CPSs. Fifty-nine of these (68%) had seizures originating in the temporal lobes. It is therefore not surprising that the clinical characteristics of temporal lobe CPSs include many of those that have been reported for CPSs in general over the years (7).

We have compared our findings with more recent reports, particularly those using video/EEG, and conclude that a temporal lobe CPS syndrome can be defined by considering the overall characteristics of the seizure. This concept avoids including many of the specific symptoms and signs associated with these seizures.

1. Mean seizure frequency for the last 20 patients with temporal lobe CPSs in our series was 4.7 per month (range 3–9). Multiple seizures per day are uncommon. This frequency estimate may be too high since it is predicated on patients referred for surgery.
2. Mean seizure duration in the same 20 patients, calculated from the time of clinical onset to complete mental clearing, was 3.8 min (range 1–20 min). This is comparable to recently reported durations of CPSs (8, 50). However, one study found 14% of seizures lasted less than 30 sec (50). We have observed CPSs that short commonly with extratemporal but not temporal origin.
3. There are ictal and postictal phases with the former usually being the shorter, lasting about 1 min. In many seizures these two phases are clinically apparent, but in others the two phases blend imperceptibly. Level of responsiveness is not a reliable indicator of ictal versus postictal phase (50). Some patients are partially responsive during the ictal phase and others can remain unresponsive during the initial postictal phase. Depth electrode recording combined with clinical evaluation establishes the two phases (Fig. 3).
4. Seizure onset is usually bland with a progressive development of signs. Wieser (53) reported a progressive evolution with most temporal lobe CPSs.

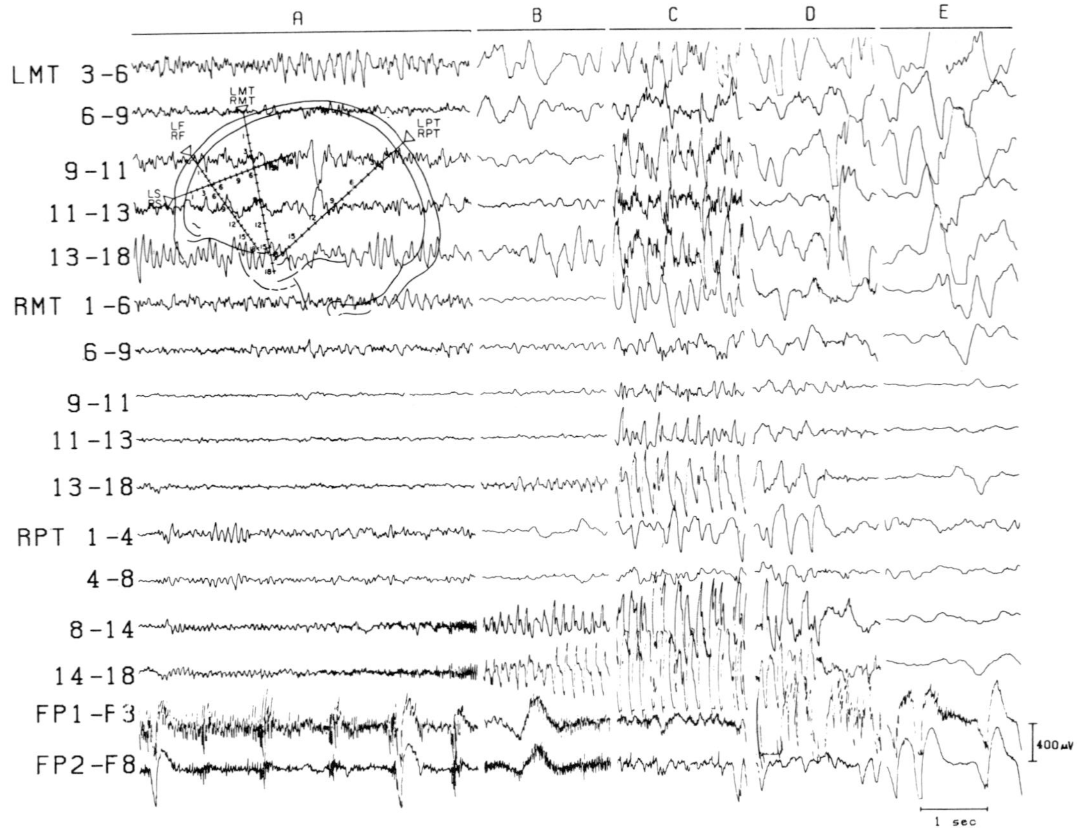

FIG. 3. Five segments of surface and depth EEG during a typical CPS. (A) Seizure onset with low amplitude rhythmic then high frequency activity right anterior hippocampus (RPT 14). (B) Pattern changes to repetitive sharp activity, and (C) then spreads to involve both sides. (D) Seizure stops, followed by postictal slowing and voltage suppression (E). Patient was totally unresponsive at B and remained so until 30 sec after end of seizure.

A motionless stare (8) is not a reliable localizing finding as it does not occur consistently in temporal lobe CPSs (50) and does occur with extratemporal CPSs (56).

5. Automatisms during the ictal phase are initially stereotyped and simple but may become more complex as the seizure evolves. Others have emphasized simple automatisms at the beginning of temporal lobe CPSs (50, 53). Since Delgado-Escueta and his colleagues emphasize the relationship between complex motor automatisms and type II extratemporal CPSs (51), we assume they associate simple automatisms with type I seizures.
6. Generalized muscular rigidity is common and may resemble tonic posturing. Automatisms emerge through this "coat of rigidity" (1).
7. Warnings or auras occurred in approximately 80% of our patients with temporal lobe CPSs. The frequency of auras in previous reports ranged from 24% (50) to 83% (28). Most auras were adequately described and included such well recognized symptoms as epigastric rising sensations, fear, and déjà-vu experiences. The localizing value of most auras has been questioned (28).
8. Complex partial status epilepticus is extremely rare even when anticonvulsant drugs are withdrawn. We have not observed it during depth electrode evaluations of 59 patients with temporal lobe CPSs but have documented it repeatedly with extratemporal CPSs (57). There has been only one case report of temporal lobe complex partial status epilepticus documented with intracranial recording (52).

Frontal Lobe CPSs

Although most reports on frontal lobe epilepsy emphasize tonic and/or clonic motor activity (3, 14, 25, 41, 42), CPSs of frontal lobe origin have been recognized for over 30 years (37). Some reports suggest frontal lobe CPSs can be differentiated from CPSs originating elsewhere (18, 19, 31, 33, 49, 53), but a consistent syndrome of frontal lobe CPSs has not been defined. We have documented frontal lobe origin in ten patients with CPSs studied with depth electrodes. Seizures did not spread beyond the frontal lobes in eight patients while secondary temporal lobe involvement occurred in two (Fig. 4). Seizures began in the medial or orbital frontal regions and not the convexities. The syndrome of frontal lobe CPSs, defined by the following clinical characteristics, is a very distinctive condition that is frequently misdiagnosed (56). The citations with each characteristic refer to reports that mentioned the characteristic, usually in case descriptions without further comment.

1. Seizures are frequent, often occurring in clusters of many per day, but there may be days or weeks without seizures (5, 6, 16–19, 27, 31, 49).
2. Seizures are brief, usually lasting under 1 min. When secondary spread to the temporal lobe occurs, seizures are more prolonged, similar to temporal lobe CPSs (5, 6, 18, 27, 31, 49) (Fig. 4).

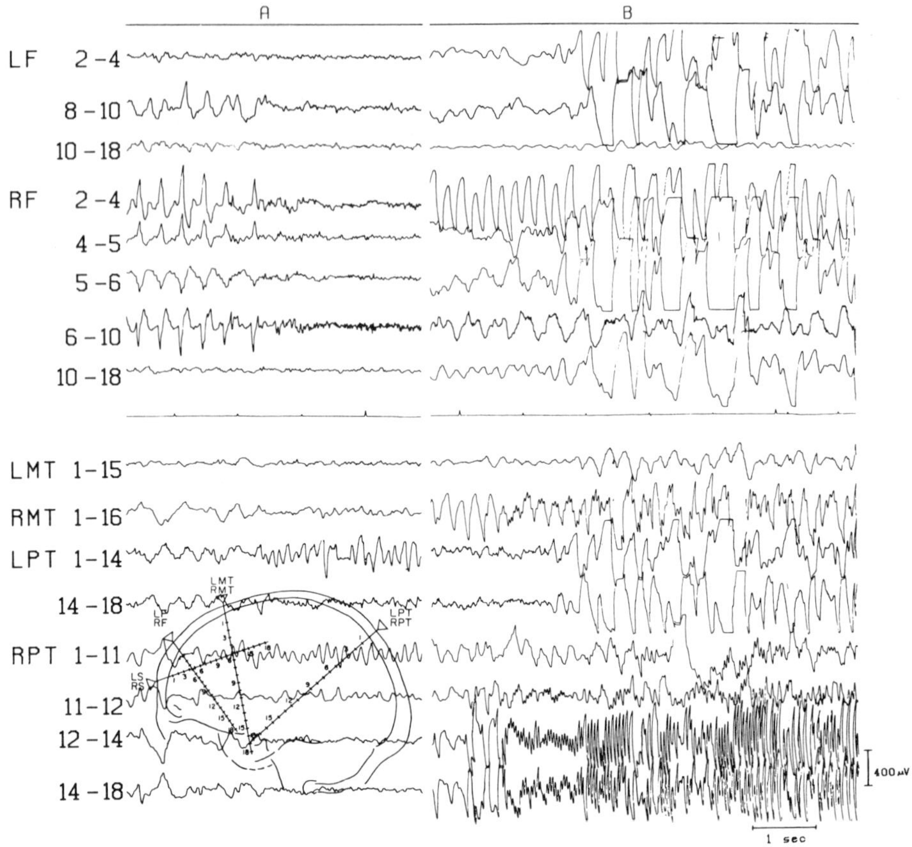

FIG. 4. Two segments of depth EEG during a frontal lobe CPS with secondary temporal spread. (A) Onset with repetitive sharp activity and high frequency low amplitude activity right medial frontal (RF 4–6). Clinical onset out of sleep; patient awakened suddenly and began to thrash, shout obscenities, and aggressively manipulate genitals. (B) Twenty-five sec after frontal lobe seizure onset, high amplitude seizure discharge developed in right mid to anterior hippocampus (RPT 14). During temporal seizure discharge, patient was lying quietly in bed, smacking lips, and uttering snorting sounds.

3. Seizures confined to the frontal lobes end abruptly with little if any postictal confusion. Clinically there are no discernible ictal and postictal phases (31, 49).
4. Motor automatisms are prominent. They begin suddenly at seizure onset or after a stare or change in facial expression. Motor automatisms are complex and semipurposeful and include thrashing, rolling, kicking, and bicycling movements. They are the most consistent finding reported in frontal lobe CPSs (2, 5, 6, 16–19, 27, 31, 37, 49, 53).
5. Sexual automatisms frequently accompany other motor automatisms (17, 18, 27, 47).

6. Vocalization is common. It is of variable complexity from simple humming to shouted obscenities (2, 6, 17, 18, 49).
7. Warnings are frequent but usually nonspecific such as a feeling of tightness. Some patients report complex warnings with psychic and illusional qualities (18, 27, 31, 49).
8. Complex partial status epilepticus was documented during evaluation in four of our ten patients. All four had histories of prolonged confusion. Two additional patients reported prolonged episodes of confusion, but did not develop complex partial status epilepticus during evaluation (5, 17, 57).
9. The clinical seizures are often bizarre resulting in the frequent erroneous diagnosis of hysteria (16, 27, 31, 37).
10. Seizures are stereotyped for individual patients (16–19, 27, 31, 34, 49).

Occipital Lobe CPSs

Ajmone-Marsan and Ralston predicted that seizures beginning in the occipital lobe could spread below the sylvian fissure and secondarily involve the temporal lobe (1). This has subsequently been verified with depth electrode studies (4, 35, 55). Eight patients from our series had some or all of their CPSs originate in the occipital lobes. Although these seizures may be indistinguishable from seizures originating in the temporal lobes, most have findings that suggest occipital onset. Occipital lobe CPSs do not constitute a specific syndrome but, rather, are temporal lobe CPSs that begin extratemporally (Fig. 5). This agrees with the earlier concept that all CPSs beginning extratemporally secondarily involve temporal lobes (44). The clinical features listed below, therefore, emphasize findings at seizure onset with the understanding that the complex partial parts of the attack resemble temporal lobe CPSs.

1. Elemental visual symptoms are an obvious indication of occipital lobe onset (30, 37). Unformed visual hallucinations occurring with original seizures may not persist and only the history of their prior existence suggests occipital lobe onset (Fig. 5).
2. Eye deviation is frequently cited as an unreliable localizing sign (46, 53). When other evidence suggests occipital onset, consistently lateralized eye deviation may help lateralize the seizure onset to the contralateral side (4, 30, 48).
3. Sensation of eye movement with no detectable movement has been reported with occipital lobe seizures (21) and we have observed this in one patient.
4. Blinking occurs frequently in all types of CPSs. Rapid forceful blinking or eyelid flutter at seizure onset has proven a reliable indication of occipital onset (4, 58).
5. Black-outs or white-outs at the beginning of seizures have been associated with occipital lobe onset (11, 22, 35, 43). One of our patients described both symptoms during different seizures.
6. Homonymous hemianopsias during seizure onset or postictally are seen

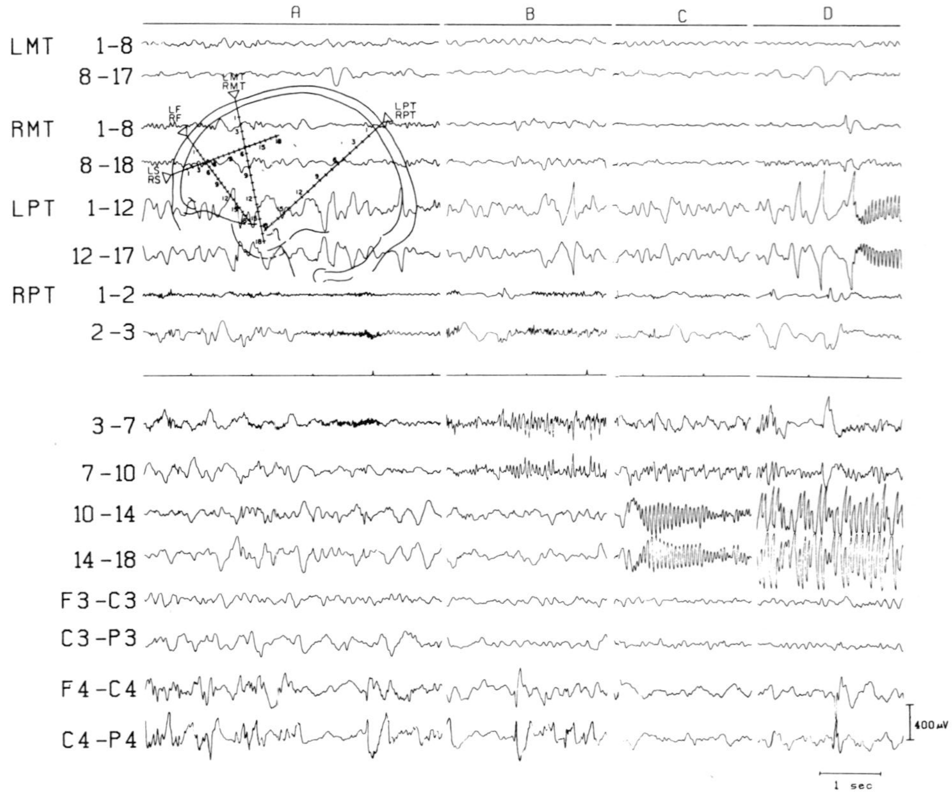

FIG. 5. Four segments of surface and depth EEG during a CPS with occipital lobe onset. (A) Onset in right occipital lobe with high frequency low amplitude activity (RPT 1–3). (B) Seizure spreads anteriorly first to medial parietal region (RPT 7), then (C) to right hippocampus (RPT 14). (D) Thirty sec after onset, seizure spreads to left hippocampus (LPT 12). Occipital onset accompanied by no objective or subjective findings. History of seeing orange ball before seizures 10 years previously.

with occipital lobe seizures (13, 35). Static visual field defects also occur and suggest occipital lobe disease particularly when the inferior homonymous quadrants are involved (30, 36, 43).

Summary of Subclassification

Although individual characteristics may not be diagnostic, the overall patterns have proven very useful in identifying different CPS subtypes. This is particularly true for frontal lobe CPSs. These seizures, when confined to the frontal lobes, can be distinguished from temporal lobe CPSs easily, but differentiating them from pseudoseizures is often difficult. The patient described previously probably has frontal lobe CPSs. When seizures secondarily spread to the temporal lobes, the diagnosis is not as obvious, but the initial features should suggest frontal origin (Fig. 4). We suspected Delgado-Escueta and his colleagues were observing frontal lobe CPSs secondarily involving temporal lobes with some of the type II seizures initially reported (12). Their subsequent reports and conclusions verify this (9, 51). Occipital lobe CPSs, when studied with depth electrodes, have always involved spread to temporal lobes (4, 35, 55). As with frontal lobe seizures that spread temporally, careful attention to the initial clinical features will help identify these seizures. Finally, when complex partial status epilepticus develops, extratemporal seizure origin is likely (57).

Clinical seizure characteristics help to define seizure subtypes and suggest possible regions of origin, but overlap among different seizure types exists. Patient evaluations include much more than seizure characterization and all the pertinent data is needed. This is obviously necessary when surgery is being considered. Other reports suggest that CPSs can be further subdivided (49, 53) but this needs to be verified.

CONCLUSION

The use of video/EEG monitoring has proven a valuable technique when used to evaluate patients with presumed CPSs. When the diagnosis of CPSs is established, careful examination of videotaped seizures has better defined these seizures particularly during depth electrode studies. Separation into different types related to region of seizure onset is beginning to be realized.

REFERENCES

1. Ajmone-Marsan, C., and Ralston, B.L. (1957): *The Epileptic Seizure. Its Functional Morphology and Diagnostic Significance.* Thomas, Springfield, Illinois.
2. Ajmone-Marsan, C., and Goldhammer, L. (1973): Clinical ictal patterns and electrographic data in cases of partial seizures of fronto-central-parietal origin. In: *Epilepsy.*

Its Phenomena in Man, edited by M.A.B. Brazier, pp. 235–258. Academic Press, New York.
3. Bancaud, J. (1969): Physiopathogenesis of generalized epilepsies of organic nature (stereo-electroencephalographic study). In: *Physiopathogenesis of the Epilepsies,* edited by H. Gastaut, pp. 158–185. Thomas, Springfield, Illinois.
4. Bancaud, J. (1969): Les crises épileptiques d'origine occipitale (étude stereo-electroencephalographique). *Rev. D'oto-Neuro-Ophthalmal.,* 41:299–315.
5. Bladin, P.F., and Woodward, J. (1974): Epilepsy and the frontal lobe. *Proc. Aust. Assoc. Neurol.,* 11:229–237.
6. Crandall, P.H. (1973): Developments in direct recordings from epileptogenic regions in the surgical treatment of partial epilepsies. In: *Epilepsy: Its Phenomena in Man,* edited by M.A.B. Brazier, pp. 287–310. Academic Press, New York.
7. Daly, D.D. (1975): Ictal clinical manifestations of complex partial seizures. In: *Advances in Neurology, Vol. 11,* edited by J.K. Penry and D.D. Daly, pp. 57–83. Raven Press, New York.
8. Delgado-Escueta, A.V., Bacsal, F.E., and Treiman, D.M. (1981): Complex partial seizures on closed-circuit television and EEG: A study of 691 attacks in 79 patients. *Ann. Neurol.,* 11:292–300.
9. Delgado-Escueta, A.V., Nashold, B., Freedman, M., Keplinger, M.D., Waddell, G., Miller, P., and Carwille, S. (1979): Videotaping epileptic attacks during stereoelectroencephalography. *Neurology,* 29:473–489.
10. Delgado-Escueta, A.V., Mattson, R.H., King, L., Goldensohn, E.S., Spiegel, H., Madsen, J., Crandall, P., Dreifuss, F., and Porter, R.J. (1981): Special Report. The nature of aggression during epileptic seizures. *N. Engl. J. Med.,* 305:711–716.
11. Engel, J., Ludwig, B.I., and Fetell, M. (1978): Prolonged partial complex status epilepticus: EEG and behavioral observations. *Neurology,* 28:863–869.
12. Escueta, A.V., Kunze, U., Waddell, G., Boxley, J., and Nadel, A. (1977): Lapse of consciousness and automatisms in temporal lobe epilepsy: A videotape analysis. *Neurology,* 27:144–155.
13. Fay, M.L., and Mattson, R.H. (1980): Clinical testing during intensive monitoring of ictal events. In: *Advances in Epileptology: The Xth Epilepsy International Symposium,* edited by J.A. Wada and J.K. Penry, pp. 65–68. Raven Press, New York.
14. Fegersten, L., and Roger, A. (1961): Frontal epileptogenic foci and their clinical correlations. *Electroencephalogr. Clin. Neurophysiol.,* 13:905 913.
15. Gastaut, H. (1970): Clinical and electroencephalographic classification of epileptic seizures. *Epilepsia,* 2:102–113.
16. Geier, S., Bancaud, J., Bonis, A., and Enjelvin, M. (1973): Non-motor frontal epilepsy: study of electrographic and clinical features using tele-EEG and tele-stereo-EEG. *Electroencephalogr. Clin. Neurophysiol.,* 34:699.
17. Geier, S., Bancaud, J., Talairach, J., Bonis, A., Szikla, G., and Enjelvin, M. (1975): Clinical Note: clinical and tele-stereo-EEG findings in a patient with psychomotor seizures. *Epilepsia,* 16:119–125.
18. Geier, S., Bancaud, J., Talairach, J., Bonis, A., Enjelvin, M., and Hossard-Bouchaud, H. (1976): Automatisms during frontal lobe epileptic seizures. *Brain,* 99:447–458.
19. Geier, S., Bancaud, J., Talairach, J., Bonis, A., Szikla, G., and Enjelvin, M. (1977): The seizures of frontal lobe epilepsy: a study of clinical manifestations. *Neurology,* 27:951–958.
20. Gloor, P. (1984): Electroencephalography and the role of intracerebral depth electrode recordings in the selection of patients for surgical treatment of epilepsy. In: *Advances in Epileptology: XVth Epilepsy International Symposium,* edited by Roger J. Porter et al., pp. 433–437. Raven Press, New York.
21. Holtzman, R.N.N., and Goldensohn, E.S. (1977): Sensations of ocular movement in seizures originating in occipital lobe. *Neurology,* 27:554–556.
22. Huott, A.D., Madison, D.S., and Niedermeyer, E. (1974): Occipital lobe epilepsy: A clinical and electroencephalographic study. *Eur. Neurol.,* 11:325–339.
23. Jackson, J.H. (1931): Case of tumor of the right temporo-sphenoidal lobe, bearing on the localization of the sense of smell and on the interpretation of a particular variety of epilepsy. In: *Selected Writings of John Hughlings Jackson, Vol 1,* edited by James Taylor, pp. 406–411. Hodder and Stoughton, London.

24. Jackson, J.H. (1931): Epileptic attacks with a warning of a crude sensation of smell and with the "intellectual aura" (dreamy state) in a patient who had symptoms pointing to gross organic disease of right temporo-sphenoidal lobe. In: *Selected Writings of John Hughlings Jackson, Vol. 1,* edited by James Taylor, pp. 464–473. Hodder and Stoughton, London.
25. Janz, D. (1964): Status epilepticus and frontal lobe lesions. *J. Neurol. Sci.,* 1:446–457.
26. Jovanovic, U.J. (1974): *Psychomotor Epilepsy: A Polydimensional Study.* Thomas, Springfield, Illinois.
27. Kennedy, W.A. (1959): Clinical and electroencephalographic aspects of epileptogenic lesions of the medial surface and superior border of the cerebral hemisphere. *Brain,* 82:147–161.
28. King, D.W., and Ajmone-Marsan, C. (1977): Clinical features and ictal patterns in epileptic patients with EEG temporal lobe foci. *Ann. Neurol.,* 2:138–147.
29. Klass, D. (1975): EEG manifestations of complex partial seizures. *Adv. Neurol.,* 11:113–140.
30. Ludwig, B., and Ajmone-Marsan, C. (1975): Clinical ictal patterns in epileptic patients with occipital electroencephalographic foci. *Neurology,* 25:463–471.
31. Ludwig, B., Ajmone-Marsan, C., and Van Buren, J. (1975): Cerebral seizures of probable orbitofrontal origin. *Epilepsia,* 16:141–158.
32. Mattson, R.H. (1980): Value of intensive monitoring. In: *Advances in Epileptology: The Xth Epilepsy International Symposium,* edited by J.A. Wada and J.K. Penry, pp. 43–51. Raven Press, New York.
33. Neidermeyer, E. (1974): Special types of epilepsy according to the site of the focus. In: *Compendium of the Epilepsies,* edited by E. Neidermeyer, Chapter 5, pp. 106–144. Charles C. Thomas, Springfield.
34. Neidermeyer, E. (1982): Depth electroencephalography. In: *Electroencephalography. Basic Principles, Clinical Applications and Related Fields,* edited by E. Neidermeyer and F. Lopes da Silva, pp. 519–533. Urban and Schwarzenberg, Baltimore.
35. Olivier, A., Gloor, P., Andermann, F., and Ives, J. (1982): Occipitotemporal epilepsy studied with stereotaxically implanted depth electrodes and successfully treated by temporal resection. *Ann. Neurol.,* 11:428–432.
36. Paillas, J.E., Vigouroux, R., Darcourt, G., and Naquet, R. (1959): Considerations sur l'épilepsie occipitale (a propos de 12 observations de lesions occipitales operées). *Neuro-Chirurgie,* 5(1):3–16.
37. Penfield, W., and Jasper, H. (1954): *Epilepsy and the Functional Anatomy of the Human Brain.* Little, Brown, Boston.
38. Penry, J.K., and Dreifuss, F.E. (1969): Automatisms associated with the absence of petit mal epilepsy. *Arch. Neurol.,* 21:142–149.
39. Penry, J.K., Porter, R.J., and Dreifuss, F.E. (1975): Simultaneous recording of absence seizures with video tape and electroencephalography. A study of 374 seizures in 48 patients. *Brain,* 98:427–440.
40. Porter, R.J., Penry, J.K., and Lacy, J.R. (1977): Diagnostic and therapeutic reevaluation of patients with intractable epilepsy. *Neurology,* 27:1006–1011.
41. Rasmussen, T. (1963): Surgical therapy of frontal lobe epilepsy. *Epilepsia,* 4:181–198.
42. Rasmussen, T. (1983): Characteristics of a pure culture of frontal lobe epilepsy. *Epilepsia,* 24:482–493.
43. Remillard, G.M, Ethier, R., and Andermann, F. (1974): Temporal lobe epilepsy and perinatal occlusion of the posterior cerebral artery. A syndrome analogous to infantile hemiplegia and a demonstrable etiology in some patients with temporal lobe epilepsy. *Neurology,* 24:1001–1009.
44. Schneider, R.C., Crosby, E.C., and Farhat, S.M. (1964): Extratemporal lesions triggering the temporal-lobe syndrome. *J. Neurosurg.,* 22:246–263.
45. Spencer, S.S., Spencer, D.D., Williamson, P.D., and Mattson, R.H. (1981): Ictal effects of anticonvulsant medication withdrawal in epileptic patients. *Epilepsia,* 22:297–307.
46. Spencer, S.S., Spencer, D.D., Williamson, P.D., and Mattson, R.H. (1982): The localizing value of depth electroencephalography in 32 refractory epileptic patients. *Ann. Neurol.,* 12:248–253.
47. Spencer, S.S., Spencer, D.D., Williamson, P.D., and Mattson, R.H. (1983): Sexual automatisms in partial complex seizures. *Neurology,* 33:527–533.

48. Takeda, A., Bancaud, J., Talairach, J., Bonis, A., and Bordas-Ferrer, M. (1970): Concerning epileptic attacks of occipital origin. *Electroencephalogr. Clin. Neurophysiol.*, 28:644–649.
49. Tharp, B.R. (1972): Orbital frontal seizures. An unique electroencephalographic and clinical syndrome. *Epilepsia,* 13:627–642.
50. Theodore, W.H., Porter, R.J., and Penry, J.K. (1983): Complex partial seizures: Clinical characteristics and differential diagnosis. *Neurology,* 33:1115–1121.
51. Walsh, G.O., and Delgado-Escueta, A.V. (1984): Type II complex partial seizures: Poor results of anterior temporal lobectomy. *Neurology,* 34:1–13.
52. Wieser, H.G. (1983): Temporal lobe or psychomotor status epilepticus. A case report. *Electroencephalogr. Clin. Neurophysiol.*, 48:558–572.
53. Wieser, H.G. (1983): *Electroclinical Features of the Psychomotor Seizure.* Fischer, Stuttgart.
54. Williamson, P.D., Spencer, D.D., Spencer S.S., and Mattson, R.H. (1980): Presurgical intensive monitoring using depth electroencephalography in temporal lobe epilepsy. In: *Advances in Epileptology: The Xth Epilepsy International Symposium,* edited by J.A. Wada and J.K. Penry, pp. 73–81. Raven Press, New York.
55. Williamson, P.D., Spencer, S.S., Spencer, D.D., and Mattson, R.H. (1981): Complex partial seizures with occipital lobe onset. *Epilepsia,* 22:247–248.
56. Williamson, P.D., Spencer, D.D., Spencer, S.S., Novelly, R.A., and Mattson, R.H. (1985): Complex partial seizures of frontal lobe origin. *Ann. Neurol.*, 18:497–504.
57. Williamson, P.D., Spencer, S.S., Mattson, R.H., and Spencer, D.D. (1985): Complex partial status epilepticus: a depth electrode study. *Ann. Neurol.*, 18:647–654.

Advances in Neurology, Vol. 46: Intensive Neurodiagnostic Monitoring, edited by R. J. Gumnit. Raven Press, New York © 1986.

Intensive Neurodiagnostic Monitoring with Intracranial Electrodes

Jerome Engel, Jr.* and Paul H. Crandall**

**Department of Neurology and Anatomy and **Division of Neurosurgery, Reed Neurological Research Center, University of California at Los Angeles School of Medicine, Los Angeles, California 90024*

HISTORICAL PERSPECTIVE

Surgical resection of epileptogenic lesions has been used as a treatment for epilepsy since Horsley (34), based initially on localization from neurologic examination and intraoperative inspection of the cerebral cortex. Localization of the epileptogenic lesion for surgical resection, based on electrophysiological evidence alone, was first published by Bailey and Gibbs (6), and EEG studies subsequently became an essential part of the presurgical evaluation. Direct recording from the brain itself, as well as electrical stimulation of the brain, was initially performed intraoperatively using electrodes placed on the cortical surface (electrocorticography or ECoG), and inserted free-hand into deeper structures such as amygdala and hippocampus (45). Chronic intracranial recordings were subsequently obtained using flexible bundles of electrodes inserted into the epidural or subdural space through burr holes (45), or placed free-hand directly into the brain with a rigid introducer (15). The latter approach was initially undertaken to evaluate patients for frontal leukotomy and only later applied to epilepsy surgery by Bickford et al. (8). Talairach et al. (50) developed the technique for stereotaxic implantation of rigid electrodes into specific intracerebral structures in order to obtain more anatomically precise localization of epileptiform EEG discharges (stereotaxic EEG or SEEG). Most recently, chronic placement of large multi-electrode grids over a wide surface of the cerebral cortex, exposed by craniotomy, has made it possible to obtain well organized recordings from the lateral and basal convexities, and also carry out direct cortical stimulation and recording of evoked potentials to obtain functional cortical mapping in awake, unrestrained patients (31, 35).

Intraoperative ECoG provides a few minutes to approximately an hour of recording time and allows interictal abnormalities, as well as patterns of electrical stimulation-induced afterdischarge, to be characterized. More prolonged chronic recording initially lasted a few days and some spontaneous ictal events, as well as pharmacologically induced epileptic seizures, could usually be captured. The combination of chronically implanted intracranial electrodes and EEG telemetry (17) subsequently made it possible to record continuously, 24 hr a day, for weeks. This approach, plus video monitoring, now provides an opportunity to capture and examine numerous spontaneous ictal EEG events and correlate them with ictal clinical behavior during the routine evaluation for resective surgery of epilepsy (1, 21, 29). Although intraoperative ECoG remains an important form of intracranial recording, the following discussion of intensive monitoring will be limited to chronic recording procedures performed outside the operating theater.

CURRENT INDICATIONS

Intensive neurodiagnostic monitoring with intracranial electrodes is only justified, on a routine basis, for evaluation of patients who are candidates for surgical resection of an epileptogenic lesion. These recording procedures are extremely important for localization and delineation of the epileptogenic tissue to be removed. They serve to map cerebral function in order to identify areas of functional deficit that confirm the presence of a lesion, and to define areas of essential primary function that limit the boundaries of the resection. Chronic EEG recording from intracranial electrodes offers the most accurate means of obtaining this essential information (49). SEEG is currently believed to be the most useful recording procedure for patients with complex partial seizures when the epileptogenic lesion is suspected to be in mesial temporal structures such as hippocampus, whereas epi- or subdural electrode grids may provide more valuable information when a neocortical lesion is suspected, particularly if this is believed to lie in or near areas of primary cortical function.

Since the safest and most effective resective surgery for epilepsy is anterior temporal lobectomy (21, 28, 35, 46), and the results of this procedure are most beneficial when mesial temporal epileptogenic lesions are present (28), SEEG recording carried out to survey mesial temporal and other forebrain limbic structures remains the most commonly employed technique for chronic intracranial recording. Multi-electrode grids have now been modified, however, to record from the basal surface of the temporal lobe, and the value of this technique for detecting mesial temporal lesions is under investigation (40).

Because all intracranial recording procedures are associated with a low but serious risk of injury, careful consideration should be given to their use. In some patients, localization of the epileptogenic lesion using noninvasive techniques may be achieved with sufficient confidence to allow resective surgery without the benefit of chronic intracranial recording (21). When a patient is considered a surgical candidate, however, and reasonable doubt concerning the location of the epileptogenic lesion persists after appropriate noninvasive evaluation, chronic intracranial recording should be considered only when prior evaluation (a) suggests that the patient is very likely to benefit from surgical treatment, and (b) has limited the possible locations for the epileptogenic lesion to a number that can be reasonably surveyed with intracranial electrodes.

At the University of California, Los Angeles (UCLA), chronic intracranial recordings are not considered necessary for anterior temporal lobectomy when scalp and sphenoidal EEG telemetry reveals a consistent ictal onset and a preponderance of interictal spikes in one temporal lobe, and other tests demonstrate focal functional deficit in the same temporal lobe (21, 27). Focal functional deficit of one temporal lobe is defined by the current UCLA criteria as hypometabolism with positron emission tomography (19, 24, 25), and any two of the following: inability to support memory following contralateral intracarotid amytal injection (21, 26), focal attenuation of thiopental-induced fast activity (21, 22), appropriate neuropsychological disturbances (21), or nonspecific structural changes on radiological examination such as atrophy, temporal horn enlargement, or intratemporal calcification. Patients with suspected extratemporal epileptogenic lesions may bypass intracranial monitoring when the location of interictal and ictal EEG abnormalities coincides with a radiologically demonstrated structural disturbance of cerebral cortex.

The most common reasons for requiring SEEG include the following: (a) to determine the side of the epileptogenic lesion when bilateral independent frontotemporal interictal spikes are present and clear lateralization of ictal EEG onset has not been obtained; (b) to differentiate between temporal and extratemporal epileptogenic lesions when EEG-recorded onsets are well lateralized but equally prominent in well defined extratemporal and temporal regions; (c) to confirm the presence of an epileptogenic lesion in one temporal lobe when EEG-recorded ictal onsets are well localized in this area, but evidence of focal functional deficit is missing or conflicting, or other data, including characteristics of the behavioral seizures, suggest an extratemporal lesion; and (d) to determine whether an epileptogenic lesion localized to one temporal lobe might extend beyond the limits of the standard *en bloc* anterior temporal lobectomy.

Reasons for requiring placement of a multi-electrode grid or other cortical surface electrodes are less well defined, but should include: (a) to precisely identify the site of a neocortical epileptogenic lesion when interictal and ictal EEG recordings localize the abnormality to a relatively broad cortical zone on one side; (b) to delineate the limits of a neocortical epileptogenic lesion when it has been well localized by interictal and ictal EEG recordings, but its extent is not certain; (c) to determine if there is a single primary epileptogenic lesion when interictal and ictal EEG recordings have localized two or three neocortical areas of epileptogenicity; and (d) to map areas of primary cerebral function adjacent to an identified epileptogenic lesion in order to determine the safe boundaries of the resection. This last functional mapping technique may become the most useful application of chronic multi-electrode grid recording, particularly in children who are unable to cooperate during long procedures carried out under local anesthesia in the operating room. Because placement of the multi-electrode grid requires a craniotomy, it is preferable to use this technique when the suspected epileptogenic lesion is well lateralized by noninvasive studies. Bilateral grid placements can be used, however, in exceptional situations.

CONTRAINDICATIONS

Intensive neurodiagnostic monitoring with intracranial electrodes should never be undertaken as a "fishing expedition." It is inappropriate when prior noninvasive evaluation has failed to limit potential locations of a resectable epileptogenic lesion to a number that can be reasonably explored by the technique to be used. Chronic recording with intracranial electrodes over weeks is also contraindicated in patients who have serious multiple illnesses or active infections that could lead to intracranial infections, or who are otherwise poor surgical risks. Stereotaxic implantation is not possible in patients with skull defects that would make electrodes unstable. Intensive surface EEG monitoring of patients prior to consideration for intracranial EEG recording is useful not only to help localize the epileptogenic lesion, but also to observe the patients in the hospital for emotional instability, psychiatric disorders, or unusually violent ictal behavior that would prevent them from fully cooperating during intracranial monitoring studies.

TECHNIQUES

Types of Electrodes

A great variety of electrode types are used for chronic intracranial recording. Although a large selection is commercially available, many centers that carry out these procedures make or design their own electrodes. Consequently, a detailed description of all the various electrodes that can be used for direct brain recording is beyond the scope of this chapter. Brief mention of some of the more commonly used electrode types is appropriate, however.

Intracerebral electrodes that can be stereotaxically implanted may be rigid or flexible. Flexible electrodes are inserted with the aid of a stylet or introducer which is subsequently withdrawn (15). Rigid electrodes are usually inserted through hollow guide pins that are securely screwed into the skull (21). Intracerebral electrodes may have closely spaced bipolar recording tips for recording from small areas of tissue, or may be multicontact with many recording tips spaced at appropriate intervals along the shaft. Fine-wire microelectrodes can be introduced through cannulae, or can be laminated onto the surface of any rigid electrodes; however, this remains a research procedure (2).

Subdural electrodes that can be inserted through burr holes are usually made of a layer of thin wires with their exposed surfaces regularly spaced along the long axis, or strips of disk electrodes embedded in silicon elastomer (57). Multi-electrode grids consist of several regularly spaced rows of small disk electrodes imbedded in sheets of silicon elastomer (41). Electrodes are equidistant, usually 10 mm center-to-center. Sheets of multi-electrode grids can be cut into appropriate sizes and fixed over the exposed surface of the brain, either over the dura (32), or under it (36). The bone flap is then replaced.

The most precise intracerebral recordings are obtained from stereotaxic implantation of rigid electrodes. Although there is less risk of cerebral injury due to electrode movement when flexible electrodes are used, these may retract when the stylet is withdrawn and placement within specific anatomical structures is less accurate. Free-hand insertion of depth electrodes for chronic recording is not recommended. Multi-electrode grids provide the most comprehensive sampling of neocortex, but require a craniotomy for placement. Although subdural electrodes inserted through burr holes provide much more limited sampling, they may still be indicated in certain patients since craniotomy is not required for their introduction. It is not possible to use standard laterally inserted SEEG electrodes and multi-electrode grids simultaneously, since the craniotomy required for the latter renders the bone too unstable for depth electrode implantation. SEEG electrodes can still be inserted from the back or top of the head, however. Simultaneous SEEG and neocortical recordings may also be obtained easily when subdural electrodes are inserted through burr holes.

Postoperative Care

Insertion of intracranial electrodes, whether by stereotaxic means, through burr holes, or with a craniotomy, requires a major neurosurgical procedure carried out under general anesthesia, and appropriate precaution must be taken in the immediate postoperative period. Patients should be discharged from the recovery room to the neurosurgical service, but can be transferred to a specialized telemetry unit or neurology ward as soon as they are ambulatory, usually within 2 days. Points of exit of electrodes or wires from the scalp are kept covered with a sterile head dressing which must be changed at least weekly, when the scalp is shaved and cleaned and the wound edges inspected under the supervision of the neurosurgeon. Evidence of superficial inflammation or infection may be treated topically, but persistent infection of the scalp, or indications of intracranial infection, require immediate removal of the electrodes and systemic antibiotic treatment.

Skull-fixed intracranial electrodes are removed under general anesthesia. The therapeutic cortical resection can be performed during the same craniotomy required to remove multi-electrode grids.

Recording

Intensive neurodiagnostic monitoring with intracranial electrodes can be carried out under a variety of conditions. Recording may be limited to several hours a day, with the patient brought to a special recording suite for this purpose, or it may be performed continuously, 24 hr a day, for days or weeks on a special inpatient monitoring unit (42). Electrodes may be connected directly into an EEG jack-box to produce a "hard-wire" recording written out on paper, or signals may be amplified and multiplexed on or near the head and transmitted via radio or cable telemetry to be stored in a variety of analog or digital modes for later review (23, 33). Direct connection to the EEG machine is the simplest means of recording a large number of channels, but requires a technician to monitor the EEG tracing, and signals are susceptible to artifactual distortion due to cable movement during seizures. With telemetry, the patient not only has increased freedom of movement, but movement artifact is markedly reduced and the constant attention of an EEG technician is not necessary. On a typical telemetry unit, patients are under constant observation by the nursing staff, either directly or via a video monitor placed at the nursing station, while combined video and EEG information is continually recorded and stored on tape or disk. Identified seizures, and other periods of interest, are then selectively reviewed by writing the appropriate segments of the EEG data out on paper and correlating this EEG with the simultaneously videotaped behavior (42).

The number of channels available for recording varies considerably depending on the system used. Due to the complex nature of intracranially recorded data, the accuracy of interpretation depends on access to an adequate number of channels. It has been suggested that 12 channels is an absolute minimum for adequate interpretation (23), but 16 to 32 are recommended.

Montage selection depends on the type of electrodes used, the specific information required, and the number of channels available. With the commonly used, multicontact, stereotaxically implanted depth electrodes, a good routine screening procedure is to use relatively equally spaced bipolar chain linkage montages, either proceeding up the shaft from tip to superficial cortex, or connecting equivalent contacts on adjacent electrodes in a reasonable configuration. Information may be lost with this approach, however, due to cancellation (30). Consequently, the montage configuration should be changed several times during the period of study.

Recordings from closely spaced tips of bipolar electrodes are useful for monitoring small volumes of tissue. They can give more precise information about local abnormalities and supplement bipolar chain linkage data, but the area sampled by this technique is too restricted to rely on solely for localization.

Common reference montages are also useful for confirmation of localized abnormalities. With some systems it is possible to record with a common reference exclusively and reconstruct any desired montage on playback, using the active electrodes included in the original montage (48). Montage reconstruction is preferable when available, since the same event can be reviewed in as many different montages as desired; however, one recording channel is necessary for every electrode and initial screening from many sites may be carried out more easily using bipolar chain linkage montages when the number of recording channels is limited.

When recording from depth electrodes, it is important to use some montages that also contain surface derivations (e.g., scalp, skull nails, neocortex) to aid in determining whether depth-recorded ictal onsets may indicate secondary spread from sites distant from the recording electrode tips.

Montage selection for epidural electrode tresses and multi-electrode grids usually consists of logical bipolar chain linkages chosen to best display the suspected abnormality, or common reference to an inactive electrode. Again, with some systems it is possible to record with a common reference and reconstruct bipolar montages on playback.

As with all intensive monitoring, it is important to obtain direct "hard-wire" recordings from all available electrodes before the patient is connected to specialized recording equipment, such as telemetry. This is usually performed the day following surgery and the tracing is necessary for initial survey of abnormalities, selection of electrodes for inclusion in subsequent montages, and as a baseline reference to assess changes in recording characteristics of particular electrodes during the course of the monitoring studies. When telemetry is used and data are stored on tape or disk, it is necessary to obtain a paper write-out at least once a day in order to check the recording system. All other approaches for assuring the integrity of the telemetry system that are discussed in this volume and elsewhere (23, 33) are appropriate for intracranial monitoring, with the exception of electrode impedance measurements. Impedance measurements for electrodes in direct contact with the brain can be performed safely with currents in the range of 10 nA.

Safety Considerations

The major risks associated with implantation of intracerebral electrodes are bleeding at the time of insertion, injury to adjacent brain tissue due to toxic properties of the electrodes (3), infection, movement of the electrodes during seizures, and current leakage (4). Mortality reported in the literature from depth electrode implantation has resulted solely from intracranial bleeding, and is less than 1% for the world's experience. Statistics on morbidity are more difficult to assess but, at UCLA, morbidity from all complications of depth electrodes is less than 3%, and has not resulted in permanent or delayed neurological deficit (11).

Electrodes intended for insertion directly into the brain must be sufficiently small to avoid serious mechanical disruption of brain tissue, but large enough to push blood vessels aside, rather than tear them. For this purpose also, the tips of these electrodes should be blunt and the shafts smooth. Electrodes have been safely used with diameters that range from 0.5 to 3.0 mm. Fine wire microelectrodes with diameters of less than 70 μm produce holes in vessels that then self-seal when the electrodes are withdrawn.

Preoperative angiograms are essential to allow surgeons to avoid major vessels when implanting intracerebral electrodes, but contact of electrodes with small vessels cannot be avoided. The greatest danger from vessel puncture during electrode insertion is continued slow bleeding, such that the volume of accumulated blood is too small to be identified on postoperative roentgenograms but increases over many hours until it eventually ruptures into a ventricle. Although no unequivocal data exist to implicate valproic acid or aspirin as a cause of persistent slow bleeding from cerebral vessels following depth-electrode implantation, anecdotal evidence suggests that this may be the case and these drugs should be discontinued several weeks prior to chronic insertion of electrodes directly into the brain. In order to attempt early identification of slow bleeding, each patient at UCLA receives an intravenous injection of technetium-labeled red blood cells prior to surgery, and a rectilinear gamma camera scan is obtained immediately after operation (21).

Most electrodes used for direct brain recording are constructed of medical grade stainless steel coated with a nonreactive insulating material. Noble metals, with the exception of silver, can also be used. Platinum and platinum-iridium alloy are ideal for microelectrodes because of their rigidity, and also for routine use when simultaneous intracranial EEG and magnetoencephalography are contemplated. Gold has been used either for SEEG, or for oxygen measurements (16). Polyurethane tubing and silicon elastomer are commonly used for flexible intracerebral and subdural electrodes, respectively.

Infection is avoided by adherence to aseptic technique, and regular inspection and cleaning of the scalp during the period of monitoring. At UCLA, electrodes have had to be withdrawn prematurely due to scalp infection in less than 5% of cases, and evidence of intracranial infection has occurred in less than 1%.

Electrode movement presents a potential risk to the patient, particularly when rigid electrodes are used. This risk is negligible when rigid electrodes are inserted through short, hollow screws that eliminate the fulcrum for movement at the skull. It is additionally necessary, however, to carefully pad these screws and electrodes where they protrude from the skull, and insure a safe environment for the patient that eliminates the opportunity for the patient's head to forcibly contact any hard object during a seizure. Patients are kept in a Posey restraint while in bed or seated in a chair, and ambulation requires two people to be in attendance, on either side of the patient. Although a few electrode blocks have come loose at UCLA, and one patient actually managed to deplant herself on one side during a seizure before present precautions were initiated, no permanent injury has resulted from movement of electrodes within the brain.

Patients with intracranial electrodes should be considered in the high-risk category (U_L type A patient) with respect to electrical safety. Patients should be isolated from ground and the recording instrument. Current leakage of any devices attached to the indwelling electrodes should be less than 10 μA. If electrical stimulation is carried out as part of the diagnostic procedure, the safe limits of stimulation intensity are determined by both instantaneous and total charge density, which reflect current passed per area of tissue at each stimulation, and over the entire testing period (4). Consequently, it is safer to pass current through electrodes with large exposed surface areas than through electrodes with small exposed surface areas. Electrical stimulation should be delivered with a current-regulated patient-isolated stimulator (5) and pulses should be biphasic to prevent polarization of the stimulating electrode. Tissue damage should not occur if instantaneous and total charge densities are kept below 60 $\mu C/cm^2$ and 9 C/cm^2, respectively (4). In practical terms, most stimulation protocols cannot be carried out if the exposed electrode surface area is smaller than 0.1 cm^2.

Some diagnostic procedures include repeated direct electrical stimulation of the brain and this has aroused concern about the possibility of inducing increased epileptogenicity similar to kindling (31). Since kindling is believed to occur only if repeated stimulation trains are delivered, single-pulse stimulation is considered to be safe. Although high frequency (60–100 Hz) trains are commonly used for kindling in animals, kindled seizures can occur with 3 Hz stimulation (12) and the use of low frequency stimulus trains in patient studies may not offer protection. Any stimulation that produces an afterdischarge should be considered capable, if repeated, of inducing enhanced epileptogenicity. Although hundreds of stimulation-induced afterdischarges, even in the amygdala, are required before kindled seizures appear in the primate (51), excitability changes undoubtedly occur earlier and no data are available to assess the risk of kindling from stimulation of human brain tissue that may already be epileptogenic. Despite the common practice of direct brain stimulation as part of the preoperative evaluation for resective surgery in epilepsy, however, no definitive evidence of kindling has been reported. Consequently, this technique can still be considered safe when used within reasonable limits (e.g., stimulation that produces afterdischarge is not repeated more than 2 or 3 times at the same site).

INTERPRETATION

Data analysis is aimed at identifying and delineating cerebral areas that demonstrate epileptiform and nonepileptiform abnormalities and, when necessary, mapping normal cerebral functions to determine safe limits of excision. Interpretation demands recognition of artifacts as distinct from ongoing interictal disturbances and ictal electrical discharges; primary electrical epileptiform events generated at or near the electrode tips must be differentiated, with reasonable confidence, from activity propagated from a distance; and appropriate physiological and electrical stimulation techniques may be employed to identify cortical areas of normal and abnormal function.

Recognition of Artifact

Common EEG artifacts such as muscle activity and electrode pops are not encountered with intracranial recording. Furthermore, movement artifacts are greatly reduced when telemetry systems are used. Consequently, combining intracranial recording with either radio- or cable telemetry results in a relatively artifact-free tracing even during epileptic seizures. A number of artifactual transients can be introduced, however, due to the complexity of the recording and reproduction procedures, and these vary considerably from one recording situation to another. It is necessary, therefore, for all workers in each individual laboratory to be familiar with the patterns of artifacts common to that laboratory. To this end, it can be useful for a laboratory to accumulate examples of all the various artifact patterns encountered and keep them in a file for future reference and training of new personnel. In addition to noncerebrally generated transients that might be confused with epileptiform discharges, more continuous asymmetries may be present throughout the study, or develop over time, that reflect aberrant recording characteristics of electrodes rather than true differences in ongoing baseline cerebral activity. An amplitude asymmetry of baseline rhythms is valid evidence of a lateralized or focal disturbance only when it can be definitively ascertained that interelectrode distances for homologous bipolar pairs are equal, and the same structures are sampled on both sides. An amplitude asymmetry generally indicates a cerebral disturbance when this occurs at several adjacent derivations. Focal frequency asymmetries must also be interpreted with caution. A slower frequency observed from only one electrode contact may be attributed to location near a blood vessel, atypical tissue reaction at the recording tip, or other problems with recording characteristics of that particular electrode.

Interictal Abnormalities

Abnormalities in ongoing baseline activity can be useful for localizing nonepileptiform focal functional deficits which are commonly encountered at the site of, and adjacent to, epileptogenic lesions (21, 26). At times, baseline EEG activity directly recorded from the brain is so abnormal that there is no problem in identification. However, due to the great variation between electrical signals recorded from one part of the brain to another, and from one patient to another, it may be difficult to recognize abnormal attenuation, or slowing, unless homologous areas from both sides of the brain can be compared. This is usually possible when bilaterally symmetrical SEEG recordings are obtained. In this case, asymmetries observed from several adjacent derivations in a single region, for instance the mesial temporal lobes, can be extremely useful for confirming the site of an epileptogenic lesion (Fig. 1). When such an asymmetry is not apparent or is equivocal in the baseline recording, it can be accentuated by

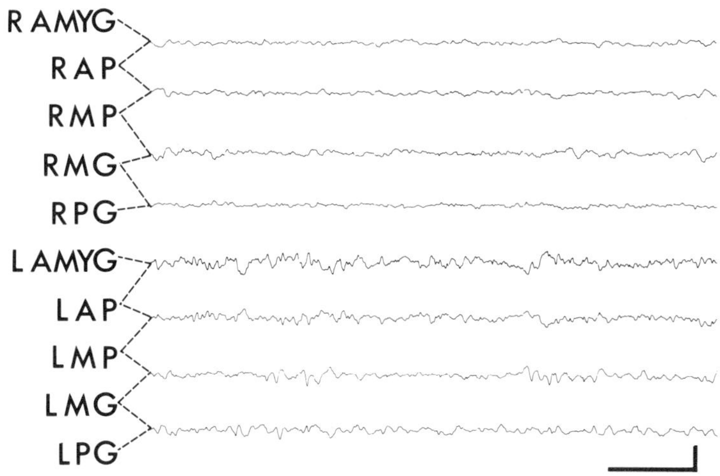

FIG. 1. Interictal SEEG recording revealing an attenuation of normal rhythmic activity in all right mesial temporal derivations. R, right; L, left; AMYG, amygdala; AP, anterior hippocampal pes; MP, midhippocampal pes; MG, midhippocampal gyrus; PG, posterior hippocampal gyrus. Calibration 1 sec, 500 μV.

giving thiopental intravenously, and recording the barbiturate-induced fast activity (21, 26).

The location of interictal epileptiform spikes using intracranial electrodes is not as reliable an indicator of the site of the epileptogenic lesion as the location of other intracranially recorded findings such as ictal onset and continuous nonepileptiform baseline abnormalities, or the location of scalp and sphenoidal recorded interictal EEG spikes (27). Particularly when the epileptogenic lesion is in mesial temporal or other limbic structures, multiple ipsilateral and contralateral sites of independent epileptiform spike generation can be identified. There is currently no way to differentiate between primary and propagated interictal spikes. In 10 to 20% of patients evaluated with SEEG, interictal epileptiform spikes are more prominent contralateral to the epileptogenic lesion (27). Interictal epileptiform spikes may have more localizing significance when the epileptogenic lesion is in the neocortex, and it is possible that multi-electrode grids will provide more reliable information when used in this situation. Differentiation between primary neocortical spikes, however, and those propagated from mesial temporal or other limbic structures that are not sampled by the grid configuration continues to be a problem.

Ictal Abnormalities

Interpretation of ictal EEG recordings obtained with intracranial electrodes is complicated by necessary restrictions on the number of cerebral structures monitored. With SEEG recording, it is possible to obtain a good bilateral representation of those mesial temporal sites most often associated with epileptogenic lesions, the hippocampus, amygdala, and hippocampal gyrus. However, only limited sampling of other mesial and basal surfaces of the brain, such as the mesial and orbital frontal cortex, and also of the neocortical convexities, is possible with this technique. Consequently, SEEG derivations may completely miss large regions of epileptogenic tissue. Although multi-electrode grids provide excellent coverage for large areas of the neocortex, including inferior temporal lobe, they are also inadequate for mesial and orbital frontal cortex, cannot sample important limbic structures such as the amygdala and hippocampus, and are usually only applied to one hemisphere. Therefore, when obtaining ictal recordings using intracranial electrodes, it is important that some tracings also include simultaneously recorded scalp and sphenoidal derivations. With SEEG, this may include bilateral recordings from disc electrodes or skull nails placed according to the International 10–20 System, as well as bilateral sphenoidal derivations, while with the multi-electrode grid this may include recordings from electrodes placed on the contralateral scalp, and bilateral sphenoidal electrodes. Within these limitations, there are a number of clues that are used to determine whether the site of an intracranially recorded ictal onset represents the location of the epileptogenic lesion, or activity propagated from a lesion distant from the tips of the recording electrodes.

When the ictal discharge initially arises in an area that is sampled by multiple electrode contacts, the pattern of electrical ictal onset provides important localizing information. With SEEG recording, ictal onsets in mesial temporal structures can be considered focal, or regional (52). Focal onsets refer to ictal discharges that begin at one or two adjacent electrode sites and are seen to propagate over time to other electrodes in the same temporal lobe. Regional onsets begin simultaneously from most or all electrode derivations in one mesial temporal lobe. In practice, there is a continuum between focal and regional patterns (Fig. 2) and clear distinctions cannot always be made. Nevertheless, it is useful to know that focal ictal onsets are a highly reliable indicator of the site of an epileptogenic lesion while regional ictal onsets, although strongly correlated with the location of the epileptogenic lesion, may also reflect ictal activity propagated from a distance (38, 39). When a regional pattern of ictal onset is identified, it is necessary to attempt to find additional evidence of focal functional deficit in that temporal lobe. Consequently, sufficient electrodes must be inserted to sample multiple sites in mesial temporal structures, and sufficient channels must be recorded simultaneously to identify the site of ictal onset and recognize whether it has a focal or regional pattern of development. In practice, this approach is not usually possible with SEEG recording from extratemporal brain structures, but focal ictal onsets may be identified from lateral neocortex using multi-electrode grids (Fig. 3).

Evidence that surface-recorded ictal EEG changes precede or are synchronous with SEEG-recorded ictal onset indicates that the SEEG electrodes are not actually at the site of ictal generation (38, 39). Ictal onsets recorded with multi-electrode grids from one hemisphere and simultaneously reflected in scalp derivations over the other hemisphere should be considered equally non-localizing. Consequently, it is important that at least some of the ictal recordings be obtained with montages that include scalp electrodes or skull nails.

The pattern of propagation of ictal discharge from one hemisphere to the other appears to have some localizing significance. Due to poor direct connections between contralateral hippocampi (56), ictal discharges in one mesial temporal area may continue for many seconds, or even minutes, without evidence of spread to the other side. A long delay between ictal onset on one side and spread to the other is correlated with an epileptogenic lesion in the mesial temporal lobe on the side of ictal onset, whereas rapid spread to the contralateral side may indicate that the epileptogenic lesion is extratemporal (37). Consequently, it is important that tracings of SEEG-recorded ictal onsets contain bilateral homotopic derivations.

In order for a recorded ictal electrical discharge to be considered responsible for observed clinical ictal behavior, it is necessary to temporally relate the EEG to videotaped behavioral data. Accurate correlation can easily be achieved when a time code generator is employed, or other mechanisms are used to synchronize EEG and videorecorded information. Two features of this correlation are necessary in order to confirm that a particular ictal EEG pattern indicates the site of the epileptogenic lesion. First, the ictal EEG discharge must precede, or be synchronous with, the onset of experiential or behavioral ictal phenomena. Although this does not prove that the EEG-recorded activity is responsible for the behavioral epileptic seizure, when this condition is not met it definitely can be concluded that the EEG-recorded activity is not responsible for the initial ictal behavioral manifestations. Second, the observed clinical ictal behavior must be typical of the patient's habitual epileptic seizures. This can be verified, if necessary, by asking relatives or close friends to review the videotape and identify the behavior. Atypical epileptic seizures may occasionally occur during intracranial recording (20) and can lead to false localization of an epileptogenic lesion if appropriate attention is not paid to the behavioral characteristics of the ictal event.

In order to apply all the approaches described here for differentiating between primary and propagated ictal onset, it is essential to be able to identify the exact time of initiation of the ictal electrical discharge. This can occasionally be extremely subtle with intracranial recording. Most focal ictal onsets begin with a change in baseline frequency in one or two channels that may be difficult to differentiate from the pre-ictal pattern (21). These are commonly low-voltage fast rhythms that are more regular than the ongoing frequency, and demonstrate an evolution that consists of increasing amplitude and decreasing frequency as propagation to other channels appears. At times, a focal onset may take the form of suppression of ongoing baseline activity, or irregular spiking, in one or two channels. On the other hand, regional onsets may also

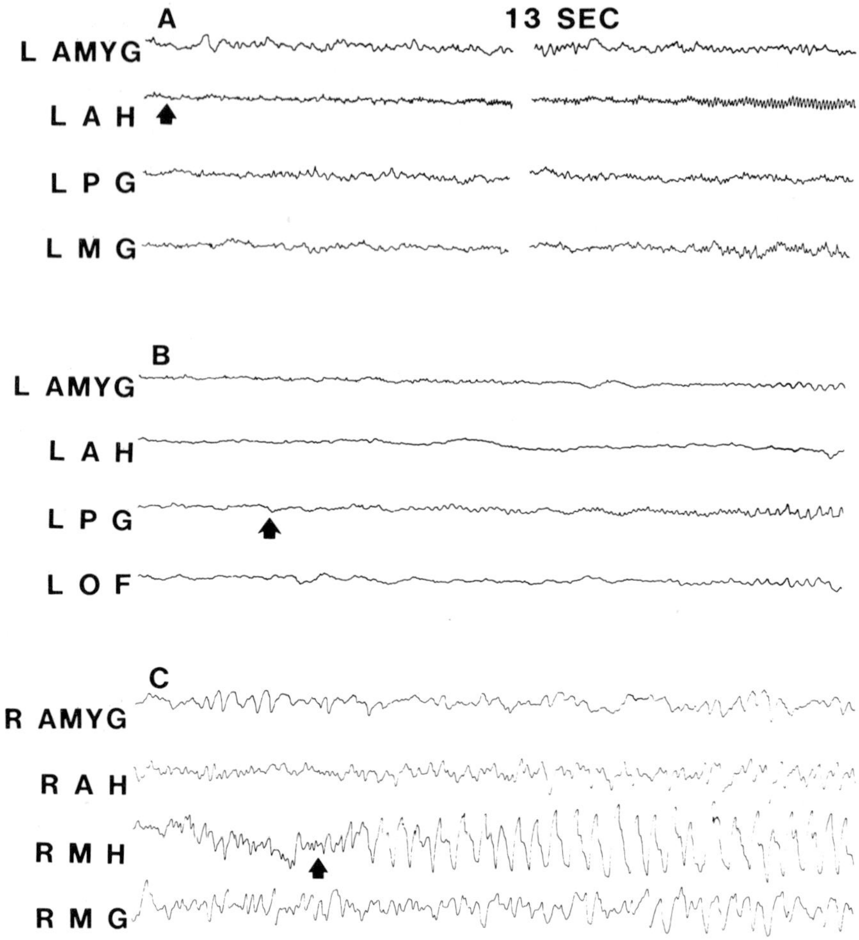

FIG. 2. Segments showing selected channels of SEEG telemetry-recorded ictal onsets from six patients, representing examples of progressively decreasing localizing value. **A–C** demonstrate focal onsets beginning in one channel (*arrow*) and gradually spreading over several seconds to other derivations in the same mesial temporal area. **D–F** demonstrate regional onsets beginning in all channels at once (*arrow*) without evidence of local spread. H refers to hippocampal pes, otherwise, abbreviations as in Fig. 1. Calibration 1 sec. (From ref. 21.)

appear as diffuse suppression of baseline activity in one area and the regional nature of such a pattern may be overlooked if a subsequent more obvious ictal discharge appears with a focal distribution. In order to accurately interpret ictal EEG recordings, it is often necessary to spread out a minute or more of tracing and carefully review the transition from pre-ictal to ictal patterns in an attempt to identify the exact time that ictal electrical changes begin. For this

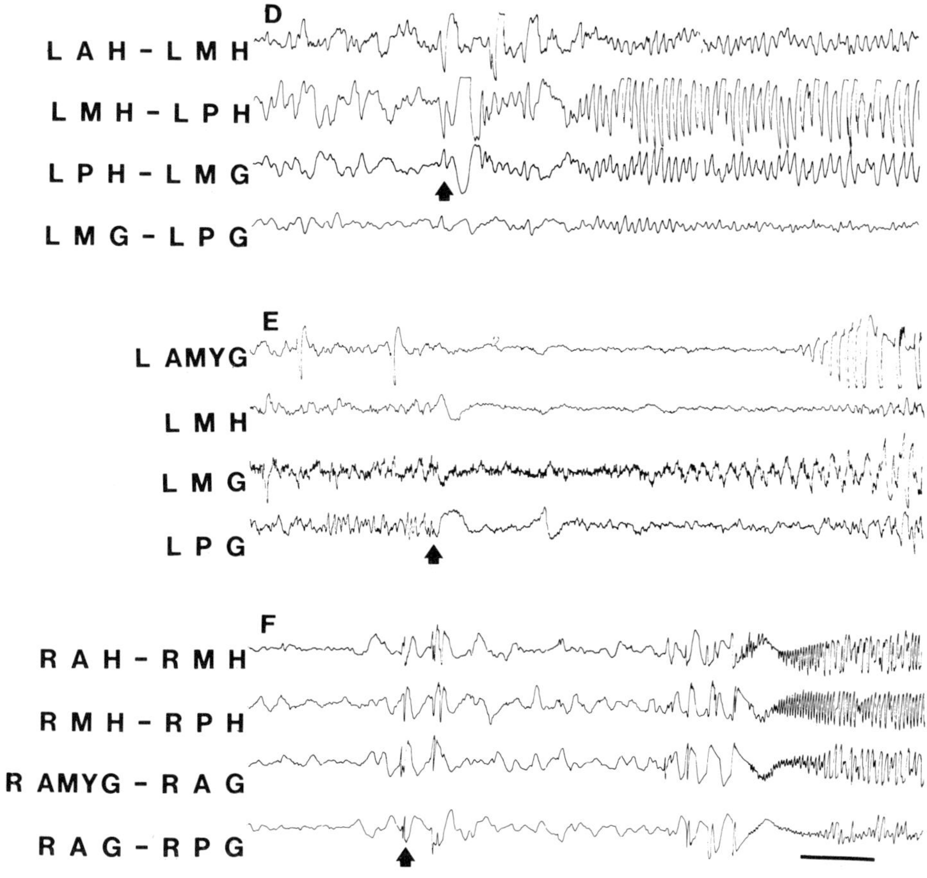

FIG. 2. (*cont'd*)

reason, it is essential that ictal data be read from paper records, since this temporal progression cannot always be easily identified from the limited period of time displayed on the screens of oscilloscopes and video monitors.

Although intracranially recorded ictal onsets are regarded as the most accurate means of identifying the location of an epileptogenic lesion, all available clinical data must be taken into consideration when interpreting the results of these electrophysiological studies. For instance, clear focal ictal onsets may occasionally be falsely localizing, while propagated ictal onsets may reflect the presence of an epileptogenic lesion distant from the electrode tips, but still within the area of a standard resection (20). It is important, therefore, that many independent measures of epileptiform and nonepileptiform cerebral functions be undertaken. Only when results of several of these tests agree can localization of an epileptogenic lesion be made with confidence.

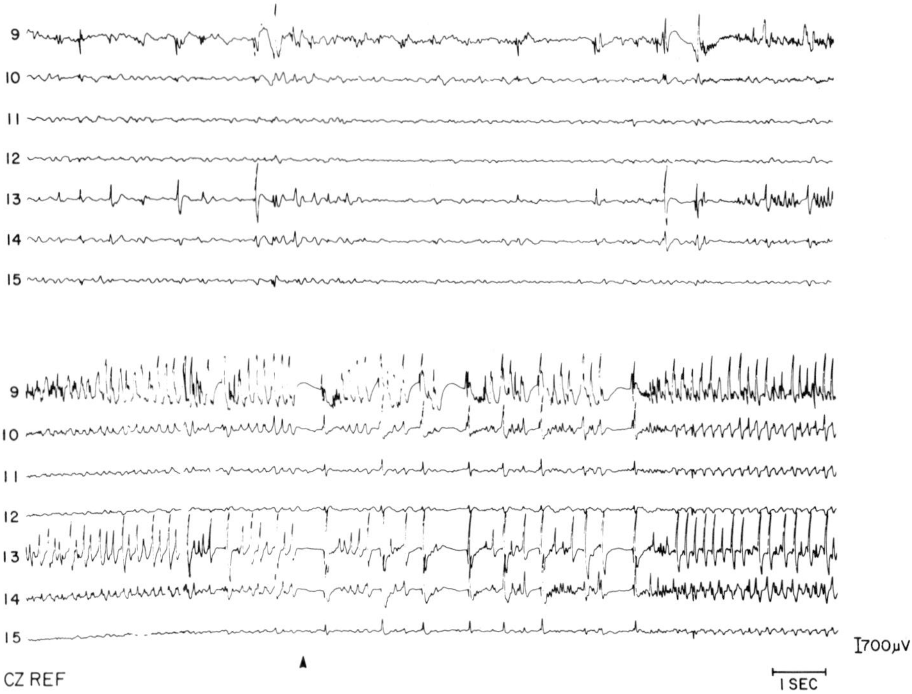

FIG. 3. Continuous recording from a grid of subdural electrodes placed under the base of the temporal lobe demonstrating a focal onset from the anterior medial aspect. Low-voltage fast activity begins only at electrodes 9 and 13 which are the most anterior of the mesial row in a 4 × 4 array with center-to-center distances of 1 cm. All electrodes are recorded with reference to CZ. *Arrow* indicates the onset of clinical symptoms. Calibration 1 sec, 700 μV. (Figure courtesy of R. P. Lesser, H. Lüders, D. S. Dinner, and H. H. Morris, Cleveland Clinic.)

Stimulation Studies

Visual, auditory, and somatosensory stimulation can be performed during intensive intracranial monitoring in order to record evoked potentials and map the boundaries of primary cortical areas that limit the extent of resection. Direct electrical stimulation of cortex is also useful for identifying cortical areas involved in motor and language function. The latter is particularly important when cortical resections are planned for the language dominant hemisphere, since the cortical representation of language varies considerably from patient to patient (44). Demonstration that stimulation does not alter language function provides reasonably reliable evidence that removal of the stimulated cortex will not result in disruption of language, and may allow a more generous resection of an epileptogenic lesion to be performed than might be indicated according to standard concepts of the location of language areas in the brain.

The converse, however, is not always true. That is, when stimulation of parts of the brain generally not felt to contain structures important to language function does cause a temporary disruption of language, inclusion of that area in the resection does not necessarily result in permanent aphasia. When the standard *en bloc* anterior temporal lobectomy (14, 21) is performed without complication in the language dominant hemisphere, permanent aphasia has not been a problem and there appears to be no need for careful mapping of language distribution. This procedure is necessary, however, when the patient might benefit from more posterior extension of this standard resection and when any nonstandard cortical resection is contemplated near areas associated with language function in the language dominant hemisphere.

Direct electrical stimulation of the brain has also been used to aid in identifying the site of the epileptogenic lesion. Although electrical stimulation of the neocortex can occasionally produce habitual seizures, the initial electrical patterns may be different from those observed with spontaneous ictal events (54), and such stimulation-induced epileptic seizures may be caused by propagation of electrical discharge from the site of stimulation to a distant epileptogenic lesion, perhaps even in the contralateral hemisphere (22). Consequently, ictal events induced by electrical stimulation of the brain must be interpreted with caution. When the epileptogenic lesion is in mesial limbic structures, however, there is a good correlation between the site of the epileptogenic lesion and an *elevation* of the afterdischarge threshold (13). That is, it is more difficult to obtain an afterdischarge by electrical stimulation of a sclerotic hippocampus that is the site of habitual seizure initiation than it is to produce afterdischarge in the contralateral, more normal, hippocampus.

FUTURE RESEARCH QUESTIONS

Although there is no doubt that intensive neurodiagnostic monitoring with intracranial electrodes can provide the most accurate information concerning the location of an epileptogenic lesion, errors can still be made with this technique and there are serious risks inherent in all of the invasive procedures that are necessary to obtain this information. Research is directed at improving the accuracy of localization based on intracranial recording, modifying the techniques to reduce risk, and devising noninvasive evaluation protocols that will reduce the number of patients for whom intracranial recording is necessary.

The techniques of SEEG and multi-electrode grid recording each have strengths and weaknesses that are complementary. An approach that would allow some form of both electrode types to be easily used simultaneously would be extremely useful. In addition, more information is needed concerning the most common sites of epileptogenic lesions in mesial and orbital frontal cortex, and other cortical areas that are not easily sampled by either technique. It would be ideal if logical patterns of intracranial electrode arrays could be used in a standard fashion that would allow adequate screening for extratemporal epileptogenic lesions, and also provide experience with normal EEG patterns encountered in these areas in order to better recognize abnormalities. Information obtained from patients, and perhaps also from primates, may provide insights into common patterns of spread that will be useful for identifying sites of seizure generation in temporal and extratemporal regions and lead to more logical sampling procedures (53).

In addition to modifications of surgical techniques for electrode insertion and of electrode design which will improve the safety of intracranial monitoring, the risks associated with intracranial recording can also be reduced if the period required for such studies can be shortened. At the present time, it is necessary to record a number of spontaneous seizures and, depending on the seizure frequency and the degree of similarity between ictal events captured, this may take 2 to 6 weeks of intensive monitoring. Attempts to provoke epileptic seizures by rapid reduction of antiepileptic medication, the use of pharmacological activation techniques, or electrical stimulation, greatly enhances the chance of obtaining information that is falsely localizing (20, 54). It may be possible, however, to identify or provoke epileptiform transient or nonepileptic continuous abnormalities in the interictal record that correlate highly with the location of the epileptogenic lesion. If such abnormalities could be identified, it might not be necessary to wait for spontaneous seizures to occur and adequate information might be obtained from intracranial monitoring over a few hours or days. Studies in progress that may ultimately identify indicators of the site of the epileptogenic lesion with a high degree of reliability include investigations of specific patterns of multi-unit activity within the primary epileptic focus (2), and characteristic responses to paired pulse stimulation (55).

Other important research involves correlating data obtained by intracranial monitoring with a variety of noninvasive techniques used for localizing cerebral dysfunction in epilepsy (18). If localizing information derived from these new diagnostic techniques compared well with localizing information obtained from intensive intracranial monitoring, and ultimately with pathological diagnosis of resected brain tissue and outcome following surgery, it would be possible to devise protocols for noninvasive presurgical evaluation that would increase confidence in identification of a resectable epileptogenic lesion and reduce the number of patients who require invasive procedures. Examples of some of the new techniques that are currently being investigated with respect to localization of epileptogenic lesions for resective surgery include: positron emission tomography (19, 24, 25), which will be able to employ a variety of positron-labeled tracers to identify local cerebral abnormalities, not only in glucose and oxygen metabolism and blood flow, but also in protein synthesis, pH, blood-brain barrier integrity, and specific neurotransmitter function; magnetic resonance which can produce high resolution structural images that may eventually provide some functional information (10), and spectroscopic information that can analyze changes in high-energy phosphates and other indicators of cerebral function in large regions of the brain (47); magnetoencephalography which is able to localize sources and directions of current flow in the brain in three dimensions (7); single photon emission tomography that is currently being used to produce images of cerebral blood flow with a resolution that is somewhat less than that of positron emission tomography (9); and applications of X-ray computed tomography that may reveal functional, rather than structural, disturbances (43).

CONCLUSIONS

The single indication for routine intensive neurodiagnostic monitoring with intracranial electrodes is localization of a resectable epileptogenic focus in patients with partial epilepsy who are considered candidates for surgery. This is achieved by combined intracranial EEG recording and video monitoring in order to describe the electrophysiological correlates of typical ictal events. Intensive monitoring with intracranial electrodes should only be performed in centers where there is a multi-specialty team experienced in the surgical therapy of epilepsy.

Although intracranial monitoring is believed to be the most accurate diagnostic procedure for localizing resectable epileptogenic lesions, not all patients with partial epilepsy who are candidates for resective surgery require these invasive studies. When noninvasive evaluation suggests that a patient would be likely to benefit from resective surgery, definitive localizing information has not been obtained, and the number of potential sites for the epileptogenic lesion are limited to a reasonable number, intracranial monitoring is appropriate. The most commonly used intracranial monitoring technique is SEEG, which is particularly suited for identifying epileptogenic lesions in mesial temporal areas prior to anterior temporal lobectomy. A multi-electrode grid has recently been devised for recording from the cortical surface, and is better suited for neocortical epileptogenic lesions on the lateral and basal aspects of the brain. Intensive monitoring with intracranial electrodes may be carried out for prolonged periods of time on a daily basis with direct connection to a standard EEG machine, but is best performed continually, 24 hr a day, on a specialized monitoring unit, ideally utilizing EEG telemetry to minimize movement artifact. Appropriate precautions are necessary to continue to record from a patient over days or weeks with intracranial electrodes, particularly with respect to possible injury from movement of electrodes, infection, and electrical current. Interpretation of interictal and ictal recordings requires familiarity with the variety of artifacts that are encountered due to the complex equipment involved; the use of sufficient electrode placements, and sufficient channels on the EEG recording to recognize spatial and temporal patterns of nonepileptiform, as well as epileptiform abnormalities, differentiation of these events from artifact, and differentiation of primary from propagated phenomena; and careful correlation of electrophysiological data with videotaped clinical behavior. Electrical and physiological stimulation may also be useful to confirm focal functional deficit, and map areas of primary cortical function that may determine the limits of resection of the epileptogenic lesion. Research in the area of intensive neurodiagnostic monitoring with intracranial electrodes is aimed at improving the accuracy of this procedure for identifying a resectable epileptogenic lesion, reducing the risks associated with these invasive procedures, and ultimately identifying those combinations of data obtained by noninvasive localizing techniques that can determine the site of a resectable epileptogenic lesion with sufficient confidence to obviate the need for intracranial electrode monitoring in a substantial number of patients.

ACKNOWLEDGMENTS

Opportunities to acquire information included here were provided in part by grant NS-02808 from the United States Public Health Service.

REFERENCES

1. Ajmone Marsan, C. (1980): Depth electrography and electrocorticography. In: *Electrodiagnosis in Clinical Neurology*, edited by M.J. Aminoff, pp. 167–196. Churchill Livingstone, New York.
2. Babb, T.L., and Crandall, P.H. (1976): Epileptogenesis of human limbic neurons in psychomotor epileptics. *Electroencephalogr. Clin. Neurophysiol.*, 40:225–243.
3. Babb, T.L., and Kupfer, W. (1984): Phagocytic and metabolic reactions to chronically implanted metal brain electrodes. *Exp. Neurol.* 86:171–182.
4. Babb, T.L., and Kupfer, W. (1986): Phagocytic and metabolic reactions to intracerebral electrical stimulation of rat brain. *Exp. Neurol. (in press).*
5. Babb T.L., Mariani, E., Sneider, K.A., et al. (1980): A circuit for safe diagnostic electrical stimulation of the human brain. *Neurol. Res.*, 2:181–197.
6. Bailey P., and Gibbs, F.A. (1951): The surgical treatment of psychomotor epilepsy. *JAMA*, 145:365–370.
7. Barth, D.S., Sutherling, W., Engel, J., Jr., and Beatty, J. (1983): Neuromagnetic evidence of spatially distributed sources underlying epileptiform spikes in the human brain. *Science*, 223:293–296.
8. Bickford, R.G., Petersen, M.C., Dodge, H.W., Jr., and Sem-Jacobsen, C.W. (1953): Observations on depth stimulation of the human brain through implanted electrographic leads, symposium on intracerebral electrography, *Mayo Clin. Proc.* 28:181–187.
9. Bonte, F.J., Stokely, E.M., Devous, M.D., Sr., and Homan, R.W. (1983): Single photon tomographic study of regional cerebral blood flow in epilepsy. *Arch. Neurol.*, 40:267–270.
10. Buddinger, T.F., and Lauterbur, P.C. (1984): Nuclear magnetic resonance technology for medical studies. *Science*, 226:288–298.
11. Cahan, L., Sutherling, W.W., McCullough, M., Rausch, R., Engel, J., Jr., and Crandall, P.H. (1984): Review of the 20-year UCLA experience with surgery for epilepsy. *Cleve. Clin. Q.*, 51:313–318.
12. Cain, D.P., and Corcoran, M.E. (1981): Kindling with low-frequency stimulation: generality, transfer, and recruiting effects. *Exp. Neurol.*, 73:219–232.
13. Cherlow, D..G., Dymond, A.M., Crandall. P.H, et al. (1977): Evoked response and after-discharge thresholds to electrical stimulation in temporal lobe epileptics. *Arch. Neurol.*, 34:527–531.
14. Crandall, P.H., Walter, R.D., and Rand, R.W. (1963): Clinical applications of studies on

stereotactically implanted electrodes in temporal lobe epilepsy. *J. Neurosurg.*, 20:827–840.
15. Dodge, H.W., Jr., Holman, C.B., Sem-Jacobsen, C.W., Bickford, R.G., and Petersen, M.C. (1953): Technique of depth electrography, symposium on intracerebral electrography. *Mayo Clinic Proc.*, 28:147–155.
16. Dymond, A.M., and Crandall, P.H. (1976): Oxygen availability and blood flow in the temporal lobes during spontaneous epileptic seizures in man. *Brain Res.*, 102:191–196.
17. Dymond, A.M., Zweizig, J.R., Crandall, P.H., and Hanley, J. (1971): Clinical applications of an EEG radio-telemetry system. *Biomed. Instrum.*, 8:16–20.
18. Engel, J., Jr. (1983): Functional localization of epileptogenic lesions. *Trends Neurosci.*, 6:60–65.
19. Engel, J., Jr., Brown, W.J., Kuhl, D.E., Phelps, M.E., Mazziotta, J.C., and Crandall, P.H. (1982): Pathological findings underlying focal temporal lobe hypometabolism in partial epilepsy. *Ann. Neurol.*, 12:518–528.
20. Engel, J., Jr., and Crandall, P.H. (1983): Falsely localizing ictal onsets with depth EEG telemetry during anticonvulsant withdrawal. *Epilepsia*, 24:344–355.
21. Engel, J., Jr., Crandall, P.H., and Rausch, R. (1983): The partial epilepsies. In: *The Clinical Neurosciences, Vol. 2,* edited by R.N. Rosenberg, R.G. Grossman, S. Schochet, E.R. Heinz, and W.D. Willis, pp. 1349–1380. Churchill Livingstone, New York.
22. Engel, J., Jr., Driver, M.V., and Falconer, M.A. (1975): Electrophysiological correlates of pathology and surgical results in temporal lobe epilepsy. *Brain*, 98:129–156.
23. Engel, J., Jr., Ebersole, J.S., Burchfiel, J.L., Gates, J.R., Gotman, J., Homan, R.W., Ives, J.R., King, D.W., Sato, S., and Wilkus, R.J. (1985): Guidelines for long-term neurodiagnostic monitoring in epilepsy. *J. Clin. Neurophysiol.*, 2:419–452.
24. Engel, J., Jr., Kuhl, D.E., Phelps, M.E., and Crandall, P.H. (1982): Comparative localization of epileptic foci in partial epilepsy by PCT and EEG. *Ann. Neurol.*, 12:529–537.
25. Engel, J., Jr., Kuhl, D.E., Phelps, M.E., and Mazziotta, J.C. (1982): Interictal cerebral glucose metabolism in partial epilepsy and its relation to EEG changes. *Ann. Neurol.*, 12:510–517.
26. Engel, J., Jr., Rausch, R., Lieb, J.P., Kuhl, D.E., and Crandall, P.H. (1981): Correlation of criteria used for localizing epileptic foci in patients considered for surgical therapy of epilepsy. *Ann. Neurol.*, 9:215–224.
27. Engel, J., Jr., Sutherling, W.W., Cahan, L., Crandall, P.H., Kuhl, D.E., and Phelps, M.E. (1984): The role of positron emission tomography in the surgical therapy of epilepsy. In: *Advances in Epileptology: Epilepsy International Symposium*, edited by R.J. Porter, R.H. Mattson, A.A. Ward, and M. Dam, pp. 427–432. Raven Press, New York.
28. Falconer, M.A. (1976): Anterior temporal lobectomy for epilepsy. In: *Operative Surgery, Vol. 14 (2nd ed.)*, edited by R.C. Smith, pp. 142–149. Butterworths, London.
29. Gloor, P. (1975): Contributions of electroencephalography and electrocorticography to the neurosurgical treatment of the epilepsies. In: *Advances in Neurology, Vol. 8, Neurosurgical Management of the Epilepsies*, edited by D.P. Purpura, J.K. Penry, and R.D. Walter, pp. 59–105. Raven Press, New York.
30. Gloor, P. (1984): Electroencephalography and the role of depth recordings. In: *Advances in Epileptology: Epilepsy International Symposium,* edited by R.J. Porter, R.H. Mattson, A.A. Ward, and M. Dam. Raven Press, New York.
31. Goddard, G.V., McIntyre, D.C., and Leech, C.K. (1969): A permanent change in brain function resulting from daily electrical stimulation. *Exp. Neurol.*, 25:295–330.
32. Goldring, S. (1978): A method for surgical management of focal epilepsy, especially as it relates to children. *J. Neurosurg.*, 49:344–356.
33. Gotman, J., Gloor, P., and Ives, J.R. (editors) (1985): Long-term monitoring. *Electroencephalogr. Clin. Neurophysiol. (Suppl.)*, 37:444.
34. Horsley, V. (1886): Brain-surgery. *Br. Med. J.*, 2:670–675.
35. Jensen, I. (1975): Temporal lobe surgery around the world. *Acta Neurol. Scand.*, 52:354–373.
36. Lesser, R.P., Dinner, D.S., Luders, H., and Morris, H.H., III. (1984): Differential diagnosis and treatment of intractable seizures. *Cleve. Clin. Q.*, 51:227–240.
37. Lieb, J.P., Babb, T.L., Engel, J., Jr., Brown, W.J., Pretorius, J., and Crandall, P.H. (1984): Interhemispheric propagation time of hippocampal seizures: cell density and sur-

gical outcome correlates. Proceedings: *Electroencephalogr. Clin. Neurophysiol.* 58:38p.

38. Lieb, J.P., Engel, J., Jr., Brown, W.J., Gevins, A.S., and Crandall, P.H. (1981): Neuropathological findings following temporal lobectomy related to surface and depth EEG patterns. *Epilepsia*, 22:539–549.
39. Lieb, J.P., Engel, J., Jr., Gevins, A.S., and Crandall, P.H. (1981): Surface and deep EEG correlates of surgical outcome in temporal lobe epilepsy. *Epilepsia*, 22:515–538
40. Lüders, H., Hahn, J.F., Skipper, G.J., Lesser, R.P., Dinner, D.S., Morris, H.H., and Estes, M.L. (1985): Chronic basal temporal arrays of subdural electrodes in the evaluation of complex partial seizures. *Electroencephalogr. Clin. Neurophysiol.* 61:24p.
41. Maxwell, R.E., Gates, J.R., Flol, M.E., Johnson, M.J., Yap, J.C., Leppik, I.E., and Gumnit, R.J. (1983): Clinical evaluation of a depth electroencephalography electrode. *Neurosurgery*, 12:561–564.
42. Nuwer, M.R., Engel, J., Jr., Sutherling, W.W., and Babb, T.L. (1985): Monitoring at the University of California, Los Angeles. In: *Long-Term Monitoring in Epilepsy*, edited by J. Gotman, P. Gloor, and J.R. Ives, *Electroencephalogr. Clin. Neurophysiol. (Suppl.)*, 37:385–401.
43. Oakley, J., Ojemann, G.A., Ojemann, L.M., et al. (1979): Identifying epileptic foci on contrast-enhanced computerized tomographic scans. *Arch. Neurol.*, 36:669–671.
44. Ojemann, G.A. (1979): Individual variability in cortical localization of language. *J. Neurosurg.*, 50:164–169.
45. Penfield, W., and Jasper, H. (1954): *Epilepsy and the Functional Anatomy of the Human Brain*, p. 896. Little, Brown, Boston.
46. Pretroff, O.A.C., Pritchard, J.W., Behar, K.L., Alger, J.R., and Shulman, G. (1984): *In vivo* phosphorous nuclear magnetic resonance spectroscopy in status epilepticus. *Ann. Neurol.*, 16:169–177.
47. Rasmussen, B. (1983): Surgical treatment of complex partial seizures: Results, lessons, and problems. *Epilepsia*, 24(Suppl.1):S65–S76.
48. Shewmon, D.A., and Krentler, K.A. (1984): Off-line montage reformatting. *Electroencephalogr. Clin. Neurophysiol.*, 57:591–595.
49. Spencer, S.S. (1981): Depth electroencephalography in selection of refractory epilepsy for surgery. *Ann. Neurol.*, 9:207–214.
50. Talairach, J., Bancaud, J., Szikla, G., et al. (1974): Approche nouvelle de la neurochirurgie de l'épilepsie. Méthodologie stérotaxique et résultats thérapeutiques. *Neurochirurgie*,20(Suppl.1):240.
51. Wada, J.A., Mizoguchi, T., and Osawa, T. (1978): Secondarily generalized convulsive seizures induced by daily amygdaloid stimulation in rhesus monkeys. *Neurology*, 28:1026–1036.
52. Walter, R.D. (1975): Principles of clinical investigation of surgical candidates. In: *Advances in Neurology, Vol. 8, Neurosurgical Management of the Epilepsies*, edited by D.P. Purpura, J.K. Penry, and R.D. Walter, pp. 49–58. Raven Press, New York.
53. Wieser, H.G. (1983): *Electroclinical Features of the Psychomotor Seizure*, p. 242. Verlag, Stuttgart.
54. Wieser, H.G., Bancaud, J., Talairach, J., et al. (1979): Comparative value of spontaneous and chemically and electrically induced seizures in establishing the lateralization of temporal lobe seizures. *Epilepsia*, 20:47–60.
55. Wilson, C.L., Isokawa-Akesson, M., Babb, T.L., Wang, M.L., and Engel, J., Jr. (1985): Lack of functional evidence for a human hippocampal commissure in the human brain. *Electroenceph. Clin. Neurophysiol.*, 61:554.
56. Wilson, C.L., I)sokawa-Akesson, M., Babb, T.L., Wang, M.L., and Engel, J., Jr. (1985): Temporal lobe neuronal excitability in complex-partial epilepsy. Paper presented at the 16th Epilepsy International Congress, Hamburg, September 6–9.
57. Wyler, A.R., Ojemann, G.A., Lettich, E., and Ward, A.A., Jr. (1984): Subdural strip electrodes for localizing epileptogenic foci. *J. Neurosurg.*, 60:1195–1200.

Advances in Neurology, Vol. 46: Intensive Neurodiagnostic Monitoring, edited by R. J. Gumnit. Raven Press, New York © 1986.

Intensive Video/EEG Monitoring of Neonates

Barry R. Tharp

Department of Neurology, Stanford University School of Medicine, Stanford, California 94305

The intensive care of the critically ill full-term or prematurely born newborn is complicated by the multisystem failure encountered in this unique population of patients. In the years immediately after the appearance of neonatal intensive care nurseries, cardiopulmonary function was the most significant determinant of survival. As ventilatory techniques improved and neonatologists became more skilled in supporting the newborn with hyaline membrane disease and pulmonary hypertension, attention was directed towards other organ systems. Though cardiac and pulmonary failure, accompanied by renal compromise, necrotizing bowel disease, and generalized sepsis are responsible for much of the immediate mortality, cerebral dysfunction in the form of cerebral palsy is the most serious long-term sequela in the increasing number of nursery survivors.

The magnitude of this problem can be appreciated by reviewing the data collected by the National Collaborative Perinatal Project (NCPP) on approximately 54,000 infants born between 1959 and 1966 (18). The incidence of cerebral palsy for children with birthweights < 1,500 g was 90.4/1,000 live births and 3.3/1,000 for children with birthweights > 2,500 g. If we apply these figures to 1979 births (3,494,398 United States births, 93% with birthweights > 2,500 g (51), we would anticipate finding 10,700 children yearly with cerebral palsy whose birth weights were > 2,500 g.

More recent studies of smaller populations of newborns have shown an overall decrease in mortality in all gestational age groups over the last decade. This increased survival can be attributed to changes in obstetric care, including the more frequent use of fetal monitoring, the increased rate of cesarean delivery, and the development of neonatal intensive care units (3,33,57). In addition, some authors have reported a decline in the incidence of neurological sequelae in very small premature infants (27), whereas others have not been able to confirm these optimistic reports (33,38). Rothberg et al. (58) recently reported a survival rate of 36% in 69 infants weighing 1,000 g or less born between 1973 and 1976. Sixty-five percent had a good outcome. Driscoll et al. (15) reported a survival rate of 48% in 54 infants born in 1977 and 1978 weighing < 1,001 g at birth. Neurological development was normal in 83% of the survivors at follow-up at 8 months to 3 years. A report from the Stanford University Medical Center nursery (12) showed a decrease in mortality of infants weighing 751 to 1,000 g born between 1961 and 1976 and those born between 1977 and 1980 (63% and 28%, respectively).

The impact of neonatal intensive care units on infant mortality and morbidity can best be illustrated by the study of Horwood et al. (33). They assessed the contribution of a regional program for perinatal/neonatal intensive care on the outcome of all very low birthweight infants live-born to residents of an urban Canadian county. The mortality of infants with birthweights of 1,000 or 1,499 g, born between 1964 and 1969, was 37.6%. The mortality declined to 22.8% after the introduction of neonatal intensive care (1973 to 1977). Major neurological sequelae (cerebral palsy, hydrocephalus, epilepsy, and/or mental retardation), blindness, and deafness, however, were the same in both groups (11% and 13%, respectively).

The majority of follow-up studies of neonatal intensive care survivors have been limited by the young age at last examination (usually 1 to 4 years) (24). The sequelae most easily recognized at that age are usually quite obvious and consist of major neurological and cognitive deficits. More subtle cognitive and behavioral abnormalities are usually not detected and can only be recognized by extension of follow-up into the school years. It is obvious, however, that such minor sequelae as language disorders, attention deficit syndrome, behavioral abnormalities, and other cognitive deficits are socially important and need further investigation. A recent study by Janowsky and Nass (35) has shown significant expressive language delay (using the Early Language Milestone Scale) in infants who had suffered small (grade I and II) intraventricular hemorrhages in the perinatal period. Ellison et al. (19) described abnormal behaviors in a group of 6- to 7-year-olds who had been treated in an intensive care unit. The real magnitude of these "minor" sequelae in nursery graduates is unknown.

Although there have been significant advances in the understanding and treatment of neonatal neurological disorders over the last several decades, the studies just discussed clearly point out the limitations of our present-day therapy for the prevention of permanent CNS damage. It is also clear that more extensive assessment of cerebral function in the neonatal period is necessary if we are to identify those factors that contribute to neonatal brain damage and, at least, to identify the child "at risk" for subsequent sequelae. Infants with serious cerebral dysfunction should be entered into infant stimulation programs at an early age and their parents counseled on the seriousness of the brain damage. The infant destined to suffer minor sequelae should be recognized prior to the school years when early intervention can assume a preventive role and lead to proper school placement and remedial teaching, thus avoiding the stress associated with unexpected school failure and behavioral and social misconduct.

The purpose of this chapter is to identify those areas where intensive neurodiagnostic monitoring can contribute to improved neonatal care and, in turn, the long-term outcome, as well as increasing our understanding of the pathophysiological substrate underlying the major neurological syndromes of the newborn. I discuss the current status of monitoring, the research in progress, and look ahead at future developments in the field.

NEONATAL NEUROLOGICAL DISORDERS

A comprehensive review of neonatal neurological disorders is beyond the scope of this chapter. Rather, I will highlight those conditions which will most readily lend themselves to intensive neurodiagnostic monitoring. Readers who are not acquainted with the common neurological syndromes of infancy are referred to Volpe's excellent text on this subject (76). It should be emphasized that a physician must become familiar with neonatal medical and neurological disorders before undertaking clinical neonatal intensive care unit (NICU) monitoring.

The most common neonatal syndromes impacting on cerebral function are listed in Table 1. The most frequently encountered and clinically significant of these [hypoxic-ischemic encephalopathy, intracranial hemorrhage, particularly intraventricular (IVH) and periventricular leukomalacia (PVL)] are the direct or indirect result of asphyxia. The most common causes of hypoxemia in the newborn period are: (a) prenatal asphyxia caused by alterations in the intrauterine environment, e.g., placental insufficiency, and cord compression during delivery; (b) postnatal respiratory syndromes, e.g., hyaline membrane disease; and (c) severe right-to-left shunts from congenital cardiac disease or persistent fetal circulation (pulmonary hypertension).

Infants suffering from these syndromes also have very unstable cardiovascular systems due to the direct effect of hypoxemia on the heart or primary heart disease secondary to irreversible (congenital malformation) or reversible (patent ductus arteriosus) shunting leading to decreased cardiac output, worsening hypoxia, and marked fluctuations in blood pressure, including long periods of

TABLE 1. *Common neurological syndromes*

Hypoxic-ischemic encephalopathy (23)
Intracranial hemorrhage (28)
Intraventricular
Intraparenchymal
Subarachnoid
Subdural
Infection—primarily meningitis
Periventricular leukomalacia (39)
Metabolic encephalopathy other than asphyxia
Developmental defects—i.e., congenital CNS malformations
Toxic syndromes including drug withdrawal
Cranial trauma

hypotension. It has recently been suggested that asphyxiated infants lack the autoregulation of cerebral blood flow that normally maintains cerebral perfusion constant during wide swings of systemic blood pressure (42). Thus, changes in blood pressure are directly transmitted to the cerebral vascular bed causing an increase or decrease in local perfusion. It is for this reason that an ischemic injury usually complicates the primary hypoxic insult and the term hypoxic-ischemic encephalopathy (HIE) used to describe the clinical and pathological syndromes caused by perinatal asphyxia. IVH is thought to result from marked swings in mean arterial pressure. Initial hypotension causes ischemia to the lateral ventricular germinal matrix overlying the caudate nucleus, followed by systemic hypertension and hyperperfusion resulting in rupture of the friable, already damaged, capillary walls, and hemorrhage into the ventricles. PVL is the result of a similar process on the distal end-arterioles and capillaries supplying the periventricular white matter (81). Ischemic infarction in the "watershed" areas surrounding the frontal and occipital horns of the lateral ventricles represents the initial insult, occasionally followed by hemorrhage and cystic degeneration of the white matter.

Infants with cerebral hypoxic injuries are also more subject to recurrent apnea, sepsis, metabolic disturbances such as hypoglycemia and hypocalcemia, and renal and bowel disease, all of which can lead to a worsening of cerebral perfusion and additional hypoxic and metabolic injury.

It is generally stated that the asphyxic insult occurs before or during delivery in 90% of infants with HIE and is purely postnatal in 10% of cases (6,29). In the past, traumatic deliveries contributed significantly to the incidence of perinatal asphyxia. Improvements in obstetric care, including more liberal use of cesarean section, and the almost universal application of fetal heart monitors during labor, have reduced the incidence of serious intrauterine hypoxia, and have probably led to a reduction in the incidence of intrauterine causes of asphyxia. There are, however, no recent studies directly addressing the issue of timing of the hypoxic-ischemic insult. The majority of newborn infants who suffered intrauterine asphyxia have low Apgar scores and evidence of prior hypoxia manifested by acidosis, hyper- or hypotension, hypovolemia, and elevated creatine phosphokinase (CPK)-BB levels (63,73). The contribution of additional postnatal hypoxia and/or ischemia to the severity of the encephalopathy, the incidence of neonatal seizures, and the ultimate outcome is unknown.

It is well known that the Apgar score alone is only a rough predictor of outcome. In an analysis of the Apgar scores recorded for the National Collaborative Perinatal Projects of NINCDS (NCPP) on approximately 49,000 singleton births, Nelson and Ellenberg (53) found that although low Apgar scores were risk factors for cerebral palsy, 73% of children with later cerebral palsy had good Apgar scores (> 7) at 5 min. The incidence of cerebral palsy in infants who survived after an Apgar of 0 to 3 at 10 and 15 min. was 16.7% and 36%, respectively. This apparent discrepancy in Apgar score and outcome had been pointed out earlier by Thomson et al. (72) in a smaller group of severely asphyxiated infants. Ninety-three percent of 31 severely asphyxiated infants (Apgar of 0 at 1 min or < 4 at 5 min) had no serious neurological or mental handicap at follow-up at age 5 to 10 years.

The infant who develops HIE during the neonatal period begins to show signs of neurological compromise within the first 24 hr of life (74). These consist of a depressed level of consciousness, tone abnormalities, weakness, episodic apnea, increased intracranial pressure, seizures, and an abnormal EEG (10,70,71). The outcome of HIE is quite variable and obviously depends on the criteria for inclusion in the study and the definition of HIE. Two recent studies revealed an average mortality of 10%, and a 22% incidence of neurological sequelae in the survivors (14,59).

Intraventricular hemorrhage occurs in approximately 40% of premature infants weighing less than 1,500 g (2). It is divided into periventricular (PVH) (germinal matrix bleed with or without parenchymal spread) and intraventricular (IVH) hemorrhage (rupture of the germinal matrix hemorrhage into the ventricles or, in older infants, rupture of the choroid plexus), thus the abbreviation PVH/IVH (shortened to IVH in the subsequent discussion). It is commonly preceded by asphyxia and an unstable cardiovascular system (75). Ment et al. (45) used the xenon-133 inhalation technique to study hemispheric blood flow in 15 preterm infants weighing $< 1{,}250$ g at birth. They measured increased hemispheric blood flows in the hemisphere with the largest hemorrhage and suggested that this represented a response of the cerebral vasculature to the hemorrhage or was an indication of loss of autoregulation. Perlman et al. (55) measured relative cerebral blood flow in the anterior cerebral arteries with a Doppler technique and found that 21 of 23 infants with fluctuating blood flows in the first 24 hr of life developed IVH as compared to 7 of 27 infants with stable blood flow patterns.

As mentioned earlier, the apparent loss of normal autoregulation of the cerebral vasculature may predispose the premature neonate to a pressure passive state leading to intracerebral hemorrhage and infarction. Ahmann et al. (1) cautioned that impaired autoregulation, per se, does not appear to be directly related to the occurrence of IVH. In their study there was no difference in the incidence of IVH in 15 infants who were pressure passive (as measured by a Doppler technique) and 17 infants who were autoregulated (9 and 8 infants with IVH, respectively). The stability of systemic blood pressure was not systematically and serially studied in these infants.

IVH is often accompanied by ventricular dilatation which may resolve spontaneously or progress rapidly to symptomatic hydrocephalus requiring a shunting procedure in the first few weeks of life. In addition, more slowly progressive "normal pressure" hydrocephalus occurs in approximately 23% of infants with IVH (28). It is unknown, at present, if such ventricular dilatation, particularly if it resolves spontaneously, has a detrimental effect on cerebral function. There are no known EEG correlates of this post-IVH syndrome. The incidence of severe hydrocephalus has been decreasing over the last few years concomitant with the reduction of serious IVH with massive ventricular bleeding (63).

IVH, per se, may be relatively innocuous (10). The severity of the encephalopathy appears to be related more to the extent of the HIE, the degree of intraparenchymal spread of the blood, and the accompanying cerebral infarction which may occur in the ipsilateral hemisphere at sites remote from the IVH (77). The latter is thought to reflect the severity of hypoperfusion prior to the hemorrhage or the consequence of posthemorrhagic spasm.

In our experience the CT scan is not a reliable predictor of long-term prognosis, particularly with the milder degrees of IVH. The EEG, which reflects more clearly the severity of cortical dysfunction, is highly correlated with neurological outcome and is invaluable in assessing the child receiving neuromuscular paralyzing agents (71). The neurological exam is of no value in these latter infants and transportation to a radiological facility is logistically difficult. Unfortunately, EEGs are usually of short duration, done infrequently and randomly, and often miss the peak severity of the HIE.

PVL occurs most commonly in premature infants (65), though some authors have been impressed by its predilection for somewhat older infants (39). In the former study it was noted that PVL was more likely to be seen at autopsy in infants who had survived more than 6 days, suggesting an evolution of the process from the initial perinatal asphyxic episode. Ultrasound studies have also clearly shown the evolution of PVL over the first weeks of life (4). Echogenic foci appear at the external angle of the lateral ventricles during the first week of life. The echo intensity may then disappear by 2 to 4 weeks of age or evolve into hypoechoic cystic lesions which are most striking at the level of the trigone of the lateral ventricles and commonly associated with long-term sequelae. Echodense periventricular lesions, called intraparenchymal echodensity (IPE) by McMenamin et al. (43), were seen in 36% of premature infants with IVH. These authors considered the pathological substrate of these lesions to be unresolved but suggested that they may represent hemorrhagic infarctions in the periventricular white matter. Infants with large IPE had a higher mortality and morbidity than those with small or absent IPE. Ultrasonography is helpful in identifying these lesions and is more accurate than conventional CT scans. A recent autopsy study (68), however, revealed that cerebral ultrasound identified only 63% of PVL lesions (as compared to a 92% accuracy in IVH).

Until recently it was thought that the EEG abnormalities seen in PVL were nonspecific. Recent observations by R. Coen and R. Bejar (*personal communication*) and ourselves (E. Novotny and B. Tharp, *unpublished observations*) have revealed an apparently high correlation between PVL and positive rolandic sharp waves, a distinctive EEG abnormality previously described by us in 30% of infants with IVH (9). We are now investigating the possibility that these latter infants may correspond to those with IVH and IPE described by McMenamin et al. (43).

There are many metabolic, toxic, infectious, and developmental conditions which occur in the neonate, are associated with compromised CNS function and abnormal EEGs, and are followed by neurological sequelae. Seizures are frequent in this population. In some cases, i.e., herpes encephalitis (48) and CNS malformations (13,22), characteristic EEG patterns have been described. In the majority, the EEG changes are nonspecific. The interested reader is referred to more thorough reviews of neonatal EEG for descriptions of the various EEG abnormalities encountered in the neonatal age group (41,70).

The ultimate goal of monitoring of the asphyxiated newborn will be to continuously assess the state of cerebral function and, as now occurs with fluctuations in blood pressure and O_2, alert the staff when an unacceptable level of dysfunction occurs. A monitoring unit should perform its task automatically, unencumbered by the ink and paper problems of conventional EEG, and with an acceptable number of falsely identified patterns or missed data. Unfortunately, at the present time the state of neonatal EEG is such that the range of normal EEG patterns, particularly for small premature infants, is not established. We also do not know which EEG patterns or background abnormalities are the most sensitive indicators of asphyxia and altered cerebral perfusion.

Over the past several years we have approached this issue by recording conventional EEGs on a group of prematures with uncomplicated neonatal courses. These "normal" infants were neurologically intact and had normal ultrasound or CT studies. All infants had some degree of hyaline membrane disease and some required brief periods of assisted ventilation. None were considered to have been significantly hypoxemic. They are seen in follow-up at 1 and 2 years of age.

Among the many EEG patterns being analyzed we have selected the interburst intervals (IBI) for quantification and application to long-term monitoring. We have chosen the IBI because it is easily measured and undergoes progressive lengthening as the asphyxiated premature infant deteriorates. The prolongation of the IBI occurs at a time when the transients expected for the conceptional age (brushes, temporal theta, and occipital theta) are still present during bursts.

An IBI is defined as a period during which there is no EEG activity $> 15\ \mu V$ in all or only one channel of a routine 16-channel EEG at sensitivity $7\ \mu V/mm$ and LLF of 0.3 sec. We allow activity in one channel because we have found that it is quite common for background delta rhythms to persist in one occipital region or the central parasagittal area at a time when the rest of the tracing is extremely low voltage. The IBI for the entire tracing, regardless of sleep state, are measured by hand and the mean, median, and longest interval calculated. Fig. 1 illustrates the mean IBI intervals of the first 12 "normal" infants studied. The gestational ages ranged from 25 to 30 weeks; some infants had several tracings during the neonatal period. All were healthy at a 1-year follow-up except one infant who died at 4 months of age from bronchopulmonary dysplasia. This latter infant had one EEG early in life at a time when blood gases were normal. Infants 13 and 14 had severe perinatal asphyxia and are in-

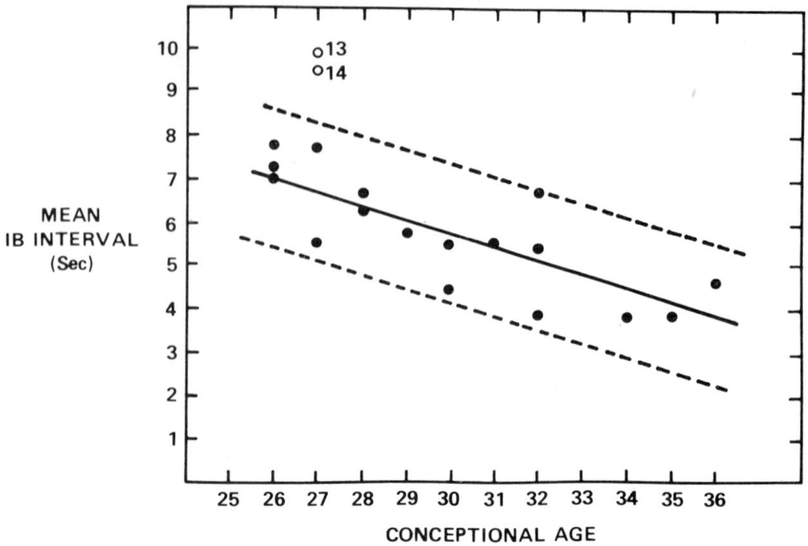

FIG. 1. Mean interburst intervals (*solid line*) in routine EGGs (30–60-min duration) recorded on 12 newborns without evidence of encephalopathy and normal at follow-up. Several infants had more than one tracing. Patients 13 and 14 had severe hypoxic-ischemic encephalopathy. *Dotted lines:* 2 standard deviations from mean.

cluded to illustrate the deviation of the IBI from normal in HIE, and thus the utility of this measurement. We anticipate adding more infants to the study even though the slope of the fitted curve is already statistically significant ($p < 0.001$).

We have just started long-term monitoring of critically ill infants. Figure 2 illustrates the EEG of a 29-week conceptional age (CA) infant with severe hyaline membrane disease and pulmonary hypertension. In addition to the EEG, transcutaneous po_2, central venous pressure, mean arterial pressure, ECG, and respirations were recorded. Figure 3 shows the results of serial IBI measurements (mean IBI/5 min) and the mean $tcpo_2$/5 min. It appears that the initial hypoxemia resulted in a gradual increase of IBI above the accepted norm for age. When the child's ventilation and cerebral perfusion were improved by a change in ventilator settings and IV albumin, the $tcpo_2$ improved and the mean IBI decreased.

These preliminary studies are presented to illustrate one approach to continuous monitoring of cerebral function in neonates. Other EEG parameters may ultimately prove more useful for measurement such as compressed spectral array techniques and pattern recognition programs for significant transients such as positive rolandic sharp waves, but, for the moment, IBI measurements appear to provide a useful measure of CNS function that could easily be adapted to automated systems.

From this brief discussion of the major neurological syndromes of the neonatal period it is apparent that they are associated with multisystem disease

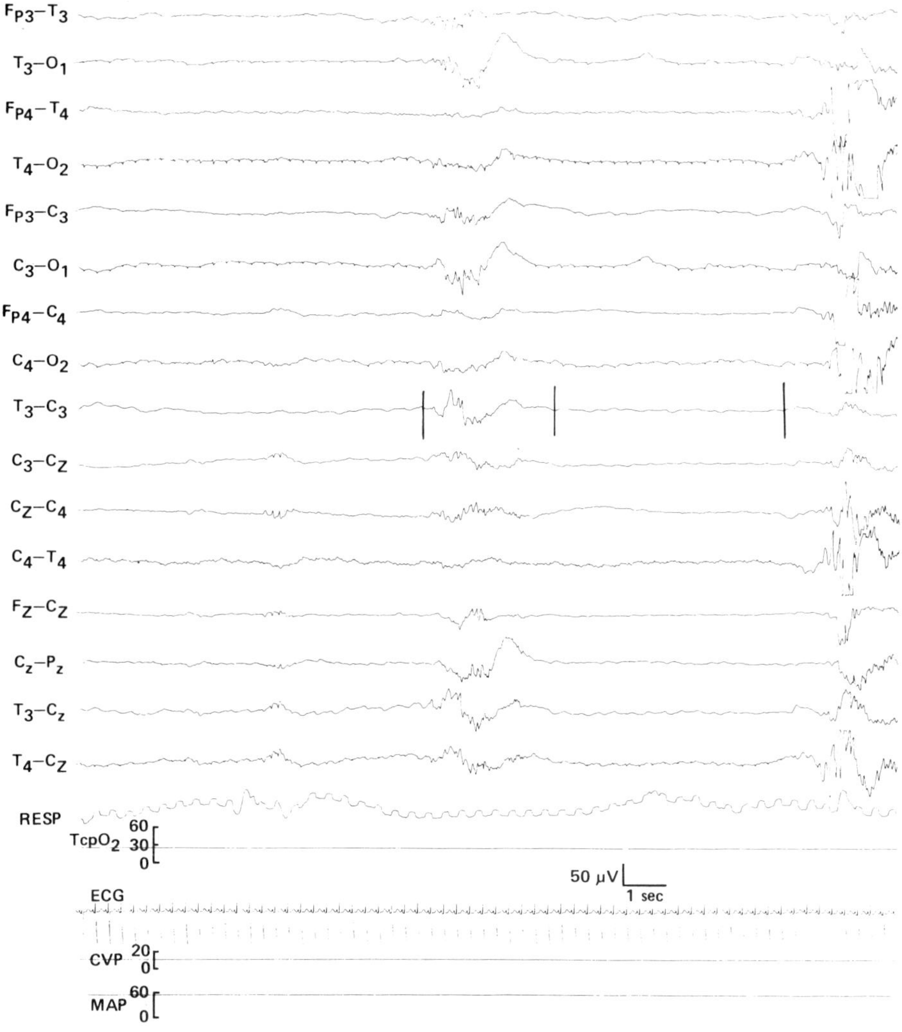

FIG. 2. Twenty-second segment of EEG of premature infant with moderately severe hypoxic-ischemic encephalopathy and pulmonary hypertension. EEG discontinuous; *vertical lines* indicate boundaries of 2 IBI; first began on previous page. Resp, respirations (piezo crystal); $Tcpo_2$, transcutaneous po_2; ECG, electrocardiogram; CVP, central venous pressure; MAP, mean arterial pressure, umbilical artery line.

and are often progressive. The initial perinatal asphyxic insult is often compounded by altered cerebral perfusion from fluctuations in systemic blood pressure and increased blood viscosity, persistent hypoxemia from chronic lung disease (16), increased intracranial pressure secondary to cerebral edema, hydrocephalus, acute pulmonary deterioration due to pneumothoraces, and sepsis, to name but a few.

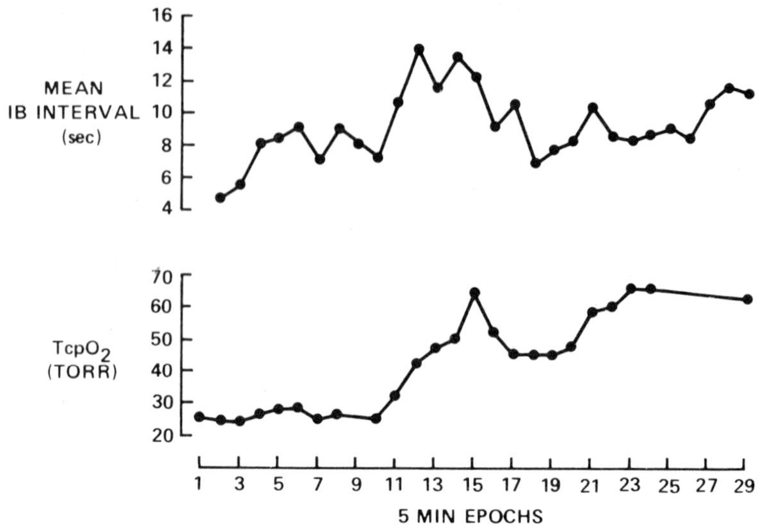

FIG. 3. Same infant as in Fig. 2. Mean IBI/5 min plotted in *upper tracing*. Mean $tcpo_2$/5 min plotted in *lower tracing*. Total duration of recording 145 min (twenty-nine 5-min epochs plotted).

SEIZURES

The incidence of seizures in the neonate has been reported to be from 1.5/1,000 (20) to 14/1,000 (5). In the large National Collaborative Perinatal Project the incidence was 5/1,000 (30). In an analysis of seizure incidence on a month-to-month basis throughout infancy, Kellaway and Hrachovy (37) reported that 80% of infants had the onset of seizures during the first 2 months of life and, of these, 85% occurred within 2 weeks of birth. The analysis of the data from the NCPP confirmed the peak incidence of infantile seizure onset in the first month of life, and in addition showed that 20% of infants with neonatal seizures had one or more nonfebrile seizures later in life, 75% of which occurred within the first year (17).

It should be emphasized that the majority of studies of neonatal seizures lack the EEG confirmation that the events are indeed cerebral in origin. It has recently been shown by Kellaway and Hrachovy (37), Mizrahi and Kellaway (47), and Shewmon (62) that many of the abnormal movements noted in critically ill newborns that resemble seizures are not associated with electrographic seizures and probably represent "brainstem release" phenomena. Abnormal behavior referred to in earlier publications as subtle seizures, myoclonus, and generalized tonic seizures were often not accompanied by cerebral seizure discharges in these recent studies, even though the EEG background was abnormal and reflected cortical depression from the severe encephalopathy. These studies have dramatically altered our thinking about the clinical spectrum of neonatal seizures. Clonic, focal tonic, and various types of shifting or multifocal clonic events with eye deviation and buccal automatisms are often seizures but should be verified electrographically in future studies before excepting them as cerebral seizures (P. Kellaway, *this volume*). It is obvious that any study of neonatal seizures must be suspect if clinical description alone is relied upon to make the diagnosis.

Seizures can accompany any of the neurologic conditions discussed in the previous section. In addition, transient metabolic disturbances such as hypocalcemia and hypoglycemia may provoke seizures which are often clonic in type. Advances in neonatal medicine over the last two decades have virtually eliminated these latter seizures which, for the most part, had benign outcomes. Seizures due to more serious encephalopathies, particularly those secondary to asphyxia, hemorrhage, and infection, are now predominant. They are more difficult to treat, require large doses of potentially toxic anticonvulsant drugs, and are associated with poor long-term outcomes.

If seizures complicate HIE, the mortality is higher and long-term prognosis poorer than in asphyxiated infants without seizures (71). Outcome is also related to the gestational age; premature infants with seizures fare less well than term infants (40). The explanation for the poorer outcome of infants with seizures is multifactorial. It is generally thought that the encephalopathy is worse in these infants and that the seizures are merely a reflection of the severity of cerebral dysfunction. On the other hand, there is very convincing evidence in the experimental animal literature that seizures, per se, cause pathological alterations that cannot be explained solely on the basis of the hypoxemia and systemic acidosis secondary to increased motor activity (44,78). Recent nuclear magnetic resonance studies of bicuculline-induced seizures in paralyzed and ventilated neonatal dogs showed a significant reduction in brain phosphocreatine as a percentage of total mobile phosphates and a decline of intracellular brain pH due, at least partially, to a local accumulation of lactic acid (82). It must be assumed that similar changes are occurring in the human neonate with status and lead to additional nerve cell loss beyond that due to the asphyxia, per se. In addition, seizures are known to increase cerebral blood flow in adults (25) and infants (56), raise intracranial pressure, cause systemic hyper- or hypotension (26), elevate or lower po_2 (49,70,71), and cause tachyarrhythmias, tachycardia (26,71), and apnea in neonates. When considered in the context of the previous discussion of the pathophysiology of HIE and PVL, it is obvious that repeated seizures will most likely extend the asphyxic encephalopathy by further compromising cerebral perfusion and neuronal metabolism and altering systemic hemodynamics in ways that promote intracranial hemorrhage and worsen cerebral edema.

The EEG is a valuable tool in the assessment of cerebral function in neonates with abnormal behavior and those immobilized by neuromuscular blocking agents. The EEG patterns associated with seizures have been well described. There is much less information on what connotes a truly interictal or pre-ictal record, e.g., what EEG patterns or transients are highly correlated with neonatal seizures and, if seen in a nonseizing infant, should alert the electroencephalographer that seizures are imminent or that the abnormal behavior in question is very likely due to cerebral seizures?

Spikes-and-sharp waves occur frequently in the EEGs of infants with normal outcomes (50). Karbowski and Nencka (36) found that the right midtemporal region was the preferential location for these normal transients. Clancy (7) and Clancy and Spitzer (8) also reported that sharp transients (mono-, di- or polyphasic sharply contoured waves, less than 300 to 500 msec, and clearly distinguishable from the background activity) were abundant in the temporal regions, but that they were equally distributed in both hemispheres.

Several recent studies have described the characteristics of transients which are more commonly seen in infants with seizures. Hughes et al. (34) found that "burnt-out" sharp waves ("blunted in form, low in voltage, repetitive but slow in frequency and at times dicrotic in morphology") and positive sharp waves (central and temporal) were frequently associated with seizures. Eighty percent and 75%, respectively, of infants whose EEGs contained these transients had seizures. This study unfortunately relied on a clinical diagnosis of seizures. Positive sharp waves in the central areas (PRS) are often seen in premature infants with IVH and PVL. In our experience there is a negative correlation between PRS and electrographic seizures (9). It is possible that the incidence of seizures in the study of Hughes et al. is inflated by the inclusion of premature infants with tonic posturing and other types of abnormal motor activity, which are particularly common in prematures with IVH and usually not accompanied by electrographic seizure activity (37,47).

Shewmon (61), using long-term video/EEG monitoring techniques, has recently described rhythmic stereotyped and repetitive waveforms in neonates with seizures. These events were brief (one-half to several seconds) and in several cases were noted to evolve over time into electrographic seizures.

These studies represent the first steps towards the development of a classification of EEG patterns and transients which are truly "epileptiform," i.e., highly correlated with neonatal seizures. Such a classification will be necessary before investigators can embark on studies of the prophylactic value of anticonvulsant drugs in the neonatal period (66). In order to identify infants at risk for the development of seizures in the first few days of life for inclusion in such studies, EEG patterns highly predictive of seizures must be discovered by continuous EEG monitoring. In addition, the identification of "epileptiform" transients will enhance the value of brief random EEGs. Many nurseries do not have long-term EEG monitoring capabilities and must rely on routine clinical recordings in the investigation of infants with questionable seizures. All too often the seizures do not occur during the tracing and the electroencephalographer is confronted with the question: "Does this EEG contain patterns consistent with an interictal tracing?" The development of a classification of potentially epileptiform discharges by long-term monitoring studies will provide the answer to this important and frequently asked clinical question.

Video monitoring of newborns will be a necessary complement to the EEG in the development of a neonatal seizure classification. Ictal EEG patterns are relatively few in type and have only a rough correlation with clinical behavior (41,79,80). A clinically useful classification must be oriented towards infant behavior, particularly if it is to be used by neonatologists and neurologists lacking access to continuous EEG and polygraphic monitoring. Video surveillance will also be helpful when monitoring asphyxiated, nonseizing infants. These infants are handled frequently and a variety of EEG artifacts are produced (69). We have found that visual observation of the patient by a technologist or physician, or storage of infant behavior on videotape is necessary when trying to decipher the source of unusual patterns encountered during off-line review. Mizrahi has recently described a portable video/polygraphic system which meets some of these criteria (46). More compact and unobtrusive systems will probably be needed before monitoring becomes a readily acceptable technique in busy and often crowded neonatal ICUs.

SELECTION OF INFANTS FOR VIDEO/EEG MONITORING

Ideally, monitoring for clinical and research purposes should commence as soon as possible following birth if it is to be of value for the prediction of seizures, and as a guide to the management of the asphyxiated infant. Criteria for patient selection have not been established. Obviously the severely asphyxiated infant, identified by low Apgar scores, the need for assisted respiration, and the presence of profound hypotonia and coma is a candidate because of the high risk for seizures, increased intracranial pressure, intracerebral hemorrhage, and progressive encephalopathy. The selection criteria for less severely affected infants is more problematic. It is known that Apgar scores, blood gas and pH measurments in cord blood or infant blood obtained immediately postpartum, and the obstetrical history have relatively little value in predicting the severity of the subsequent perinatal encephalopathy in the individual child (53,54,71, 73). I do not intend to ignore the well-known fact that many perinatal events, when studied in large populations of infants, can be statistically correlated with outcome (52,53), but to emphasize what was discussed earlier, i.e., some infants who appear moderately to markedly compromised in the first few hours of life may have totally benign courses.

It has also been shown that infants requiring iatrogenic paralysis are at risk to develop HIE, PVL, and hemorrhage, which are often followed by seizures (11,21,26,66,71). Studies using routine random and more continuous EEG polygraphic recordings have yielded a high incidence of clinically unsuspected seizures and other EEG abnormalities in this selected population (Fig. 4).

Until more specific criteria are developed it would seem prudent to monitor

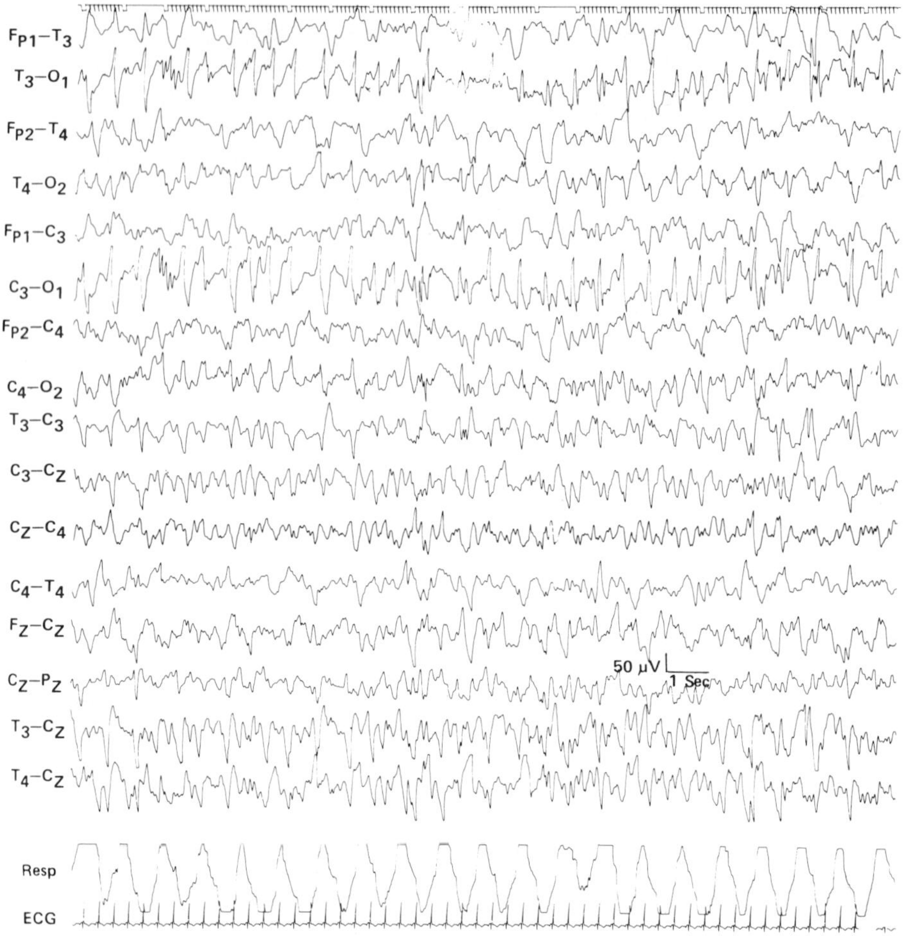

FIG. 4. Full-term newborn with mild asphyxic encephalopathy paralyzed with pavulon. Focal seizure in left occipital region. Background EEG was only moderately abnormal and child was normal at 1-year follow-up.

all severely asphyxiated infants (Apgar at 5 min. $\lesssim 3$, persistent hypotonia, coma, and need for assisted ventilation), those requiring muscle relaxant drugs, and those manifesting intermittent abnormal behavior which might be seizures, including unexplained autonomic symptoms (flushing, hypertension, acute fluctuations of serum or transcutaneous blood gases, and tachycardia). Infants with deteriorating neurological status, CNS infections, very unstable cardiovascular function, and evidence of IVH and PVL on ultrasound studies should be considered for continuous, or at least intermittent, monitoring.

Monitoring should ideally include, in addition to the EEG, other physiologic functions including respiration, ECG, and heart-rate variability, po_2, pco_2, mean arterial blood pressure, and, if indicated, intracranial pressure (subarachnoid bolt or a transfontanelle pressure transducer), esophageal pH, temperature, and other pulmonary functions (see ref. 31 for details of infant monitoring for apnea, gastroesophageal reflux, and other disorders not discussed in this chapter). The interested reader should refer to recent reviews for the technical details of recording the EEG (41,68,70) and other physiologic functions in this age group (32).

Continuous video/EEG monitoring is of proven value in the detection of neonatal seizures and the investigation of neonatal apnea. We still know very little about the value of continuous EEG in the assessment of the critically ill neonate. It is hoped future studies will provide data for the establishment of clinical criteria for selection of infants for monitoring and give us a better understanding of the contribution of postnatal events including seizures and cardiovascular fluctuations to the severity of neonatal encephalopathy and the long-term neurological outcome.

TECHNICAL CONSIDERATIONS

Continuous long-term polygraphic monitoring of critically ill newborns presents many logistical and technical problems. Experience with this procedure is still limited and standardization of the technical aspects of long-term recording is not yet practical. The following discussion reflects the techniques being used at our medical center, in addition to published and unpublished input from colleagues involved in similar work elsewhere.

In most intensive care nurseries, continuous monitoring of blood pressure, pulse, respirations and transcutaneous po_2 are performed routinely. Additionally, transcutaneous pco_2, intracranial pressure via a subarachnoid bolt or a transfontanelle pressure transducer, central venous pressure, and esophageal pH may also be recorded. The EEG/polygraphic machine must, therefore, be relatively unobtrusive if it is to join this myriad of equipment which occupies the limited space around the isolette.

A standard EEG machine can be placed next to the isolette. Cables can be connected to the other monitoring equipment and provide a continuous printout of mean blood pressure, $tcpo_2$, and central venous pressure on the EEG paper using the available AC amplifiers. Alternatively, one can use a less obtrusive recording system which digitizes and multiplexes the polygraphic data and records onto a 6-hr videocassette with a standard commercial recorder (see ref. 60 for more details of this system). This compact unit does not require paper printout and, therefore, avoids all the problems of a pen-and-ink system. A digital time code generator has recently been added to the system and a television camera and VHS recorder will be interfaced in the near future. The data may be reviewed on a screen with variable gains and time scale and all or portions of the data printed out on paper at a later time using a standard EEG machine.

The addition of the closed-circuit television system is crucial, particularly if one wishes to rely on nursing staff observations during segments of the recording. It is not practical to have a qualified EEG technologist at the infant's bedside for the entire 24- to 48-hr recording. Artifacts generated by handling, suction, etc. will appear on the video cassette tape printout of the polygraphic data and can be verified by review of the time-synchronized video recording of the infant's behavior. Additionally, infant behavior during seizures can be reviewed in detail at a later time and stored indefinitely for future research or clinical recall.

The system can be activated by the technologist. When he/she is satisfied that the equipment and electrodes are functioning satisfactorily, subsequent observation can be performed by the infant's nurse or other responsible nursery personnel. Periodic electrode checks can be made by the technologist during regular working hours and when needed during the night by on-call laboratory personnel. A detailed log should be kept by the infant's nurse to include staff interventions, such as drug administration, changes in respirator settings, unusual behavior, results of blood gases (with concomitant $tcpo_2$ and $tcpco_2$ recordings), infant's position in the isolette, comments on technical maneuvers such as calibrating of equipment, and attachment of new electrodes. When the nursery personnel becomes familiar with EEG patterns, major changes in the EEG background can be noted in the log by the nursery personnel. A microphone should be placed near the infant to record infant sounds as well as the voice of the nurse who can "dictate" comments onto the videotape.

Recording systems will obviously vary according to the problem at hand and the limitations and demands of the neonatal nursery. The system just described is primarily used when studying EEG background changes in relation to hemodynamic and respiratory fluctuations. Mizrahi and colleagues have developed a system using a standard EEG machine to study neonatal seizures (46). Those interested in infant behavior during sleep have used still different recording systems (31,32).

A major technical limitation of any recording system is the scalp electrode. We have relied on electrodes attached with standard EEG paste, particularly in premature infants. We are reluctant to keep electrodes attached for more than 24 hr because of the risk of skin breakdown. If the recording is to continue for longer periods, the electrodes are removed, the skin inspected, and the electrodes symmetrically reattached immediately adjacent to the original recording site. Some laboratories rely on collodion attachment and have noted few skin problems, at least in term babies recorded for up to 24 hr. Studies using a variety of electrode attachment materials are needed to better define the ideal method for infants of different conceptional ages.

Future developments will include more automated systems using on-line computers to monitor the EEG for changes due to compromised cerebral perfusion and oxygen supply, identify interictal transients which are predictive of imminent seizures, follow the effect of therapy on subclinical seizures, and to identify seizures occurring in iatrogenically paralyzed infants.

ACKNOWLEDGMENT

This review was supported in part by a Premature Research Center grant RR-00081.

REFERENCES

1. Ahmann, P, Dykes, F., Lazzara, A., Holt, P., Giddens, D., and Carrigan, T. (1983): Relationship between pressure passivity and subependymal/intraventricular hemorrhage as assessed by pulsed Doppler ultrasound. *Pediatrics*, 72:665–669.
2. Ahmann, P., Lazzara, A., Dykes, F., Brann, A., and Schwartz, J. (1980): Intraventricular hemorrhage in the high-risk preterm infant: incidence and outcome. *Ann. Neurol.*, 7:118–124.
3. Alberman, E., Benson, J., and McDonald, A. (1982): Cerebral palsy and severe educational subnormality in low-birthweight children: A comparison of births in 1951–53 and 1970–73. *Lancet*, 1:606–608.
4. Bowerman, R., Donn, S., DiPietro, M., D'Amato, C., and Hicks, S. (1984): Periventricular leukomalacia in the pre-term newborn infant: Sonographic and clinical features. *Radiology*, 151:383–388.
5. Brown, J., Cockburn, F., and Forfar, J. (1972): Clinical and chemical correlates in convulsions of the newborn. *Lancet*, 1:135–139.
6. Brown, J., Purvis, R., Forfar, J., and Cockburn, F. (1974): Neurological aspects of perinatal asphyxia. *Dev. Med. Child Neurol.*, 16:567–580.
7. Clancy, R. (1984): Sharp electroencephalographic transients in neonates with seizures. *Ann. Neurol.*, 14:377.
8. Clancy, R., and Spitzer, A. (1984): Cerebral cortical function in infants at risk for sudden infant death syndrome. *Ann. Neurol.*, 16:396.
9. Clancy, R., and Tharp, B. (1984): Positive rolandic sharp waves in the electroencephalograms of premature neonates with intraventricular hemorrhage. *EEG Clin. Neurophysiol.*, 57:395–404.
10. Clancy, R., Tharp, B., and Enzman, D. (1984): EEG in premature infants with intraventricular hemorrhage. *Neurology*, 34:583–590.
11. Coen, R., McCutchen, C., Wermer, D, Snyder, J., and Gluck, F. (1982): Continuous monitoring of the electroencephalogram following perinatal asphyxia. *J. Pediatr.*, 100:628–630.
12. Cohen, R., Stevenson, D., Malachowski, N., Ariagno, R., Kimble, K., Hopper, A., Johnson, J., Ueland, K., and Sunshine, P. (1982): Favorable results of neonatal intensive care for very low-birth-weight infants. *Pediatrics*, 69:621–625.
13. DeMyer, W., and White, P. (1964): EEG in Holoprosencephaly (Arhinencephaly). *Arch. Neurol.*, 11:507–520.
14. DeSouza, S., and Richards, B. (1978): Neurological sequelae in newborn babies after perinatal asphyxia. *Arch. Dis. Child.*, 53:564–569.
15. Driscoll, J., Driscoll, Y., Steir, M., Stark, R., Dengman, B., Perez, A., Wung, J., and Kritz, P. (1982): Mortality and morbidity in infants less than 1,001 grams birthweight. *Pediatrics*, 69:21–26.
16. Ellison, P., and Farnia, M. (1980): Progressive central nervous system deterioration: A complication of advanced chronic lung disease of prematurity. *Ann. Neurol.*, 8:43–46.
17. Ellenberg, J., Hirtz, D., and Nelson, K. (1984): Age at onset of seizures in young children. *Ann. Neurol.*, 15:127–134.
18. Ellenberg, J., and Nelson, K. (1979): Birthweight and gestational age of children with cerebral palsy or seizure disorders. *Am. J. Dis. Child.*, 133:1044–1048.
19. Ellison, P., Prasse, D., Siewart, J., and Browning, A. (1984): Behavioral outcomes in children from the neonatal intensive care unit. *Ann. Neurol.*, 16:389.
20. Eriksson, M., and Zetterstrom, R. (1979): Neonatal convulsions. Incidence and causes in the Stockholm area. *Acta Paediatr. Scand.*, 68:807–811.
21. Eyre, J., Oozeer, R., and Wilkinson, A. (1983): Continuous electroencephalographic recording to detect seizures in paralyzed newborn babes. *Br. Med. J.*, 286:1017–1018.

22. Fariello, R., Chun, R., Doro, R., Buncic, J., and Prichard, J. (1977): EEG recognition of Aircardi's syndrome. *Arch. Neurol.*, 34:563–566.
23. Fenichel, G. (1983): Hypoxic-ischemic encephalopathy in the newborn. *Arch. Neurol.*, 40:261–266.
24. Finer, N., Robertson, C., Richards, R., Pinnell, L., and Peters, K. (1981): Hypoxic-ischemic encephalopathy in term neonates: Perinatal factors and outcome. *J. Pediatr.*, 98:112–117.
25. Gabor, A., Brooks, A., Scobey, R., and Parsons, G. (1984): Intracranial pressure during epileptic seizures. *EEG Clin. Neurophysiol.*, 57:497–506.
26. Goldberg, R., Goldman, S., Ramsey, R., and Feller, R. (1982): Detection of seizure activity in the paralyzed neonate using continuous monitoring. *Pediatrics*, 69:583–586.
27. Hagberg, B. (1971): Epidemiological and preventive aspects of cerebral palsy and severe mental retardation in Sweden. *Eur. J. Pediatr.*, 130:71–78.
28. Hill, A., and Volpe, J. (1981): Normal pressure hydrocephalus in the newborn. *Pediatrics*, 68:623–629.
29. Hill, A., and Volpe, J. (1981): Seizures, hypoxic-ischemic brain injury and intraventricular hemorrhage in the newborn. *Ann. Neurol.*, 10:109–121.
30. Holden, K., Mellits, E., and Freeman, J. (1982): Neonatal seizurs. 1. Correlation of prenatal and perinatal events with outcomes. *Pediatrics*, 70:165–176.
31. Hoppenbrouwers, T. (1982): Electronic monitoring in the newborn and young infant: Theoretical considerations. In: *Sleeping and Waking Disorders. Indications and Techniques*, edited by C. Guilleminault, pp. 17–59. Addison-Wesley, Menlo Park.
32. Hoppenbrouwers, T., Geidel, S., Ruiz, M., and Judson, L. (1982): Electronic monitoring in the newborn and young infant: Technical guidelines. In: *Sleeping and Waking Disorders. Indications and Techniques*, edited by C. Guilleminault, pp. 61–98. Addison-Wesley, Menlo Park.
33. Horwood, S., Boyle, M., Torrance, G., and Sinclair, J. (1982): Mortality and morbidity of 500 to 1,499 gram birthweight infants live-born to residents of a defined geographic region before and after neonatal intensive care. *Pediatrics*, 69:613–620.
34. Hughes, J., Fino, J., and Gagnon, L. (1983): The use of the electroencephalogram in the confirmation of seizures in premature and neonatal infants. *Neuropediatrics*, 14:213–219.
35. Janowsky, J., and Nass, R. (1984): Early language development in children with cortical and subcortical perinatal injury. *Ann. Neurol.*, 16:387.
36. Karbowski, K., and Nencka, A. (1980): Right mid-temporal sharp EEG transients in healthy newborns. *EEG Clin. Neurophysiol.*, 48:461–469.
37. Kellaway, P., and Hrachovy, R. (1983): Status epilepticus in newborns: A perspective on neonatal seizures. In: *Advances in Neurology, Vol. 34: Status Epilepticus*, edited by A. Delgado-Escueta, C. Wasterlain, D. Treiman, and P. Porter, pp. 93–99. Raven Press, New York.
38. Knobloch, H., Malone, A., Ellison, P., Stevens, F., and Zdeb, M. (1982): Considerations in evaluating changes in outcome for infants weighing less than 1501 grams. *Pediatrics*, 69:285–295.
39. Leviton, A., and Gilles, F. (1984): Acquired perinatal leukoencephalopathy. *Ann. Neurol.*, 16:1–8.
40. Lombroso, C. (1979): Convulsive disorders in newborns. In: *Pediatric Neurology and Neurosurgery*, edited by R. Thompson and J. Green, pp. 205–239. Spectrum, New York.
41. Lombroso, C. (1982): Neonatal electroencephalography. In: *Electroencephalography. Basic Principles, Clinical Applications and Related Fields*, edited by E. Niedermeyer and F. Lopes da Silva, pp. 599–637. Urban and Schwarzenberg, Baltimore.
42. Lou, H., Lassen, N., and Friis-Hansen, B. (1979): Impaired autoregulation of cerebral blood flow in the distressed newborn infant. *J. Pediatr.*, 94:118–121.
43. McMenamin, J., Shackelford, G., and Volpe, J. (1984): Outcome of neonatal hemorrhage with periventricular echodense lesions. *Ann. Neurol.*, 15:285–290.
44. Meldrum, B. (1983): Metabolic factors during prolonged seizures and their relation to nerve cell death. In: *Advances in Neurology, Vol. 34: Status Epilepticus*, edited by A. Delgato-Escueta, C. Wasterlain, D. Treiman, and R. Porter, pp. 261–275. Raven Press, New York.
45. Ment, L., Ehrenkranz, R., Lange, R., Rothstein, P., and Duncan, C. (1981): Alterations

in cerebral blood flow in premature infants with intracranial hemorrhage. *Pediatrics*, 68:763–769.
46. Mizrahi, E. (1984): Electroencephalographic/polygraphic/video monitoring in childhood epilepsy. *J. Pediatr.*, 105:1–9.
47. Mizrahi, E., and Kellaway, P. (1984): Characterization of seizures in neonates and young infants by time-synchronized electroencephalographic/polygraphic/video monitoring. *Ann. Neurol.*, 16:383.
48. Mizrahi, E., and Tharp, B. (1982): A characteristic EEG pattern in neonatal herpes simplex encephalitis. *Neurology*, 32:1215–1220.
49. Monin, P., Vert, P., Andre, M., and Vibert, M. (1979): Transcutaneous Po_2 monitoring in the newborn during apneic spells, convulsions, cardiac catheterizations and exchange transfusions. *Birth Defects*, 15:469–491.
50. Monod, N., Pajot, N., and Guidasci, S. (1972): The neonatal EEG: Statistical studies and prognostic value in full-term and pre-term babies. *EEG Clin. Neurophysiol.*, 32:529–544.
51. National Center for Health Statistics, (Sept. 29, 1981) *Monthly Vital Statistics Report*, Vol. 30, No. 6, Suppl. (2).
52. Nelson, K., and Ellenberg, J. (1979): Neonatal signs as predictors of cerebral palsy. *Pediatrics*, 64:225–232.
53. Nelson, K., and Ellenberg, J. (1981): Apgar scores as predictors of chronic neurologic disability. *Pediatrics*, 68:36–44.
54. Nelson, K., and Ellenberg, J. (1984): Obstetric complications as risk factors for cerebral palsy or seizure disorders. *JAMA*, 251:1843–1848.
55. Perlman, J., McMenamin, J., and Volpe, J. (1983): Fluctuating cerebral blood-flow velocity in respiratory-distress syndrome. *N. Engl. J. Med.*, 309:204–209.
56. Perlman, J., and Volpe, J. (1983): Seizures in the preterm infant: Effects on cerebral blood flow velocity, intracranial pressure, and arterial blood pressure. *J. Pediatr.*, 102:288–293.
57. Pharoah, P., and Alberman, E. (1981): Mortality of low birthweight in England and Wales 1953 to 1979. *Arch. Dis. Child.*, 56:86–89.
58. Rothberg, A., Maisels, M., Bagnato, S., Murphy, J., Gifford, K., and McKinley, K. (1983): Infants weighing 1,000 grams or less at birth: Developmental outcome for ventilated and nonventilated infants. *Pediatrics*, 71:599–602.
59. Sarnat, H., and Sarnat, M. (1976): Neonatal encephalopathy following fetal distress. *Arch. Neurol.*, 33:696–705.
60. Shewmon, A., and Krentler, K. (1984): Off-line montage reformatting. *EEG Clin. Neurophysiol.*, 57:591–595.
61. Shewmon, D. (1983): Brief interictal rhythmic discharges in newborns. *EEG Clin. Neurophysiol.*, 56:24P.
62. Shewmon, D. (1983): Dissociation between cortical discharges and fetal movements in neonatal seizures. *Ann. Neurol.*, 14:368.
63. Shields, W., and Feldman, R. (1982): Serum CK-BB isoenzyme in preterm infants with periventricular hemorrhage. *J. Pediatr.*, 100:464–486.
64. Shinnar, S., Molteni, R., Gammon, K., D'Souza, B., Altman, J., and Freeman, J. (1982): Intraventricular hemorrhage in the premature infant. *N. Engl. J. Med.*, 306:1464–1468.
65. Shuman, R., and Selednik, L. (1980): Periventricular leukomalacia. *Arch. Neurol.*, 37:231–235.
66. Staudt, F., Roth, J., and Engel, R. (1981): The usefulness of electroencephalography in curarized newborns. *EEG Clin. Neurophysiol.*, 51:205–208.
67. Svenningsen, N., Blennow, G., Lindroth, M., Gaddlin, P., and Ahlstrom, H. (1982): Brain-oriented intensive care treatment in severe neonatal asphyxia. *Arch. Dis. Child.*, 57:176–183.
68. Szymonowicz, W., Schafler, K., Cussen, L., and Yu, V. (1984): Ultrasound and necropsy study of periventricular hemorrhage in preterm infants. *Arch. Dis. Child.*, 59:637–642.
69. Tharp. B. (1980): Neonatal and pediatric electroencephalography. In: *Electrodiagnosis in Clinical Neurology*, edited by M. Aminoff, pp. 67–117. Churchill Livingstone, New York.
70. Tharp, B. (1981): Neonatal electroencephalography. In: *Progress in Perinatal Neurology, Vol. I*, edited by R. Korobkin and C. Guilleminault, pp. 31–64. Williams & Wilkins, Baltimore.

71. Tharp. B., and Laboyrie, P. (1983): The incidence of EEG abnormalities and outcome of infants paralyzed with neuromuscular blocking agents. *Crit. Care Med.*, 11:926–929.
72. Thomson, A., Searle, M., and Russell, G. (1977): Quality of survival after severe birth asphyxia. *Arch. Dis. Child.*, 52:620–626.
73. Tooley, W., Phibbs, R., and Schlueter, M. (1977): Delivery room diagnosis and immediate management of asphyxia. In: *Intrauterine Asphyxia and the Developing Fetal Brain*, edited by L. Gluck, pp. 251–261. Year Book, Chicago.
74. Volpe, J. (1977): Observing the infant in the early hours after asphyxia. In: *Intrauterine Asphyxia and the Developing Fetal Brain*, edited by L. Gluck, pp. 263–283. Year Book, Chicago.
75. Volpe, J. (1979): Intracranial hemorrhage in the newborn: Current understanding and dilemmas. *Neurology*, 29:632–635.
76. Volpe, J. (1981): *Neurology of the Newborn.* Saunders, Philadelphia.
77. Volpe, J., Herscovitch, P., Perlman, J., and Raichle, M. (1983): Positron emission tomography in the newborn: Extensive impairment of regional cerebral blood flow with intraventricular hemorrhage and hemorrhagic intracerebral involvement. *Pediatrics*, 72:589–601.
78. Wasterlain, C., and Dwyer, B. (1983): Brain metabolism during prolonged seizures in neonates. In: *Advances in Neurology, Vol. 34, Status Epilepticus*, edited by A. Delgado-Escueta, C. Wasterlain, D. Treiman, and R. Porter, pp. 241–260. Raven Press, New York.
79. Watanabe, K., Hara, K., Miyazaki, S., Hakamada, S., and Kuroyanagi, M. (1982): Apneic seizures in the newborn. *Am. J. Dis. Child.*, 136:980–984.
80. Watanabe, K., Hara, K., Miyazaki, S., Kuroyanagi, M., Asano, S., Kondo, K., Kuno, K., Jose, H., and Iwase, K. (1977): Electroclinical studies of seizures in the newborn. *Folia Psychiatr. Neurol. Jpn.*, 31:383–392.
81. Young, R., Hernandez, M., and Yagel, S. (1982): Selective reduction of blood flow to white matter during hypotension in newborn dogs: A possible mechanism of periventricular leukomalacia. *Ann. Neurol.*, 12:445–448.
82. Young, R., Osbakken, M., Briggs, R., Yagel, S., Rice, D., and Goldberg, S. (1984): ^{31}P nuclear magnetic resonance study of cerebral high-energy phosphate metabolism during prolonged seizures in neonatal dogs. *Ann. Neurol.*, 16:377.

Advances in Neurology, Vol. 46: Intensive Neurodiagnostic Monitoring, edited by R. J. Gumnit. Raven Press, New York © 1986.

Intensive Monitoring in Infants and Children

Peter Kellaway

Section of Neurophysiology, Department of Neurology, Baylor College of Medicine, and The Methodist Hospital, Texas Medical Center, Houston, Texas 77030

This book is concerned primarily with practical questions regarding the overall usefulness and cost/benefit ratio of intensive monitoring. This chapter concerns these questions as they apply specifically to the diagnosis and management of seizures in infants and young children. The role of intensive monitoring in children suspected of having seizures must be to provide specific and objective information, not otherwise available, concerning three main questions that require specific answers: (a) Are the presenting symptoms epileptic in character, and, if not, what is their true nature? (b) If the symptoms are epileptic, what specific type of epilepsy is involved? (c) What is the etiology and what is the prognosis?

Once the answers to these questions are obtained and treatment is initiated, the role of intensive monitoring must be to help determine whether the treatment is effective and, if so, when it can be discontinued.

Traditionally, routine electroencephalographic (EEG) studies have been used to help the physician make these determinations, but such studies have not always been helpful. The problems are compounded in infants and young children, who are unable to communicate their subjective symptoms effectively and whose behavior may not be witnessed.

DIAGNOSIS

Diagnosis in infants and children is often difficult because they are commonly subject to behavioral and subjective symptoms that may be misconstrued as epileptic, and because these signs and symptoms are rarely observed and documented by a trained individual. Descriptions of the critical events by parents, siblings, and other observers may be vague or distorted because of the emotional reaction to a sudden and unexpected change in behavior or consciousness. Yet, positive diagnosis is critical in this early period, probably more so than at any other time of life. Certainly, there is evidence that early, correct diagnosis may facilitate seizure control and influence prognosis. On the other hand, the lifelong social and economic consequences of a false diagnosis of epilepsy are incalculable. It is often forgotten that the determination that a child does *not* have epilepsy is as important as establishing that he *does*. Obviously, diagnosis cannot be based on limited or tenuous supporting evidence. In addition to the significant social and economic consequences of a false diagnosis, there is the important consideration of possible toxic and other undesirable side effects of anticonvulsant drugs gratuitously prescribed, and drug dosage is likely to be pushed to toxic levels when the symptoms for which the drugs are prescribed do not respond to treatment.

Because diagnosis must often be made with only vague and limited historical information, the physician is often forced to rely unduly on the routine EEG to provide definitive information. This age group is particularly prone to show normal or nonspecific EEG findings that may be misinterpreted as supporting a diagnosis of epilepsy. Conversely, the yield of the routine EEG in terms of providing specifically epileptiform findings in infants and young children who do, indeed, have epilepsy, may be disappointing. Even when techniques such as sleep, overventilation, and photic stimulation are employed to enhance the yield, detection of a specific EEG abnormality may be less than 50% in some types of epilepsy.

Because the old EEG literature indicates that nonspecific dysrhythmias are more common in epileptics than in the normal population, there has been a tendency to accept such findings as supportive of a clinical diagnosis of epilepsy—a diagnosis which may itself be tenuous due to inadequate clinical information. The fact that nonspecific dysrhythmias (slow, fast, paroxysmal slow) are common in children who do *not* have epilepsy is often overlooked. Such EEG findings neither establish a diagnosis of epilepsy nor illuminate the character of the disorder. Furthermore, a generalized slow dysrhythmia, or even a paroxysmal slow dysrhythmia, may be present in a child whose seizures, in fact, arise from a focus that may not have been demonstrated. Another important consideration is that whereas in an adult the demonstration of a specific EEG pattern (e.g., generalized spike-and-wave bursts or a focus of spike activity) implies a high probability that the abnormality and the patient's paroxysmal symptoms are related, and that the abnormality demonstrated defines the nature of the epilepsy, the situation is quite different in children. Demonstration of a spike focus in a child does not necessarily mean that the child has clinical epilepsy. Depending on the locus, spike foci have a variable association with epilepsy. In a group of 2,724 children, aged 3 to 16 years, with clear evidence of spike foci, only 38% of those with central spike foci and 54% with occipital spike foci had clinical seizures. Even multiple spike foci may not be associated with seizures; 24% of the children in the same series who had multiple foci did not have clinical seizures (8).

Another relatively common "epileptic" EEG finding in children is the abortive generalized spike-and-wave pattern. This is defined as generalized, or bilateral frontal, 3- to 4-Hz spike-and-wave bursts that occur in a series of no more than three or four complexes, even during hyperventilation, photic stimulation, or sleep. About 45% of children showing this pattern have generalized tonic/clonic seizures only; 35% have no seizures; and the remainder (20%) have seizures that are not generalized and may show a spike focus as well. For instance, abortive spike-and-wave bursts were demonstrated in the prolonged monitoring studies of ten (20%) of our last 50 patients with complex partial seizures. The clinical seizures of these patients arose focally in the temporal or frontal region on one side and at times when the spike-and-wave bursts were not present. Even though some of these patients were monitored for periods of up to 3 weeks, no seizures either initially generalized or temporally associated with the spike-and-wave bursts were recorded.

Thus, although the first essential for diagnosis is the detection of the presence of interictal epileptic activity in the brain, such a finding, alone, is insufficient. It is also necessary to prove that there is a close association between the demonstrated interictal abnormality and the patient's clinical attacks. In other words, diagnosis can be considered unequivocal only when a clinical attack is recorded in appropriate temporal relationship to electrical seizure activity. In some instances, this may require the use of sphenoidal or depth electrodes to provide access to deeply situated or mesial brain structures. The placement of such electrodes, especially indwelling depth electrodes, demands that optimal methods be employed to detect and characterize any existing abnormality. This requirement can be met only by intensive video/EEG/polygraphic monitoring.

Another important example of the need to relate a detected epileptiform EEG abnormality to the patient's clinical symptoms is the problem of diagnosis constituted by bizarre nocturnal sleep behaviors in young children. Parasomnias or pavor nocturnus may be characterized by thrashing about or struggling movements and by crying out, and the child may be confused or incoherent when approached. Nocturnal complex partial seizures may be characterized by this same type of behavior and altered cognitive state. Monitoring of a typical episode may be required to make the proper diagnosis. The complexity of the problem is compounded in this situation if a central spike focus is demonstrated in routine EEG studies. Does the presence of this focus establish that the bizarre nocturnal behavior is epileptic? As pointed out above, less than 40% of such foci are associated with seizures, so there is an equal chance that the behavior is pavor nocturnus rather than complex partial epilepsy. A third possibility also exists, namely, that the child is subject to benign rolandic seizures and that the bizarre behavior witnessed represents a postictal state. Seizures of this type tend to be nocturnal and, in fact, may occur only at night. Soon after falling asleep, the child may have a focal motor or secondarily generalized clonic seizure, and by the time the parents or others are alerted, the seizure is over and the child appears only to be confused, agitated, and, perhaps, struggling as if to climb out of bed (for review, see ref. 9).

Thus, establishment of an unequivocal diagnosis of epilepsy requires not only the *detection* of epileptiform electrical activity in the brain, but a specific correlation of the electrical seizure activity with the patient's clinical attacks. From this information is derived the *characterization*, in electroclinical terms, of the specific type of epilepsy (5).

DETECTION

The detection of an interictal electrical epileptiform event (e.g., a spike focus) is constrained by two factors: (a) interictal epileptiform discharges, particularly if confined to buried mesial or inferior cortical areas, may not be manifest at the scalp, and (b) the distribution of interictal epileptiform activity over time may be such that the timing and duration of a routine EEG study, even if it includes sleep, may not be appropriate or adequate to detect the presence of such activity. Prolonged monitoring studies have demonstrated that interictal epileptiform events are not randomly distributed over time (10) and that they tend to be modulated in a manner that suggests the interaction of ul-

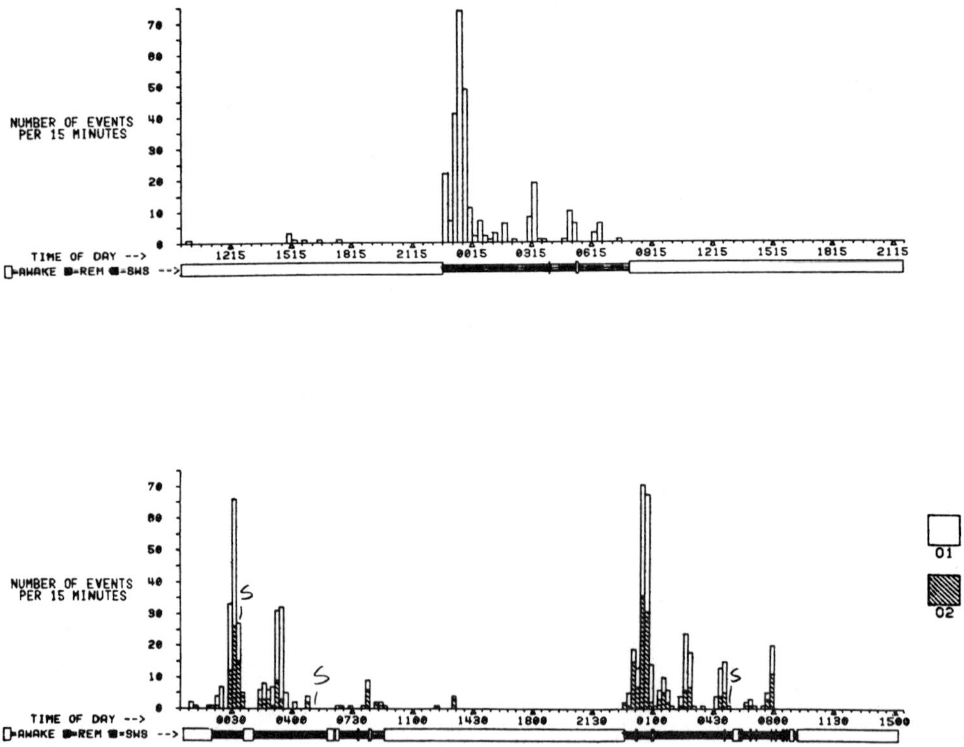

FIG. 1. Computer plot of time distribution of focal spike activity in a patient with partial and secondarily generalized seizures and independently firing foci at O_1 and O_2. Clinical seizures occurred at the points in time marked with an S.

tradian and circadian modulatory influences (9,11,13). The density of the discharges at any particular time is quite variable in the same patient, and there may be prolonged periods in which there are no discharges (10).

The time distribution of focal spike activity over a period of 72 hr in a patient with independent foci at O_1 and O_2 is shown in Fig. 1. Note that there are prolonged periods throughout the day when no focal spike activity is present. An EEG sample obtained at any time between 7:45 A.M. and 9:00 P.M. on the second day would not have shown any spike activity. This sampling error of routine EEG studies is also a problem if such studies are used to help determine if medication can be decreased or discontinued.

DEMONSTRATION OF RELATIONSHIP BETWEEN INTERICTAL DISCHARGES AND CLINICAL SEIZURES

Once the presence of specific electrical epileptiform activity has been established, it becomes necessary to demonstrate a direct relationship between the detected abnormality and the clinical seizures or symptoms for which the patient was referred. For example, even though a spike focus is detected, it is not necessarily the origin of the patient's clinical seizures. Recognition of this fact is important, particularly if a surgical approach to treating the patient's epilepsy is being considered. Children who have complex partial seizures may have bilateral independent or multiple unilateral spike foci, and it is necessary to determine which focus or foci are responsible for the clinical seizures. Monitoring may reveal that the clinical seizures originate at different times from different foci or that, for example, the most active interictal focus is not the one responsible for the child's clinical seizures.

CHARACTERIZATION

The determination of the type of epilepsy the child has often cannot be made without appropriate monitoring. Seizures in children are rarely witnessed by trained observers, and often the most dramatic aspect of the seizure (e.g., generalized jerking) may be the only feature that the observer is able to report. The initial and important localizing features may be obscured by subsequent events. In addition, the precise sequence of events may not be documented or all aspects of the onset of the seizure noted, even when witnessed by trained observers. In some children, the progression of the seizure may be so rapid that a focal onset can be determined only by analysis of time-synchronized EEG and video recordings. Furthermore, seizure types usually considered to be evidence of *generalized* epilepsy (e.g., atonic or tonic seizures) may, in young children, be associated with *focal* seizure activity in the EEG. This correlation of a generalized clinical event with focal electrical seizure activity can, in most instances, be established only by intensive monitoring. Young infants, especially newborns, may show normal, or abnormal but nonepileptic, behavior that is difficult to differentiate from epileptic phenomena without appropriate monitoring. Failure to establish the true nature of such behavior (18) may result in the infant's being treated gratuitously with potentially harmful drugs, whereas failure to recognize that the infant is having *true* seizures may have adverse clinical and prognostic consequences.

Pseudoseizures are not uncommon in older children, and intensive monitoring may be essential to distinguish between feigned or hysterical attacks and true ones, particularly in a child who has both epileptic and nonepileptic seizures (20). Intensive monitoring may also be necessary for evaluation when seizures are said to be precipitated by certain specific events and behaviors or by specific stimuli of various kinds. Reading, specific language, music, mathematical calculations, and even movements of a limb have been reported as precipitants of clinical seizures in individual patients or groups of patients. Documentation by intensive monitoring that a significant precipitant exists may be important to the patient's care. Paroxysmal behaviors of equivocal significance, such as laughing (2), aphasia (1), rotational movements (7), and running (2), may require intensive monitoring to determine their true significance. In the neonate, episodes of flushing, sweating, abrupt and transient blood pressure and respiratory changes, and pupillary dilatation or constriction have all been reported to occur in association with an electrical seizure discharge in the EEG (16,17,19). However, combined EEG/video/polygraphic monitoring studies may be required to establish that such symptoms have an epileptic basis. Unfortunately, many of the subtle and recondite symptoms that are diagnosed as epilepsy are so diagnosed on the basis of the interictal EEG findings. But although several different types of normal, and abnormal but nonepileptic, sharp transients occur in EEGs of normal and abnormal neonates, truly epileptic interictal electrical events are uncommon. Therefore, an intimate relationship must be demonstrated between the symptoms and the EEG seizure activity before a diagnosis of epilepsy can be proved.

Videotape recording permits unlimited replay of the infant's or child's behavior in real time or in slow motion, making it possible to analyze the onset and subsequent features of the behavior in time-synchronized relationship to the EEG and polygraphic data channels. The origin and spread of the electrical seizure activity can be documented in precise time relationships to the development of the various behavioral changes and to autonomic changes recorded by the polygraphic data channels.

The point of origin in the brain, and the character and spread of the electrical seizure activity, as determined by surface and, perhaps, depth electrodes, are essential to the decision-making process concerning the feasibility and chances for success of epilepsy surgery. Currently, most of the centers in which epilepsy surgery is performed require that from three to five of the patient's typical seizures be recorded arising from the same focal source before such surgery can be recommended (3,21).

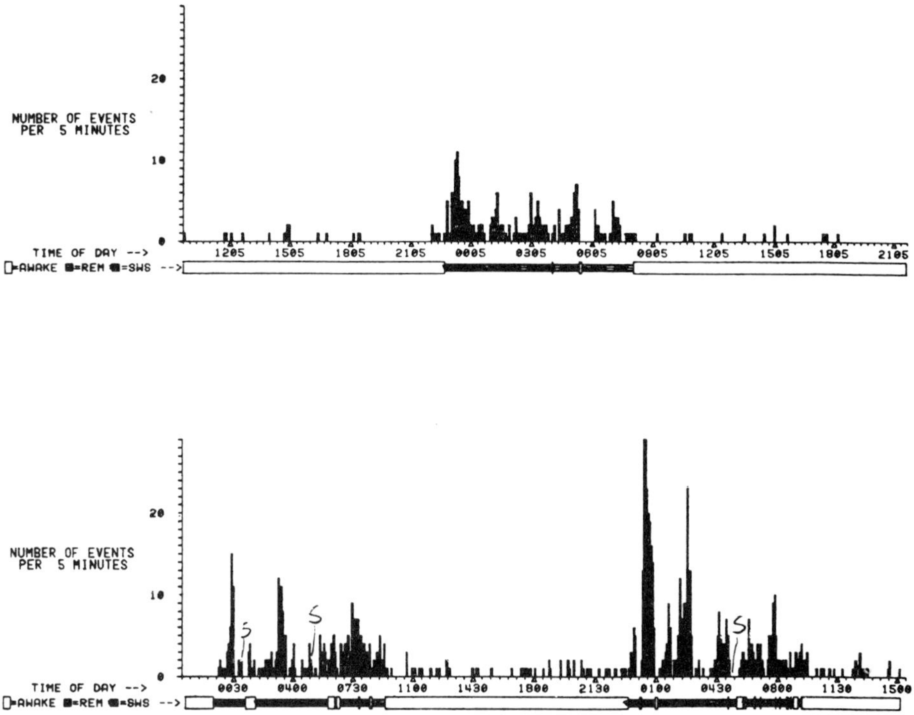

FIG. 2. Computer plot of the time distribution of focal spike discharges at F_7 over 72 hr in a patient with complex partial seizures. Clinical seizures occurred at the points in time marked with an S.

Finally, experience during the past 12 years with several thousand hours of monitoring of different types of patients and various age groups has constantly and cogently demonstrated that the characterization of the seizures by the patient, parents, or other observers is quite often deficient or inaccurate.

QUANTITATION

The concept that there is a meaningful relationship between the hazard for seizures and interictal EEG discharges is a reasonable one, but it has limitations in terms of application when routine clinical EEGs are used to assess the effects of therapy or to help in making decisions concerning discontinuance or reduction of anticonvulsant drugs.

Figure 2, which is a time plot of the spike discharges occurring over a 72-hr period in a patient with complex partial seizures and a spike focus at F_7, cogently demonstrates the limitations of making a determination of prevailing electrical epileptic activity on the basis of a routine EEG study. The time plot also demonstrates the effect that an appropriate anticonvulsant drug (carbamazepine) may have on the incidence of spike discharges. In the study shown, the patient was being evaluated as a possible candidate for surgery; the medication had been discontinued just before the monitoring study, and the blood levels decreased progressively to zero during the study. The effect of the drug on the amount of spike-and-wave activity present is clearly illustrated. However, studies of the effects of anticonvulsant drugs on the amount of spike activity present over prolonged periods of 12 to 72 hr have shown that although the amount of spike activity is decreased by effective drug treatment, there is no simple relationship between this measure and the hazard for clinical seizures (14). For example, two patients with similar amounts of spike-and-wave activity measured over 48 hr may have entirely different incidences of clinical seizures (e.g., no seizures versus many). In individual patients, although effective anticonvulsant drug treatment invariably reduces the number of electrical seizure discharges, there is no correlation with degree of seizure control. That is, the patient may show, for example, an exacerbation of seizures without a change occurring in the amount of focal spike activity measured over a period of 12 hr or more, including nocturnal sleep.

Recent evidence indicates that although overall spike activity may not be an effective measure of seizure hazard, certain specific measures of the individual spikes do appear to be correlated with seizure hazard, but only in terms of the changes in these measures that take place in response to drug treatment (4,6, 14). Serial monitoring studies of children with focal epilepsy (temporal or central spike foci) have shown that at drug levels at which clinical control is attained, there is a reduction in the amplitude of the spikes, an increase in their sharpness, and a reduction in both the duration of the spikes and the size of the potential field. A computer method of making these measurements has been devised (4) which requires only 100 spikes to be recorded in a single state (e.g., slow-wave sleep) so that relatively short periods of monitoring are all that is necessary for the determination of drug effectiveness.

In generalized epilepsy with 3-Hz spike-and-wave activity, however, such a determination requires prolonged monitoring in order to obtain significant data. Comprehensive monitoring studies over periods of 24 to 36 hr have demonstrated that (a) there is a direct quantitative relationship between the incidence of seizures of absence, atonic, and/or myoclonic type and the overall incidence of spike-and-wave activity; (b) effective drug treatment (ethosuximide) reduces, and eventually abolishes, spike-and-wave activity; (c) the rate at which the reduction of spike-and-wave activity occurs in relationship to specific anticonvulsant drug levels is a measure of drug effectiveness; (d) with effective treatment, the spike-and-wave activity is abolished first in REM sleep, then in wakefulness, and last in slow-wave sleep; (e) absence, atonic, and myoclonic seizures no longer occur at a drug level that abolishes spike-and-wave activity in REM sleep and awake; (f) generalized tonic/clonic seizures may persist as long as *any* spike-and-wave activity continues to be present in any state; (g) ethosuximide levels much greater than that specified as the top of the therapeutic range may be required to abolish spike-and-wave activity and to control seizures; levels of 200 μg/ml can be tolerated by many children without adverse side effects or toxic reactions; and (h) the curve relating the amount of spike-and-wave activity to serum drug levels flattens out to an asymptotic level in some patients, and marked increases in drug levels may be required to produce small changes in the amount of spike-and-wave activity once high drug levels are attained (15).

When these data are applied to the use of routine EEG studies to help determine whether medication can be reduced or stopped, it is clear that the presence of spike-and-wave bursts in the waking state is evidence of inadequate drug levels; but, the absence of spike-and-wave activity may merely reflect a sampling error due to a short recording. It would appear from the findings given above that in children with generalized epilepsy and 3-Hz spike-and-wave bursts, "treating the EEG" is a reasonable practice; but for this to be done effectively, intensive monitoring is required.

TECHNICAL AND OPERATIONAL PRINCIPLES

Most of the diagnostic and therapeutic problems discussed here require that the data collection and analysis be as free as possible of any factors that could lead to misinterpretation or failure to obtain interpretable data. The cost effectiveness of intensive monitoring is directly related to the quality and precision of the data obtained. Even in the best circumstances, and when optimal monitoring techniques are utilized, interpretation of the time-synchronized video and EEG data may be quite difficult and subject to uncertainties. The cost of monitoring in terms of time spent by the patient, the technicians, and the medical staff, and the actual cost in dollars to the patient or third-party payer, can be justified only if entirely accurate and precise information is obtained.

The design of the monitoring suite and the selection of equipment depends somewhat on the type and age of the patients who are to be studied (5,12). The suite should include a patient room containing a bed, chair, washbowl and mirror, and a toilet. Provision of a television set and of toys or games for the child's entertainment is essential. A long leash system is preferable to telemetry, which should be reserved for special applications. The use of telemetry increases the hazard for artifacts and instrument failure. The telemetry unit, particularly if placed on the head, is cumbersome, and it is difficult for young children to adjust to its presence. While it is true that the use of a leash decreases mobility, children are much less conscious of the tether than of a worn device, and if their movements are not significantly restricted, they generally forget about the attachment. A happy, comfortable patient is a critical factor in obtaining clean data. Parents should be encouraged to spend time with the patient and to watch television, read, and play games with the child during the periods when the child is awake.

Constant attendance by a trained technician is essential to obtaining high-quality and reliable data. The effective interaction of the technician with the child, who at various times may be anxious, bored, or irritable, is not only essential to the well-being of the patient but may determine the degree of success of the entire procedure. The possibility of the occurrence of a generalized seizure, status epilepticus, or some other emergency requires that a trained individual be immediately at hand throughout the entire monitoring session. Technicians can be trained to attend appropriately to such problems and should also be certified in cardiopulmonary resuscitation. The one-on-one attention of the technician is also required to keep the patient constantly "on camera" and in focus; otherwise, essential behavioral information may be lost. In the case of neonates or other infants or children who may be in intensive care units, the technician must be trained to interact effectively and unobtrusively with the nurses and others who are immediately responsible for the patient's care.

The constant attendance of a technician makes it possible for such problems as faulty electrodes or minor malfunctions of equipment to be immediately corrected. His or her close presence is required for the appropriate care of infants and young children in terms of their needs and comfort. Changing of diapers and occasionally the management of other secretions are some of the necessary duties of the technician, and for long-term monitoring of infants, the technician must be adept in the preparation of food and drink for the patients throughout the period of study. A small refrigerator in the monitoring suite is an asset in this regard. Auxiliary or back-up equipment should be available in case of primary equipment failure, and it is desirable to have a biomedical apparatus technician available if a major failure occurs. A house officer or one of the neurophysiology medical staff members must be immediately available at all times for consultation with the technician.

Intensive monitoring performed without around-the-clock attendance and without appropriate attention to the factors that have just been outlined is of limited value in dealing with the kinds of clinical problems that infants and young children present (12). Ambulatory cassette monitoring imposes a marked limitation on the yield of reliable and useful data because the problem of artifact is inordinately great and because of the lack of the all-important time-synchronized behavioral information (video). The limited number of data channels also places constraints on data collection and precise localizing information.

ACKNOWLEDGMENT

Supported by grant NS11535 from the National Institute of Neurological and Communicative Disorders and Stroke, National Institute of Health.

REFERENCES

1. Boudouresques, J., Roger, J., and Gastaut, H. (1962): Crises aphasiques subintrantes chez un épileptique temporal. Etude électroclinique. *Rev. Neurol.*, 106:381–393.
2. Chen, R.-C., and Forster, F.M. (1973): Cursive epilepsy and gelastic epilepsy. *Neurology*, 23:1019–1029.
3. Engel, J., Jr., Rausch, R., Lieb, J.P., Kuhl, D.E., and Crandall, P.H. (1981): Correlation of criteria used for localizing epileptic foci in patients considered for surgical therapy of epilepsy. *Ann. Neurol.*, 9:215–224.
4. Frost, J.D., Jr. (1979): Microprocessor-based EEG spike detection and quantification. *Int. J. Biomed. Comput.*, 10:357–373.
5. Frost, J.D., Jr., Hrachovy, R.A., Kellaway, P., and Zion, T. (1978): Quantitative analysis and characterization of infantile spasms. *Epilepsia*, 19:273–282.
6. Frost, J.D., Jr., and Kellaway, P. (1981): Changes in epileptic spike configuration associated with achievement of clinical seizure control. *Electroencephalogr. Clin. Neurophysiol.*, 51:20P–21P.
7. Gastaut, H., and Broughton, R. (1972): *Epileptic Seizures*, p. 127. Thomas, Springfield, Illinois.
8. Kellaway, P. (1981): The incidence, significance and natural history of spike foci in children. In: *Current Clinical Neurophysiology: Update on EEG and Evoked Potentials*, edited by C.E. Henry, pp. 151–175. Elsevier/North-Holland, Amsterdam.
9. Kellaway, P. (1984): Genetic, ontogenetic, and biorhythmic factors in epilepsy. In: *Current Neurology, Vol. 5*, edited by S.H. Appel, pp. 259–284. Wiley, New York.
10. Kellaway, P., and Carrie, J.R.G. (1977): Relationship between quantitative EEG measurements and clinical state in epileptic patients. In: *Epilepsy: the 8th International Symposium*, edited by J.K. Penry, pp. 153–158. Raven Press, New York.
11. Kellaway, P., and Frost, J.D., Jr. (1983): Biorhythmic modulation of epileptic events. In: *Recent Advances in Epilepsy*, edited by T.A. Pedley and B.S. Meldrum, pp. 139–154. Churchill Livingstone, Edinburgh.
12. Kellaway, P., and Frost, J.D., Jr. (1985): Monitoring at the affiliated hospitals of Baylor College of Medicine, Houston. In: *Long-Term Monitoring in Epilepsy (EEG Suppl., No. 37)*, edited by J. Gotman, J.R. Ives, and P. Gloor, pp. 397–408. Elsevier, Amsterdam.
13. Kellaway, P., Frost, J.D., Jr., and Crawley, J.W. (1980): Time modulation of spike-and-wave activity in generalized epilepsy. *Ann. Neurol.*, 8:491–500.
14. Kellaway, P., Frost, J.D., Jr., and Crawley, J.W. (1980): Influence of phenobarbital on C_3/C_4 spikes in rolandic epilepsy of children. *Electroencephalogr. Clin. Neurophysiol.*, 50:153P.
15. Kellaway, P., Saltzberg, B., Frost, J.D., Jr., and Crawley, J.W. (1979): Relationship between clinical state, ictal and interictal EEG discharges, and serum drug levels: generalized epilepsy/ethosuximide. *Neurology*, 29:559.
16. Lou, H.C., and Friis-Hansen, B. (1979): Arterial blood pressure elevations during motor activity and epileptic seizures in the newborn. *Acta Paediatr. Scand.*, 68:803–806.
17. Meldrum, B.S., Vigouroux, R.A., and Brierley, J.B. (1973): Systemic factors and epileptic brain damage. *Arch. Neurol.*, 29:82–87.
18. Mizrahi, E.M., and Kellaway, P. (1984): Characterization of seizures in neonates and young infants by time-synchronized electroencephalographic/polygraphic/video monitoring. *Ann. Neurol.*, 16:383.
19. Perlman, J.M., and Volpe, J.J. (1983): Seizures in the pre-term infant: effects on cerebral blood flow velocity, intracranial pressure, and arterial blood pressure. *J. Pediatr.*, 102:288–293.
20. Riley, T.L., and Roy, A. (editors)(1982): *Pseudoseizures*. Williams & Wilkins, Baltimore.
21. Spencer, S.S. (1981): Depth electroencephalography in selection of refractory epilepsy for surgery. *Ann. Neurol.*, 9:207–214.

Advances in Neurology, Vol. 46: Intensive Neurodiagnostic Monitoring, edited by R. J. Gumnit. Raven Press, New York © 1986.

Ambulatory EEG: Telemetered and Cassette-Recorded

John S. Ebersole

Department of Neurology, Yale University School of Medicine, New Haven, Connecticut 06510, and Epilepsy Center, Neurology Service, Veterans Administration Medical Center, West Haven, Connecticut 06516

RATIONALE

The evaluation of patients reporting transient episodes of altered consciousness or behavior is a common problem for neurologists. Clinical examination after such episodes is usually not revealing, and historic data may suggest an extensive differential diagnosis including epilepsy, transient ischemic attacks, cardiac arrhythmias, and psychiatric syndromes. When seizures are a possibility, one or more standard laboratory electroencephalograms (EEGs) are a routine part of the initial workup. Unfortunately, the relatively short duration of a standard EEG is not well suited to detect paroxysmal abnormalities that are infrequent. In fact studies of a population of patients with verified epilepsy have revealed that only about 50% of those patients will show epileptiform abnormalities on an initial routine EEG (1,10). Twenty additional percent may be identified on a second EEG and a slightly higher percentage with a sleep and/or sleep-deprived recording. The remaining quarter of the patients, who have or will prove to have seizure disorders, will not demonstrate epileptiform EEG abnormalities during standard EEG evaluation.

Patients such as these may present several diagnostic dilemmas. Do they in fact have a seizure disorder, or are their spells related to noncerebral organic disease or a functional disturbance? Is their EEG not really normal, but epileptiform only intermittently? Even if a diagnosis has already been made, are a patient's seizures not under good control because they have been inadequately characterized and thus improperly treated? Are new spells in a patient with previously well controlled epilepsy related to breakthrough seizures or nonepileptic disturbances, such as intermittent drug toxicity? Has the current or new medical regimen significantly altered the number of ictal discharges a patient is having? In each instance, long-term recording of EEG is needed to document, characterize, and quantify epileptiform abnormalities.

During the past 15 years specialized epilepsy centers have evolved to fulfill this need. Intensive inpatient monitoring at these facilities includes not only prolonged EEG recording, but also simultaneous video- and audiotaping of patient behavior as discussed in previous chapters (2,5,21–24,30,33). With these techniques the probability of documenting capricious clinical episodes has greatly increased. Although recognized as the most reliable means of diagnosing and clarifying epilepsy, intensive inpatient monitoring has inherent disadvantages. Chief among those are that hospitalization is required, and patient mobility and activities are restricted. The hospital setting is clearly unnatural, which may inhibit both epileptic and nonepileptic episodes (28). Such evaluations are often unavailable for only a modest number of centers exist (24), and those usually have a patient backlog on the order of several months. Finally, intensive inpatient monitoring is by its very level of sophistication an expensive proposition, and should be reserved for carefully selected patients.

Telemetered and ambulatory EEG monitoring by a variety of newly introduced techniques would appear to be at least a partial solution to these problems, since they can provide expanded temporal sampling of EEG and other physiologic parameters on a portable and outpatient basis, as well as less restricted inpatient basis. Patients may not have to be hospitalized, but are free to pursue more normal daily activities. Other advantages include a natural home or work setting, with its accompanying normal stress, to evoke the episodes in question. Potential greater availability and reduced cost relative to hospitalization can result in improved and more economical patient care.

The traditional EEG recording set-up, however, is not suited to long-term telemetered and ambulatory EEG monitoring. If the patient is to have some freedom of movement during the prolonged recording session, a different way must be found to transmit the EEG signals from the head to the recording apparatus. Likewise, if the recording is going to last many hours to several days, continuous paper write-out may not be the most appropriate or efficient means of storing the EEG. Regardless of the storage medium, review of the data collected becomes increasingly more difficult as the duration of the recording lengthens. A more efficient means of analysis is needed. Finally, since an EEG technologist or other qualified observer may not be present during much of the monitoring, behavior recording must be made differently. The following sections review telemetered and ambulatory EEG techniques for solving these problems.

TECHNIQUES

Electrode Application

Disk electrodes applied by collodion technique are currently the only means of insuring stable long-term EEG recordings from the scalp. Even with this technique, rejelling may be necessary every 24 hr or less. Electrode application using paste, needles, or head gear is not suitable. Long-term recording may also be performed with sphenoidal and intracranial electrodes during intensive inpatient evaluations. These techniques are not, however, applicable to a completely ambulatory or outpatient setting. When individual channel preamplifiers are placed on the head, they also should be secured to the scalp. Electrode wires leading to preamplifiers on the head or elsewhere on the body should be stabilized by at least one additional collodion attachment to minimize transmitted movement to the electrode disk during active wakefulness, which is the major source of extrinsic artifact.

EEG Preamplification

One of the initial hurdles in the evolution of mobile and ambulatory EEG was the necessity of preamplifying the microvolt level EEG so that it could be multiplexed, more easily transmitted over longer distances, or recorded on miniature cassette recorders (16). Theoretically, it made sense to place the amplifier as close as possible to the signal source in order to minimize lead artifact that could be prominent during active wakefulness. The on-head preamplifier chip developed by Quy (26) became the prototype for the industry. Each chip represented a single channel and had its own grid 1 and grid 2 inputs. Its size was small enough to be concealed in the patient's hair. Although these individual preamplifiers, which are glued to the scalp, have the shortest leads and are the most secure, their attachment is time-consuming and the connections become complex with an increasing number of channels. It remains necessary to have one cable for each channel lead to the recorder.

Multiple combined preamplifiers may also be head-mounted and are faster and easier to attach, but the leads are longer. As a single unit, it is not as secure; a turban is usually necessary in order to hold it in place. The total weight or size of the amplifier unit may become a comfort problem for the patient. Size and weight are less of a problem with preamplifier collections carried on the body elsewhere, for example, belt-mounted; but progressively longer leads may give an increased potential for lead movement artifacts. These preamplifier collections are more commonly used with mobile, but not completely ambulatory, EEG techniques of cable and radio telemetry (2,15). All preamplifiers mounted on the body make compromises in order to be small, light, and use small amounts of power. These include a lack of selectability of filter settings of gain, and in some instances a lesser than customary high frequency response.

It is notable, however, that most of the artifact which confounds the EEG during active wakefulness is of physiologic origin, namely electroculogram (EOG) and electromyogram (EMG), which even head-mounted preamplification cannot reduce. The major source of lead-related artifact appears to come from movement of the electrode cup relative to its scalp interface, and not from the movement of the wire itself. If additional efforts are taken to secure the electrode wire to the scalp proximal to the disk, as a form of strain relief, there is far less extrinsic movement artifact. On-head preamplification may still be superior in settings where recordings are made during periods of vigorous activity. Conversely, off-head preamplifications would clearly be well suited to inpatient and outpatient recordings where activity is restricted.

Montages are fixed at the time of hook-up, and a montage change requires a reconfiguration of the electrode inputs to the preamplifiers. Sometimes insertable cards with the prewiring of a given montage are available. Electrodes with bifurcated leads are necessary for linked montages when individual preamplifier chips are used.

Recording all channels to a common reference and creating variable bipolar derivations upon replay is one way to achieve montage flexibility (29). However, if a common reference is used with ambulatory EEG recordings, one is forced to do the initial detection of abnormalities by video scanning common reference EEG. This is far more difficult than with bipolar montages, especially if one is searching for focal features. An additional drawback is that the loss of or excessive artifact from the reference electrode(s) means that all of the EEG is lost or confounded.

EEG Multiplexing

Multiplexing the preamplified EEG signals is standard procedure for most cable telemetry, all radio telemetry, and epoch ambulatory EEG recording techniques. Multiplexers can combine a number of EEG signals, typically eight or sixteen, into one channel and thus greatly reduce the total number of individual wires in the transmission cable or the number of transmission channels necessary in radio telemetry. Demultiplexers separate out the component EEG signals before or after recording. The two main types of multiplexing methods are frequency-division and time-division. In frequency-division multiplexing, each channel is allocated a small frequency bandwidth that is a fraction of the overall transmission frequency bandwidth. Amplitude of the EEG in a given channel is encoded by the amplitude, phase, or frequency variations within its particular bandwidth. In time-division multiplexing each channel is repeatedly sampled for a short time period in a set sequence. During the time interval allocated to each channel, EEG amplitude can be encoded by the amplitude of a pulse (pulse-amplitude modulation), by the position of a pulse (pulse-position modulation), or by a digital binary code (pulse-coded modulation) (see ref. 17 for review). Of practical importance with the more common time-division multiplexing is that the sampling rate of the multiplexer per channel should be at least twice the frequency of the EEG signals of interest. One disadvantage is that multiplexing adds to the complexity of the required electronics.

EEG Transmission

The most common technology emloyed in epilepsy centers across the country is cable telemetry (2,15). After the usual preamplification and multiplexing,

EEG signals are carried by a single cable to the recording device. This allows a certain amount of patient mobility about the monitoring room, since the tethering cable can be light, flexible, and many feet in length. These systems have little problem with interference and are simple to operate.

An alternative transmission technique is radio telemetry (25,31). After initial amplification and multiplexing, the combined EEG signal is broadcast from a miniature radio transmitter worn by the patient to a receiving and decoding station in a monitoring control room nearby. Radio telemetry offers more patient mobility, since no cable is necessary, however, this is often negated by the fact that video recording of behavior requires the patient to stay on camera. Additionally, these systems have a limited range (approximately 50–100 feet), which is dependent on the power of the transmitter and ultimately on the size of the equipment and battery. Multiple antennas located in several rooms and adjoining corridors, and the use of dual diversity reception techniques, in which the stronger signal from two antennas is automatically sought, can increase the operational range of radio telemetry. Regardless, this technique is more susceptible to interference and signal dropout. Since radio telemetry systems are more complicated at both the transmission and reception sites, they can be more difficult to operate than cable telemetry.

Neither telemetry technique offers complete ambulatory freedom for the patient, however, nor can they conveniently be used on an outpatient basis. Cassette-recorded EEG offers maximum patient mobility. Patients do not need to be hospitalized, but are free to pursue normal daily activities. It is operationally simple and is not susceptible to interference, which can be advantageous in an inpatient setting, such as an ICU, as well as in an outpatient environment. EEG transmission is directly from the head or body-mounted preamplifier to the cassette recorder also worn by the patient. One thin flexible cable is used for each EEG channel in continuous record devices. Signal multiplexing permits the use of just one cable with epoch recorders. A major disadvantage with direct transmission to cassette recorders is that the EEG cannot be monitored while it is being recorded.

EEG Recording and Storage

Although paper is the most common recording and storage medium for routine laboratory EEG, it has many drawbacks in long-term telemetry monitoring—excessive bulk, expense, the necessity of round-the-clock personnel in order to attend the machine, tedious manual review of the record, and the inability to replay the electrographic record once recorded. For ambulatory EEG such methodology is out of the question. Analog magnetic tape recording of EEG data is the most common solution in both instances.

The initial cassette recorders were an offshoot of those that had been developed for Holter monitoring of ECG. After a multichannel portable tape recorder was developed (20), Ives and Wood, in 1975 (16), showed that recording EEG on it was feasible. Four-channel commercial systems became available in 1979. All 4-channel recorders are standard analog devices utilizing four recording heads with ⅛- or ¼-inch tape. Tape speed is reduced to approximately 2 mm/sec so that a standard C120 or special ¼-inch cassette can record at least 24 hr of continuous EEG. Recorders weigh approximately 1.5 pounds and are easily worn by belt or strap on most patients, including small children.

In 1983, the first 8-channel continuous recorder was introduced. In order to record eight channels of physiologic data plus real digital time and events in excess of 24 hr on standard format ⅛-inch cassettes, a new recording technology was developed called "blocked analog" recording. In essence, 1-sec segments of three channels are digitized, temporally compressed, combined into a single new 1-sec segment, converted back to analog, and recorded on one tape channel. In addition to the other EEG channels, timing and synchronizing signals make up the remainder of the 12-channel (four times three) complement. A reverse order transcription is necessary on replay. Another 8-channel system is now available which uses a special ¼-inch cassette tape. The larger size permits eight channels of physiologic data plus time to be recorded in standard analog fashion using a 9-channel recording head. Size of the 8-channel recorders is only slightly larger than the smallest 4-channel recorder.

In 1982, a 16-channel ambulatory recorder utilizing signal multiplexing was introduced, but it was limited to recording short epochs (14). The recorder is of standard "Walkman" type, and uses a standard tape speed in order to achieve the frequency response necessary to record faithfully multiplexed signals. High quality metal tapes are suggested, which have a total recording time of 45 min. Recording is done in selectable periodic epochs, e.g., 15 sec every 10 min over 24 hr. The recorder can also be turned on by a push-button, which the patient can activate when experiencing a spell. Currently being implemented is a 40- to 80-sec delay, which allows recording of EEG prior to the button push.

With cable and radio telemetry systems EEG data are also most often recorded onto magnetic tape. Since standard analog recorders seldom offer even eight channels, multiplexing of EEG signals onto one or more data channels is routine and provides the capability of recording sixteen or more channels of EEG. The trade-off made when EEG is multiplexed is that tape speed must be faster, and thus available recording time shorter, in order to achieve the higher frequency response necessary to faithfully record the combined signal. This technique allows for continuous, even unattended, monitoring for typically 6 to 10 hr per tape. Storage of data is less bulky and may be less expensive than paper, since the tapes can be reused. Multiplexed EEG data can also be recorded on one of the two audio channels of a videotape which is simultaneously recording patient activity.

The recent reduction in the size and expense of video recorders has created new possibilities for portable and mobile, if not ambulatory, EEG recording. Frequency response characteristics of portable video recorders allow 16 to 32 channels of EEG to be multiplexed upon the videotape. Six- to 8-hr recording times are possible with long-playing tapes and the extra slow recording speeds available on most units. Small videotape recorders have enough portability to be carried with the patient from one place to another.

Long-term recording of EEG in a digital format on tape or computer disks can also be done, but these have limited storage capacity and require more sophisticated technology. In a few inpatient centers computer programs have been devised to assist in the selection of EEG to be stored (11,12). Rather than a continuous storage of ongoing EEG, only pertinent segments are recorded, and those are selected by triggering from a patient-activated push-button or automatic computer programs which detect seizures and interictal epileptiform events. A time delay is available to allow the recording of a seizure onset detected by either means. Integrated computer-based systems for long-term EEG monitoring are not commercially available, however.

One problem with tape-recording EEG, either by telemetry or cassette, is that on-line monitoring of the quality of the recording requires additional effort or is unavailable. With cable or radio telemetry, the EEG being recorded can simply be printed out periodically on a polygraph. Ongoing feedback as to the status and content of taped EEG can also be provided by a waveform reformatter. This electronically produces a video image of the ongoing EEG signal which can be monitored on a television and/or recorded as a video image in a split-screen format with patient behavior.

The price that is paid for the ultimate mobility of ambulatory cassette-recorded EEG with outpatients is that there is no means of monitoring the record. Technical difficulties, such as the loss of signal from an electrode, go undetected until the tape is reviewed. In an inpatient setting, the preamplified EEG signals can be periodically obtained from the cassette recorder and monitored by the same means as above.

EEG Review and Analysis

Depending on the method of EEG storage, there are several alternative ways of analyzing EEG data recorded by cable and radio telemetry techniques. Although continuous paper recording has many disadvantages, it is immediately accessible and interpretable by traditional means. Manual analysis of a days worth of EEG recording can be tedious, however. Without the use of a special time marker, a paper record is impossible to synchronize accurately to a videotape record of patient behavior. Most importantly there is no data retrieval, replay, or additional analysis other than visual inspection at whatever setting it was originally recorded. If the quality of the tracing is inadequate, nothing further can be done.

Multiplexed EEG on analog tape, on the other hand, is retrievable, and after demultiplexing it can be written out onto hard copy repeatedly at any setting or speed desired to enhance the EEG abnormality. It is practical only when short segments are to be reproduced, however, since this replay is usually done in real time. The major problem with tape monitoring systems is not recording all the data, but reviewing it rapidly and extracting what is pertinent. Frequently, only specific segments of EEG related to clinical episodes are transcribed onto hard copy. These are usually located by means of a time code recorded with the EEG, or by an event marker actuated by the patient or monitoring staff. Subclinical electrographic events and interictal abnormalities may go unappreciated, even if random sampling of the tape is also employed. Standard tape recording of EEG, thus, has its greatest advantage in long-term monitoring when only the electrographic correlates of clinical seizures are desired.

Alternatively, some telemetry systems provide a means of reviewing the tape-recorded EEG on a video display. At present, these playbacks are either not paginated or are slower in review than ambulatory EEG systems. This form of review is also insufficient by itself for detailed EEG diagnosis. A paper copy of the EEG, written either on-line or off-line from tape after demultiplexing, is the usual standard for diagnostic purposes. For this same reason, recording the EEG signals only as a video image by means of a reformatter is not recommended, since they cannot be converted back into analog signals that can be pen-written.

For epilepsy units utilizing computer-assisted recognition of abnormalities and selective storage of EEG, only those selected segments are written out onto paper copy. Although data analysis is simplified and shortened in such a selective storage process, these automated computer detection programs are not completely accurate, resulting in false positive detections related to artifacts. These can usually be quickly identified by visual inspection. Unfortunately some genuine ictal and interictal events are also not detected in these schemes and, hence, are not recorded. Beyond detection, computer-based programs offer various additional forms of signal analyses. Equipment and software necessary for this type of automated analysis are complex and expensive. At present, their use is limited to only a few centers.

Several methods are also employed in the retrieval and review of ambulatory EEG. Paginated rapid video playback was the conceptual breakthrough that made efficient analysis of long-term ambulatory cassette tape recordings feasible (32). Initially, the EEG had to be transcribed onto paper by jet-ink writers. The first video units displayed data at selectable page lengths (8 or 16 sec) and speeds of review (20 and 60 times) and provided a simultaneous audio reproduction of one channel. At the fastest replay speed, 24 hr could be reviewed in 24 min. Four channels of physiologic data were displayed, or three channels, if an accurate digital time code occupied the fourth channel. Epochs of data displayed on the screen were written out on paper by connecting the playback unit to a standard EEG machine. A second generation of playback devices added digital time to the four data channels, as well as an automatic search mechanism to find a specific time.

The newer 8-channel playback units not only provide a means of displaying additional physiologic data, but a number of improved operational features have also been incorporated into one or both of the available systems. These include: digital real time as a separate channel, automatic search to a specific time, up to 64 sec of memory so that approximately 30 sec before and after the present screen can be viewed without tape movement, gain and filter adjustments without tape movement, alphanumeric registry of channel gain and filtering status, continuous printout of data as well as epoch printout, and stereo audio reproduction utilizing any number of channels.

Ambulatory cassette EEG possesses all the advantages of tape-recorded EEG monitoring, and suffers only from a limited number of data channels (four or eight) and some decrease in high-frequency response that is of questionable clinical significance. As with telemetry systems, hard-copy transcription of any particular segment can be reproduced in any desirable variety of gain or filter settings. In addition, however, the video playback component of the ambulatory EEG offers unique features. Long periods of EEG monitoring can be rapidly reviewed in a paginated video fashion. Interictal abnormalities and subclinical seizures, as well as clinically recognized episodes, can be detected and analyzed. Specific times and push-button-marked events can be accurately, swiftly, and automatically located. These are definite advantages over other tape-recording methods, where a major problem is how to review all of the data that is recorded. The time compression that is possible on the video unit can make seizure patterns more recognizable and the onset or laterality more perceptible. Detection of ictal discharges by their audio characteristics is a particular advantage of ambulatory EEG playback. Such analysis of seizures from various electrode derivations can be more informative than a visual analysis, particularly when the clinical seizure is accompanied by obscuring artifact. Subclinical seizures that might otherwise go unnoticed are very effectively detected by an auditory analysis of rapidly reviewed cassette EEG.

The 16-channel epoch recorder does not use a video playback device. A demultiplexer is interposed between a cassette player and a standard EEG machine upon which the recorded epochs are transcribed onto paper in real time. A time-code reading and writing device is available to transcribe onto paper the time of the recorded epochs. Analysis otherwise is like that of standard EEG, except that only short periodic epochs (e.g., 5–20 sec) are available for review, unless the recorder was activated by the push-button, which initiates a several-minute recording period. Although this greatly reduces the time necessary to read the record, the intermittent sampling can miss infrequent interictal abnormalities or seizures for which the patient has no aura. The disconnected nature of the tracing can make it difficult to assess the artifactual versus epileptiform nature of isolated paroxysms.

Behavioral Recording

A major goal of long-term monitoring is the correlation of behavior with EEG findings. Behavioral and electroencephalographic data are truly complementary. Bizarre behaviors that are not easily recognized as seizures are given credence by a simultaneous ictal discharge on EEG. Conversely, classic behavioral manifestations of a seizure may be sufficient to diagnose epilepsy even in the face of no EEG abnormality during such an episode. Although a variety of techniques for behavioral monitoring may be employed, only certain ones are applicable to telemetered and ambulatory EEG monitoring. With increasing mobility there is, by necessity, progressively less ability to document behavior objectively. This is probably the most significant trade-off ambulatory EEG makes to traditional inpatient intensive monitoring (4).

Self-reporting is the principal form of behavior monitoring used with ambulatory cassette EEG. A daily diary or log in which the patient notes the occurrence of behavioral episodes in question is the basic mechanism. A more advanced form of self-reporting includes the use of a push-button event marker for the patient to signal an event of note. The advantages of self-reporting are that: (a) it is simple, (b) it requires little special equipment, (c) it is easy to implement, and (d) it is a practical way to monitor patients with infrequent seizures. The disadvantages are that: (a) the behavioral correlation is subjective, (b) there is no objective record of behavior available for repeat or detailed analysis, (c) temporal correlation may be inaccurate, especially when an event marker is not used, and (d) self-reporting is not useful with seizures for which the patient has no warning or memory.

Observer-reporting complements self-reporting in all forms of logs and diaries and in the use of push-button event markers. Although the observations of family members and friends are often useful, those of trained medical personnel can be more objective. This is the major form of behavior monitoring in ambulatory cassette EEG recordings of young children or mentally retarded patients who cannot reliably self-report. It is also routinely used in inpatient settings with telemetered EEG when personnel are available. Behavioral data in this instance can be recorded on the EEG if a continuous hard copy is being produced, on an audio channel if the EEG is being taped, or in a log. Observer-reporting has the same advantage of simplicity as self-reporting. When performed by professional staff, more interactive assessments can also provide critical information about functional deficits accompanying episodes. It is a practical way to monitor patients as long as their seizures have a behavioral manifestation that can be recognized. The patient does not need to have a warning or memory of the event. The disadvantages, although somewhat less, are also the same as self-reporting.

Video/audio tape recording is the principal and most effective means of behavior monitoring in inpatient long-term monitoring settings. Patient activity can be continuously recorded on videotape concurrent with the taping of telemetered EEG by one of several techniques (J. Ives, *this volume*). Behavioral and EEG data are temporally correlated by means of synchronized time code or by recording both on the same tape. Video recording has the advantage that it is an objective record of behavior that is available for replay and detailed analysis. It is useful in seizures of all types, even if there are minimal behavioral manifestations, since the video record allows after-the-fact review of behavior associated with EEG changes, not just a review of EEG at times identified by behavioral events. There are, however, disadvantages. The patient has to remain "on camera" to be recorded. Mobility, even if available by cable telemetry, and especially radio telemetry techniques, is restricted by the field of the video camera. Video/audio systems can be complicated, expensive, and time-consuming to implement. When recordings are made without personnel present, interactive assessments of neurologic function are unavailable.

One of the deficiencies of outpatient ambulatory cassette-recorded EEG as compared to inpatient telemetry monitoring has always been this lack of objective behavioral information. In those instances where total patient mobility is not a necessity, the conveniences of cassette EEG recording can be combined with portable video recording to create a mobile intensive monitoring system. Outpatients can be recorded in physicians' offices, in hotel rooms, or at home, and thus avoid the inconvenience and expense of hospitalization. Compromises usually have to be made both on the part of the patient to spend most of the time on camera and on the part of the investigator to accept less than complete monitoring of all activities. Despite these negatives, the potential for additional useful information make such efforts worthwhile. The only technical necessity is that the cassette EEG tape and the videotape of patient behavior must be synchronized so that temporal correlations can be made. This is most easily done by adding a time-code generator to the video recorder system and synchronizing it to the cassette recorder time code at the beginning of a recording session. Portable video recorders can also complement cassette recording of EEG in hospitals without telemetry systems or when patients are unable to be moved to monitoring units.

Advantages and disadvantages of the three principal types of monitoring systems (cable telemetry, radio telemetry, and ambulatory cassette recording) are summarized in Table 1.

Other Uses for Ambulatory Cassette Recording

The capability of recording several channels of electrophysiologic data over long periods of time lends itself to the diagnosis or evaluation of several types of disorders other than epilepsy. The physiologic parameters other than EEG most commonly monitored are ECG, EOG, EMG, and respiration by means of strain gages, impedance pneumonography, or thermisters. Monitoring these parameters in an inpatient setting is now commonplace; their full utilization in ambulatory cassette recording is just evolving.

ECG is commonly recorded along with EEG in the evaluation of patients with sudden loss of consciousness or dizzy spells, which may be related to syn-

TABLE 1. *Advantages and disadvantages of the three principal types of monitoring systems*

Advantages	Disadvantages
Cable telemetry	
16–32 Channels Low interference Relatively simple Continuous unattended recordings for 6–10 hr Less bulky storage, tapes reusable Data can be replayed and subjected to analysis Easily adaptable to video monitoring	Limited patient mobility Inconvenience of cable Multiplexing usually required On-line monitoring requires additional device Data not easily reviewed without additional devices
Radio telemetry	
More patient mobility No tethering cable Continuous unattended recordings for 6–10 hr Less bulky storage, tapes reusable Data can be replayed and subjected to analysis	Susceptible to interference and signal dropout Limited range Multiplexing required More complicated electronics On-line monitoring requires additional device Data not easily reviewed without additional devices More difficult to use with video monitoring
Ambulatory cassette recording	
Maximum patient mobility Routine outpatient use Relatively simple Low interference Continuous unattended recordings for 24 hr Less bulky storage, tapes reusable Data can be rapidly reviewed, replayed, and subjected to analysis Data analysis by audio	Limited number of channels No on-line monitoring Additional review skills required More difficult to use with video monitoring

cope or cardiac arrhythmias rather than seizures (3,13,18). Analysis usually centers around clinical events marked in the patient diary or on the tape by an event button-push. ECG may be easily monitored in a continuous fashion during rapid playback by listening to it. Arrhythmias stand out, as they are named, from the monotonous regularity of the ongoing ECG. In one system the ECG recorded by the ambulatory EEG recorder can be analyzed on that company's ECG processor as well.

EOG and EMG monitoring are often added to EEG when evaluation of sleep cycles is desired. Sleep staging is easily performed using ambulatory EEG equipment. The temporal compression and rapid review features of ambulatory EEG systems greatly speed up this process. The dynamics of sleep are more easily appreciated as well. Such monitoring may assist in the diagnosis of narcolepsy or other sleep disorders. Measures of respiration may be added to the above parameters in order to evaluate paroxysmal disorders of respiration, such as sleep apnea or sudden infant death syndrome. The new 8-channel systems are obviously better suited to these multiparameter studies. Fewer than three EEG channels should not be used if epilepsy is one of the diagnostic considerations.

EFFICACY RELATIVE TO TRADITIONAL EEG

The overall usefulness of intensive inpatient monitoring at specialized epilepsy centers has been the subject of a number of reports. More accurate seizure classification, identification of additional seizure types, improved seizure control, and an overall improvement in the lifestyle of epileptic patients have resulted from the multifaceted services provided by epilepsy centers in the context of intensive monitoring. In addition to combined video/EEG recording, antiepileptic drug monitoring, neuropsychological testing, psychiatric, social, and occupational counseling each play an important role. Several studies have documented the superiority of intensive neurodiagnostic monitoring as compared to routine EEG in the detection of seizures among a population of epileptic patients—50 and 70% yield for long-term monitoring versus 2½ and 7% yield for baseline EEG (21,22). Most studies have concerned patients with medically refractory seizures, and among those improved seizure control following intensive inpatient monitoring was seen in 70%, 68%, and 60% in three different series (22,23,33). Some change in the classification of seizure type was seen in 48% and 84% of patients with intractable epilepsy, and a second previously unrecognized type of seizure was documented in 20% and 60% of patients in the same two studies (22,33). This added information about the patients' seizure disorders allowed a more rational and objective reconsideration of their drug therapy. In one investigation 22% of patients admitted over a 3-year period for evaluation of presumed epilepsy were found to have nonepileptic attacks of varying etiology, psychiatric and cardiovascular; sleep disorders; toxicity; and movement disorders (21). Clinically useful information was obtained in 72% of patients monitored in another study (2), including 67% in which the referral question was answered.

Although there was initially concern over the usefulness of ambulatory cassette-recorded EEG (ACR) data when restricted to three or four channels, an early large clinical study (465 patients) found that approximately 20% of patients with normal routine EEGs had abnormal findings on ambulatory recordings (27). Later controlled studies comparing 3-channel ambulatory cassette EEG to 8- or 16-channel cable telemetry showed respectable relative yields (77 and 93%) in the identification of epileptiform abnormalities (4,9). Detection of seizures was 100% for those both generalized and focal, and false positive errors were at an acceptable level. The ability of the electroencephalographer to differentiate abnormalities from artifacts and normal transients on rapid video review was found to be a greater limiting factor than the restricted number of data channels (7,8,19). This was confirmed in a recent comparison of 3- and 8-channel ambulatory EEG systems, which showed nearly comparable yield in the detection of both ictal and interictal EEG features (6). Only in detailed characterization of epileptiform events were eight channels shown to be superior to three. However, 8-channel recordings clearly had an advantage in differentiating true abnormalities from artifacts and in so doing yielded a reduced number of false positive errors. In these same studies, ambulatory EEG monitoring was shown conclusively to be superior to routine baseline recordings. Identification of epileptiform abnormalities, both interictal and ictal, was increased by ambulatory EEG over routine EEG by a factor of 1.5 to 2.5 (4,9).

In an analysis of clinical usefulness relative to the referral questions, 24 hr of ambulatory EEG was found to provide as much positive or negative information as did intensive inpatient monitoring (average 4.4 days) in 60% of diagnostic admissions (4). The greatest advantage of intensive inpatient monitoring over ambulatory EEG was not its electroencephalographic superiority, but the additional information obtained through video monitoring of behavior and the ability to withdraw antiepileptic medications under medical observation. Ambulatory EEG recordings need not, however, be limited to 24 hr or to outpatients. Its use in an inpatient or monitored outpatient setting coupled with the capability to do video recording and perhaps selective drug withdrawal could make this form of recording nearly comparable to current day intensive monitoring for many indications.

INDICATIONS

In light of the preceding discussions, the following is an outline of recommended clinical indications for mobile and ambulatory EEG monitoring. This listing is not meant to be all inclusive, since special circumstances may warrant additional considerations.

Diagnosis

1. Documentation of clinically suspected, paraoxysmal electrographic abnormalities in patients with normal or equivocal routine EEG studies. These include seizures, overt and subclinical, and interictal epileptiform discharges.

EEG abnormalities that are identified may assist in the differential diagnosis of seizure disorder from syncope, cardiac arrythmias, transient ischemic attacks, narcolepsy, other sleep disturbances, psychogenic seizures, or other behavioral disorders.

2. Verification of the ictal nature of new "spells" in a patient with previously documented and controlled seizures.
3. Documentation of clinically suspected, non-EEG, paroxysmal electrographic abnormalities. These include cardiac arrythmias via ECG, abnormalities of sleep or sleep-related respiration via EEG, EMG, EOG, ECG, and/or respiration parameters.

Classification/Characterization

1. Electrographic classification of seizure type(s) in a patient with documented but poorly characterized epilepsy.
2. Characterization (lateralization, localization, distribution) of EEG abnormalities, both ictal and interictal, associated with seizure disorders.
   The extent of characterization is dependent on the number of EEG channels available. Lateralization, but not localization, is possible with 4-channel ambulatory EEG systems.
3. Characterization of the relationship of seizures to specific precipitating circumstances or stimuli (e.g., nocturnal, catamenial, situation-related, activity-related). Verification and/or characterization of periodic seizure patterns.

Quantification

1. Quantification of the number or frequency of seizures and/or interictal discharges and their relationship to naturally occurring events or cycles.
2. Quantitative documentation of the EEG response (ictal and interictal) to a therapeutic intervention or modification (e.g., drug alteration).
   Monitoring objective EEG features is most useful in patients with frequent seizures and/or interictal discharges, and particularly with absence and other seizures having indiscernible or minimal behavioral manifestations.

There are, however, several areas where ambulatory cassette EEG recording is not adequate because of its spatial sampling restrictions and technical limitations. These are in the final evaluation of patients for possible seizure surgery and in the documentation of electrocerebral silence in those patients with possible brain death. Additionally, a negative ACR/EEG, i.e., no electrographic changes or definite epileptiform activity during a spell, cannot by itself establish a diagnosis of a nonepileptic seizure or psychiatric disturbances. True complex partial seizures may have no surface EEG manifestations. Video/

EEG monitoring is recommended for these differential diagnoses. Sixteen channel epoch recordings are also not appropriate in the evaluation of interictal features or seizures for which the patient has no aura or is too confused to push the marker button.

REFERENCES

1. Ajmone-Marsan, C., and Zivin, L.S. (1970): Factors related to the occurrence of typical paroxysmal abnormalities in the EEG records of epileptic patients. *Epilepsia*, 11:361–381.
2. Binnie, C.D., Rowan, A.J., Overweg, J., Meinardi, H., Wisman, T., Kamp, A., and Lopes da Silva F. (1981): Telemetric EEG and video monitoring in epilepsy. *Neurology (NY)*, 31:298–303.
3. Blumhardt, L.D., and Oozeer, R. (1983): Simultaneous ambulatory monitoring of the EEG and ECG in patients with unexplained transient disturbances of consciousness. In: *ISAM-GENT-1981. Proceedings of the Fourth International Symposium on Ambulatory Monitoring*, edited by F.D. Stott, S.L. Wright, E.B. Raftery, and D.L. Clement, pp. 171–182. Academic Press, London.
4. Bridgers, S.L., and Ebersole, J.S. (1985): The clinical utility of ambulatory cassette EEG monitoring. *Neurology (Cleveland)*, 35:166–173.
5. Delgado-Escueta, A.V. (1979): Epileptogenic paroxysms: modern approaches and clinical correlations. *Neurology (NY)*, 29:1014–1022.
6. Ebersole, J.S., and Bridgers, S.L. (1985): Direct comparison of 3- and 8-channel ambulatory cassette EEG with intensive inpatient monitoring. *Neurology (Cleveland)*, 35:846–854.
7. Ebersole, J.S., Bridgers, S.L., and Silva, C.G. (1983): Differentiation of epileptiform abnormalities from normal transients and artifacts on ambulatory cassette EEG. *Am. J. EEG Technol.*, 23:113–125.
8. Ebersole, J.S., and Leroy, R.F. (1983): An evaluation of ambulatory cassette EEG monitoring: II. Detection of interictal abnormalities. *Neurology (Cleveland)*, 33:8–18.
9. Ebersole, J.S., and Leroy, R.F. (1983): An evaluation of ambulatory cassette EEG monitoring: III. Diagnostic accuracy compared to intensive inpatient EEG monitoring. *Neurology (Cleveland)*, 33:853–860.
10. Ebersole, J.S., and Spencer, S.S. (1981): The efficacy of 24-hour EEG monitoring in the epilepsy diagnosis. *Epilepsia*, 22:235–236.
11. Gotman, J. (1982): Automatic recognition of the epileptic seizures in the EEG. *Electroencephalogr. Clin. Neurophysiol.*, 54:530–540.
12. Gotman, J., Ives, J.R., and Gloor, P. (1979): Automatic recognition of interictal epileptic activity in prolonged EEG recordings. *Electroencephalogr. Clin. Neurophysiol.*, 46:510–520.
13. Graf, M., Brunner, G., Weber, H., Auinger, C., and Joskowicz, G. (1982): Simultaneous long-term recording of EEG and ECG in "Syncope" patients. In: *Mobile Long-term EEG Monitoring: Proceedings of the MLE Symposium, Bonn, May 1982*, edited by H. Stefan and W. Burr, pp. 67–75. Fischer, New York.
14. Ives, J.R. (1982): A completely ambulatory 16-channel cassette recording system. In: *Mobile Long-term EEG Monitoring: Proceedings of the MLE Symposium, Bonn, May 1982*, edited by H. Stefan and W. Burr, pp. 205–217. Fischer, New York.
15. Ives, J.R., Thompson, C.J., and Gloor, P. (1976): Seizure monitoring: a new tool in electroencephalography. *Electroencephalogr. Clin. Neurophysiol.*, 41:422–427.
16. Ives, J.R., and Woods, J.F. (1975): Four-channel 24 hour cassette recorder for long-term EEG monitoring of ambulatory patients. *Electroencephalogr. Clin. Neurophysiol.*, 39:88–92.
17. Kamp, A., and Lopes da Silva, F. (1982): Special techniques of recording and transmission. In: *Electroencephalography—Basic Principles, Clinical Applications, and Related Fields*, edited by E. Niedermeyer and F. Lopes da Silva, pp. 639–654. Urban and Schwartzenberg, Baltimore.
18. Lai, C., and Ziegler, D.K. (1981): Syncope problem solved by continuous ambulatory simultaneous EEG/EKG recording. *Neurology (NY)*, 31:1152–1154.

19. Leroy, R.F., and Ebersole, J.S. (1983): An evaluation of ambulatory, cassette EEG monitoring: I. Montage design. *Neurology (Clevland)*, 33:1–7.
20. Marson, G.B., and McKinnon, J.B. (1972): A miniature tape recorder for many applications. *Control and Instrumentation*, 4:46–47.
21. Mattson, R.H. (1980): Value of intensive monitoring. In: *Advances in Epileptology. The Xth Epilepsy International Symposium*, edited by J.A. Wada and J.K. Penry, pp. 43–52. Raven Press, New York.
22. Perry, T.R., Gumnit, R.J., Gates, J.R., and Leppik, I.E. (1983): Routine EEG vs. intensive monitoring in the evaluation of intractable epilepsy. *Public Health Rep.*, 98:384–389.
23. Porter, R.J., Penry, J.K., and Lacy, J.R. (1977): Diagnostic and therapeutic reevaluation of patients with intractable epilepsy. *Neurology (Minneapolis)*, 27:1006–1011.
24. Porter, R.J., Theodore, W.H., and Schulman, E.A. (1981): Intensive monitoring of intractable epilepsy: a two year follow-up. In: *Advances in Epileptology: XIIth Epilepsy International Symposium*, edited by M. Dam, L. Gram, and J.K. Penry, pp. 265–268. Raven Press, New York.
25. Porter, R.J., Wolf, A., and Penry, J.K. (1971): Human electroencephalographic telemetry: A review of systems and their applications and a new receiving system. *Am. J. EEG Technol.*, 11:145–159.
26. Quy, R.J. (1978): A miniature preamplifier for ambulatory monitoring of the electroencephalogram. *J. Physiol* (*Lond.*), 284:23–24.
27. Ramsay, R.E. (1982): Clinical usefulness of ambulatory EEG monitoring of the neurological patient. In: *ISAM-GENT-1981. Proceedings of the Fourth International Symposium on Ambulatory Monitoring*, edited by F.D. Stott, S.L. Wright, E.B. Raftery, and D.L. Clement, pp. 234–243. Academic Press, London.
28. Riley, T.L., Porter, R.J., White, B.G., and Penry, J.K. (1981): The hospital experience and seizure control. *Neurology (NY)*, 31:912–915.
29. Shewmon, D.A. and Krentler, K.A. (1984): Off-line montage reformatting. *Electroencephalogr. Clin. Neurophysiol.*, 57:591–595.
30. Stalberg, E. (1976): Experiences with long-term telemetry in routine diagnostic work. In: *Quantitative Studies in Epilepsy*, edited by P. Kellaway and I. Petersen, pp. 269–278. Raven Press, New York.
31. Stevens, J.R., Milstein, V.M., and Dodds, S. (1969): Prolonged recording of EEG by radiotelemetry: an aid to localization and treatment of epilepsy. *Electroencephalogr. Clin. Neurophysiol.*, 27:544.
32. Stores, G., Hennion, T., Quy, R.J. (1980): EEG ambulatory monitoring system with visual play-back display. In: *Advances in Epileptology. The Xth Epilepsy International Symposium*, edited by J.A. Wada and J.K. Penry, pp. 89–94. Raven Press, New York.
33. Sutula, T.P., Sackellares, J.C., Miller, J.Q., and Dreifuss, F. (1981): Intensive monitoring in refractory epilepsy. *Neurology (NY)*, 31:243–247.

Advances in Neurology, Vol. 46: Intensive Neurodiagnostic Monitoring, edited by R. J. Gumnit. Raven Press, New York © 1986.

Ambulatory Diagnostic Monitoring of Seizures in Children

Gregory Stores

National Centre for Children with Epilepsy and University of Oxford Department of Psychiatry, Park Hospital for Children, Headington, Oxford, OX3 7LQ England

ASSESSMENT ISSUES

There are two main aspects of the diagnosis of seizures in children. The first concerns the differential diagnosis of attacks, that is, the recognition of seizures in comparison with the many other types of acute, short-lived episodes of altered behavior in children. The second aspect is the clarification of seizure type in children whose seizure disorder has been established.

The procedures available for both these diagnostic purposes consist of: clinical assessment by means of accurate documentation of the child's attacks, the child's past history and general condition; conventional EEG recordings (by which is meant standard recordings and those obtained under conditions of sleep deprivation or sleep), and intensive neurodiagnostic monitoring. The methods comprising the last of these procedures are video/EEG monitoring, telemetry, and cassette recording. Radio telemetry and cable telemetry, allowing the child sufficient freedom of movement to walk about within the hospital, are ambulatory procedures. The same is obviously true of cassette recording which permits the child to be investigated outside the hospital setting, if required.

Ideally, information would be available to allow the relative merits of these diagnostic procedures to be assessed. The most appropriate way of making these comparisons would be to investigate a cohort of patients by means of these procedures and judge them directly with each other. Such a systematic comparison has not been carried out and there must be some doubt whether it would be ethically justified to put children through such an assessment battery, irrespective of the benefit to them of the investigation. As a result, comparisons are only possible on different patient groups and must, therefore, be tentative.

Even so, by what criteria should the merits of any diagnostic procedure be judged? Fundamentally the procedure needs to be acceptable to children to obtain the information required. In the case of such investigations, findings need to be of sufficient technical merit to allow them to be evaluated meaningfully. The diagnostic yield of the procedure is the all-important clinical consideration but clearly its cost must come into the reckoning.

MISDIAGNOSIS

Before considering the respective merits of different procedures, it is appropriate to ask to what extent special investigations are necessary for accurate diagnosis. The evidence is that clinical assessment alone commonly gives rise to diagnostic doubt or error.

Episodic, brief disturbances of behavior are common in children and are of many different types, some physical, others psychological in nature. Such attacks are often confused with each other. In a recent series (6), nonepileptic attacks had been misdiagnosed as epilepsy in 25% of cases. The childhood conditions most usually misdiagnosed in this way were syncope, breath-holding attacks, aggressive outbursts, night terrors, and migraine. Panic attacks and psychogenic seizures had been mistaken for epilepsy in adolescents.

Those working in epilepsy clinics are aware of the converse problem that seizures may not be recognized as such and may well be mistaken for psychological disorders. Absences and complex partial seizures are of this type as well as nonconvulsive status. Even when a correct diagnosis of epilepsy is made, mistakes may occur in identifying precisely the child's type of seizure. Absences and complex partial seizures tend to be confused with each other because their characteristic distinguishing features are not fully appreciated or considered when seizure descriptions are obtained (7). Other diagnostic limitations include the failure to distinguish clinically between partial seizures, secondarily generalized and tonic-clonic seizures which are generalized from the outset. Similarly, insufficiently detailed descriptions may fail to identify the benign epilepsies of childhood and the opportunity for reassurance about the future course of the disorder is missed.

In general, therefore, clinical assessment of attacks probably produces diagnostic uncertainty or mistakes in a significant number of children. The solution partly lies in ensuring more accurate descriptions of attacks and the circumstances in which they occur. However, even with careful clinical documentation the nature of the child's attacks may remain unclear. This is a place for special studies to improve diagnostic accuracy.

CONVENTIONAL EEG PROCEDURES

Traditionally, in these circumstances, assistance has been sought from EEG recordings. However, the contribution of conventional EEG recordings has been largely disappointing. Interattack findings can be misleading. A normal EEG soon after an apparent convulsion is strong evidence that the attack was not organic, but outside this special situation even repeatedly normal interattack results do not exclude the possibility that the attacks are organic. On the other hand, the presence of unusual features (seen more in children's EEGs than in adults) does not necessarily have pathological significance. In retarded children the presence of interattack spikes or other pathological features may be a reflection of brain dysfunction, rather than convincing evidence that the attacks in question are seizures. If children with seizures have epileptic features in their interictal recordings, again this does not necessarily imply that the new attacks about which diagnostic uncertainty exists are epileptic. Further interattack recordings under conditions of sleep or sleep deprivation may increase the confidence with which brief recordings are interpreted (at least in nonretarded children without a history of seizures), but the ability to record during a patient's attack is highly advantageous. The possibility of doing so increases significantly with the use of intensive neurodiagnostic monitoring.

SPECIAL CONSIDERATIONS CONCERNING INTENSIVE NEURODIAGNOSTIC MONITORING IN CHILDREN

Intensive monitoring in children is generally a more difficult proposition than in the case of adult patients. What characteristic features of children are of special relevance?

1. Children do not easily understand the nature and importance of investigations. They are more likely to become frightened, bored, or otherwise intolerant of the monitoring procedure, especially where restrictions are imposed on their activities or some degree of discomfort is involved. Young or retarded children are more likely to interfere with the recording system.
2. Children are smaller than adults. This has implications for the size of the equipment, a point of special relevance when component parts have to be attached to, or carried by, the patient. At least some children are very sensitive about wearing recording equipment that is obvious to others. Although it may sometimes be possible to present wearing recorders or transmitters as part of an interesting game, unobtrusive recording is more acceptable for general use.
3. Children are generally more active than adults. In particular, they play, sometimes roughly, so that equipment for use throughout these activities needs to be robust and to remain securely attached.
4. Children are less able to provide accurate reports of their experiences or activities over long periods. Therefore investigators have to be more reliant on observers for objective information on these points. Schoolchildren may well move through several different situations during the recording period, at least from home to school and back again. During hospital investigations they are likely to encounter a wide variety of different circumstances and staff, intensifying the need to ensure accurate and consistent observational reporting.
5. Most children prefer home to hospital. Long admissions for monitoring purposes are undesirable for this reason alone. Purposes of short, planned

admissions for monitoring may well be frustrated because of the apparent universal experience that patients' attacks, including definite seizures, occur less frequently or stop completely on admission.

Overall, when working with children, much attention has to be paid to these practical problems as well as technological considerations. An essential part of pediatric EEG practice is the skills of careful, caring, and patient technicians, able to secure and maintain the child's cooperation. The help of parents, teachers, nursing and other staff in intimate contact with the child, over what might be a prolonged recording period, cannot be overestimated.

VIDEO/EEG MONITORING

The considerable diagnostic potential of video/EEG monitoring of attacks in patients of all ages is evident from the reviews in this volume. In a sense, video/EEG monitoring represents the ideal in that it can provide information for repeated review of the simultaneous clinical and EEG features during the episode in question. In this way recognition of seizures may be greatly facilitated and the precise nature of a child's seizures may become evident. Tapes produced by this means are of considerable teaching value in providing a compelling demonstration of the attacks. A high level of technical merit is easily possible with current video recording systems which need not be expensive.

In our own center, video monitoring is used when practicable. Over the last several years 37 children with attacks of an uncertain nature have been investigated this way. In 26 children attacks occurred during the recording period. On the basis of the recorded information a firm diagnosis of epilepsy was possible in 14 children. In the remaining 12, the absence of EEG changes at the time of the attacks, taken with other details of each case, was considered to infer that the child's attacks were not epileptic in nature. The diagnostic yield in this series was therefore in the order of 70%.

Over the same period video/EEG monitoring was performed on an additional 25 children who were known to have epilepsy and in whom the prime purpose of the investigation was to clarify their seizure type. Attacks were recorded in 19 of this group and additional information was obtained in all, representing a diagnostic yield, in terms of accurate seizure classification, of 76%.

However, video/EEG monitoring of children carries some disadvantages. In particular, it is an inpatient procedure in which the child has to be confined to a recording studio, the unfamiliar nature of which may well inhibit the attacks in question. Restriction of free movement over a long period is often not possible with young or disturbed children. In other, more compliant children, boredom and distress are common consequences. Greater freedom of movement can be provided by the combined use of a portable video system and a radio telemetry system. By this means, split-screen recording of children playing in the hospital grounds can be achieved (G. Stores, *unpublished data*). Although equipment is not costly, video/EEG monitoring is an overall expensive exercise because it is staff intensive. With children the procedure often requires the continuous presence of an EEG technician and an additional staff member to accompany the child.

AMBULATORY MONITORING SYSTEMS

Although reference has sometimes been made to the use of "ambulatory" (cassette) EEG monitoring in relatively immobile infants and in sleep studies, for the purposes of the present discussion ambulatory monitoring will be defined literally, that is, monitoring of the fully mobile patient. Binnie (1) has provided a thoughtful review of monitoring procedures that fall within this definition but his discussion of portable cassette recording systems did not include the recently developed 8-channel Medilog system.

Although cable telemetry can be specially adapted to extend its range within the hospital setting (3), such a system still restricts the patient's freedom of movement within one area of the hospital. The ambulatory monitoring systems (for fully mobile patients) currently available therefore consist of: radio telemetry which requires the patient to be within the hospital precincts in proximity to the EEG receiver, although the use of multiple aerials in different parts of the hospital extends the patient's range of movement as described by Porter et al. (8); cassette recorders with normal tape speed but with limited recording duration (2); and cassette recorders of low tape speed but long recording duration. The last type of system, in 4-channel form, has been used for the past several years. Recently, an 8-channel system has been developed.

8-Channel Medilog System

In 1975 Ives and Woods (4) described the adaptation of the Medilog EEG recorder for prolonged EEG monitoring. Three years later this 4-channel system became commercially available and has been used extensively in children and adults for various clinical purposes (10,12), although the main use has been in the differential diagnosis of attacks.

The main reservations about the system were the availability of only 4 channels, one of which was often sacrificed to allow the occurrence of clinical events to be marked on the cassette tape. The recent development of an 8-channel system has been of particular interest in the increased versatility of use that it offers. The main features of the two commerically available systems have been described by J. Ebersole (*this volume*). A particular feature (from the point of view of monitoring children) is that they preserve the quality of being relatively unobtrusive and therefore they are appropriate for outpatient use. In addition the recorders are robust and capable of withstanding rough handling. Although the 8-channel recorder is rather heavier and bigger than its 4-channel counterpart, it is still acceptable to most children.

8-Channel Ambulatory Cassette EEG Recordings at the Park Hospital for Children

Over the past 3 years a total of 5,906 hours of 8-channel (Medilog) recording has been carried out on 86 children at the Park Hospital in Oxford. The age of the children has ranged from 4 to 16 years. They were referred to the Park Hospital EEG Unit which provides a service as part of the National Centre for Children with Epilepsy, although it is mainly a service for children's hospitals in the Oxford region. Thirty-two percent of this series were investigated as part of the latter, nonspecialist EEG service. The intellectual level of these children ranged from severe retardation to above average, 23% being retarded to some extent.

Eighty-four recordings consisted of EEG alone, the remainder combined EEG with ECG. The recordings were carried out at home or at school in 34 cases. The rest were performed either at the Park Hospital itself or in general pediatric wards elsewhere. During this evaluation period one additional recording with early equipment failed and no information was obtained at all. The recording period ranged from 24 hr to 18 days. Twenty-two recordings were restricted to 24 hr and 30 lasted 25 to 48 hr, 20 continued from 49 to 72 hr and 14 were extended beyond 72 hr.

The main purpose of the recordings was the investigation of attacks (47 patients), the next most frequent indication being the need to clarify the child's seizure type (26 patients). In eight children, the possibility of subtle seizures affecting their mental state (especially performance at school) had been raised. In the remaining five children, monitoring was carried out with the intention of quantifying the child's seizure discharge in relation to changes in drug treatment. This last use will not be considered further here other than to say that it was a valuable means of objectively assessing nonconvulsive seizure frequency, especially in children with communication problems.

Of the 47 children with attacks of an uncertain nature, 27 had a past history of definite epilepsy. The question arising in this subgroup was whether or not their new attacks were an additional form of seizure manifestation. This was shown to be so in seven children by the presence of seizure activity at the time of their attacks. Fifteen had no EEG accompaniments of their attacks. The remaining five children in this subgroup did not have attacks during the recording period.

The 20 children with attacks and no past history of definite epilepsy were characteristically referred by child psychiatrists rather than pediatricians. Twelve of these children had no attacks during the recording period. Of the eight who did have attacks, none showed EEG changes at the time.

In the eight children in whom subtle seizures had been suspected as a cause of poor school performance, this was confirmed in four. This included one child with periods of absence status occurring several times every day, but manifested by only mild clouding of consciousness. As such, the occurrence of such seizures had been overlooked by parents, teachers, and ward staff. Combining those children with attacks and those investigated for subtle seizures (total 55 children) it was considered that EEG findings had contributed significantly to diagnosis in 34 (62%). Of those, a confident diagnosis of seizures was made in 11 including the occurrence of partial seizures in five.

Twenty-six children with known epilepsy were monitored in the hope that recording during their seizures would clarify their seizure type. In this group conventional, interictal recordings (including sleep EEGs) had produced uncertain results. In particular, the main seizure source was unclear. Twenty-three had attacks during the recording period and it was considered that significant new information, relevant to this issue, was obtained in 20 of these children, an overall yield of 70%. Five had attacks accompanied by generalized seizure activity alone, nine showed evidence of localized discharge only, and the remaining six showed both localized and generalized seizure activity. Three of the other six children produced no additional information to that already obtained from conventional recordings. Interestingly, the remaining three children had no seizure discharge at the time of their recorded attacks, raising the possibility that they had a combination of seizures and nonepileptic attacks.

PRACTICAL ASPECTS OF AMBULATORY CASSETTE RECORDING WITH CHILDREN

Experience with this system at the Park Hospital suggests the following factors are important in its use: patient selection, contact with parents, fitting the recorder, length of recording, and interpretation of negative findings.

Patient Selection

New technologies often attract inappropriate referrals. Ambulatory monitoring is likely to justify its use if restricted to patients for whom clinical assessment of their problems has been diagnostically insufficient or where conventional EEG procedures have not provided a solution. In the case of children with attacks, careful clinical assessment is a prerequisite. For practical purposes, their attacks need to be occurring several times a week to provide a reasonable prospect of recording during such episodes.

Contact with Parents

Before the child attends the hospital for the recorder to be fitted, a check should be made with the parents that the attacks are still occurring frequently enough to justify the procedure. Parents, teachers, and others involved should have the precise nature of the procedure explained. It should also be made clear that the recording may need to be continued for several days if the attack frequency falls below that which is expected.

Fitting the Recorder

The increased size and weight of the 8-channel recorder over its 4-channel counterpart makes it somewhat unsuitable for use in children under the age of 4 years. For younger children above this age level, it is probably best to wear the recorder in a satchel rather than on a belt. Parents should be instructed on the importance of carefully kept records of the child's activities over the recording period, especially regarding timing and description of attacks. Diaries specially provided for this purpose are advisable, requiring entries or descriptions to be made at specified intervals.

Length of Recording

The procedure is best continued until several attacks have been recorded, especially where attacks of different types have been described. The possibility of a combination of epileptic and nonepileptic attacks needs to be considered. For recordings above 24 hr, inpatients can return to the EEG department for replacement of cassettes and batteries and re-jelling of electrodes.

Capable parents of outpatients can be supplied with the materials required to continue recording. Removal of electrodes may be necessary at intervals of several days to allow the patient to bathe, with reattachment afterwards to avoid skin reactions. Acetone fumes in the removal of the electrodes can be unpleasant for the child and adequate ventilation and protection of the eyes is strongly recommended.

Interpretation of Negative Findings

Seizure activity at the time of attacks is a valuable finding. Interpretation of the absence of EEG change at this time is contentious. The frequency with which undoubted seizures are unaccompanied by scalp-recorded EEG change is not known, but estimates as high as 20% have been made in patients with partial seizures (1,5). In such patients the negative EEG changes have to be considered in conjuction with information about the attacks and the patient in general, and a judgment made about the likely nature of the attacks. In general, it seems that negative findings significantly increase the chance that the attacks are not epileptic in type. In a recent follow-up over a 3-year period of 25 children with such negative findings during attacks in 4-channel Medilog recordings, only one child had been subsequently shown to have epilepsy (G. Stores, *unpublished*). The importance of follow-up in such cases is obvious.

INDICATIONS FOR AMBULATORY CASSETTE RECORDING, ADVANTAGES AND DISADVANTAGES

On the basis of Park Hospital experience and preliminary reports (P. Plouin, *personal communication*) and Powell et al. (9) it appears that the 8-channel cassette-recording system can be profitably used for the diagnosis of attacks in children and for the clarification of seizure type in children with established epilepsy. The procedure is of special value where admission of the child to hospital for video/EEG or telemetry investigation is not feasible, where inpatient video/EEG or telemetry investigation is not available, or when no attacks occur during the period of inpatient admission. Outpatient cassette recording may be the only realistic way of investigating the influence of real life environmental factors on attack occurrence.

The procedure generally allows more prolonged recording periods than other intensive monitoring systems. With a sympathetic approach to the child and care in fitting the recorder, the system is acceptable to children and parents, largely because of its unobtrusive nature. In our experience, it has rarely been significantly interfered with by children and is capable of a high degree of technical reliability and good quality traces. In contrast to video/EEG and telemetry monitoring, the system does not require the constant attention of a technician, although clear instructions to parents and others in close contact with the child are essential to ensure continuity of good observational recording, especially over long periods. The system is versatile, allowing the detection of both partial and generalized seizures as well as investigation of other aspects of seizure disorders, such as response to antiepileptic drugs and the identification of other patterns of occurrence (11). Other applications outside the field of epilepsy include sleep studies with patients sleeping at home.

A potential difficulty with a cassette recording is the reliance that must be placed on accurate reporting of the child's behavior during the recording period. Parents, nurses, and others vary greatly in the ease with which they will be able to provide the necessary clinical detail. The provision of observation sheets or diaries helps to standardize observations, but explicit instruction is required. The prospect of variable standards of reporting as the child moves from one situation and observer to another, especially during the school day, was mentioned earlier.

At present the main cost of cassette recording lies in the initial purchase of equipment and the time the technician or electroencephalographer must spend in reviewing the large amount of information collected in this way.

FUTURE RESEARCH

Automated analysis is the next logical step in the development of a self-contained cassette-recording system. The prospect of achieving this has been discussed by J. Gotman (*this volume*). A further area in which greater effort is required is the translation into practical advantages to the patient (usually by devising or altering the treatment strategies) of the results of cassette recording or any other form of intensive monitoring. The rarity with which this translation has been demonstrated empirically is emphasized by C. Binnie (*this volume*).

SUMMARY

Considerable scope still exists for more accurate recognition of childhood seizures and the definition of their precise type. Careful clinical observation is generally the most appropriate way of achieving these objectives. However, in a proportion of patients even detailed clinical evaluation will leave this issue unclear. Intensive neurodiagnostic monitoring carries the advantage over conventional EEG recordings in generally increasing the likelihood of recording during the child's attacks.

Special consideration has to be given to children in carrying out intensive monitoring, largely because of their limited understanding of investigatory procedures and lessened ability to cooperate compared with adults, including adjustment to hospital admission. Equipment design must acknowledge the smaller size of children and the fact that they are generally more active than adult patients. In order to help interpretation of the EEG findings, great reliance has to be placed on the observation by parents and other observers in achieving adequate behavioral accounts.

The comparative acceptance by children of the different recording procedures and their relative diagnostic yield are difficult to evaluate objectively. No systematic comparison has been made on the same group of children undergoing the various procedures. Consequently, comparisons have to be made on different patient groups investigated in different centers where it is likely there will be differences in selection criteria for investigation as well as the details of the procedure followed.

Video/EEG, telemetry, and cassette recording are best seen as complementary procedures from which a choice is made depending on the child's problem and circumstances and, in particular, whether admission to hospital for video or telemetry is possible or likely to provide the opportunity for studying the clinical phenomena in question. All are capable of high levels of technical merit and a high degree of diagnostic yield when used with appropriate indications. However, especially for EEG services outside special centers and without extra staff resources, it is likely that cassette recording in its 8-channel form has distinct advantages, both in terms of acceptability to children and of operating costs.

REFERENCES

1. Binnie, C. D. (1983): Telemetric EEG monitoring in epilepsy. In: *Recent Advances in Epilepsy,* edited by T. A. Pedley and B. S. Meldrum, pp. 155–178. Churchill Livingstone, Edinburgh.
2. Ives, J. R. (1982): A completely ambulatory 16-channel cassette recording system. In: *Mobile Long-term EEG Monitoring,* edited by H. Stefan and W. Burr, pp. 205–217. Fischer, Stuttgart.
3. Ives, J. R., Thompson, C. J., and Gloor, P. (1976): Seizure monitoring: a new tool in electroencephalography. *Electroencephalogr. Clin. Neurophysiol.,* 41:422–427.
4. Ives, J. R., and Woods, J. F. (1975): 4-Channel 24 hour cassette recorder for long-term EEG monitoring of ambulatory patients. *Electroencephalogr. Clin. Neurophysiol.,* 39:88–92.
5. Ives, J. R., and Woods, J. F. (1980): A study of 100 patients with focal epilepsy using a 4-channel ambulatory cassette recorder. In: *ISAM 1979: Proceedings of the Third International Symposium on Ambulatory Monitoring,* edited by F. D. Stott, E. B. Raftery, and L. Goulding, pp. 383–392. Academic Press, London.
6. Jeavons, P. M. (1983): Non-epileptic attacks in childhood. In: *Research Progress in Epilepsy,* edited by F. C. Rose, pp. 224–230. Pitman, London.
7. Penry, J. K., Porter, R. J., and Dreifuss, F. E. (1975): Simultaneous recording of absence seizures with video tape and electroencephalography. *Brain,* 98:427–440.
8. Porter, R. J., Wolf, A. A., and Penry, J. K. (1971): Human electroencephalographic telemetry. *Am J. Med. Technol.,* 11:145–159.
9. Powell, T. E., Jeavons, P. M., and Harding, G. F. A. (1984): An evaluation of 3 and 8 channel ambulatory monitoring. *Acta Neurol. Scand.,* 70:204–256.
10. Stefan, H., and Burr, W. (editors) (1982): *Mobile Long-term EEG Monitoring.* Fischer, Stuttgart.
11. Stores, G., and Brankin, P. (1982): Recent developments in ambulatory EEG monitoring. *Br. J. Clin. Pract. (Suppl.),* 18:10–14.
12. Stott, F. D., Raftery, E. B., Clement, D. L., and Wright, S. L. (editors) (1981): *ISAM-Gent 1981. Proceedings of the Fourth International Symposium on Ambulatory Monitoring.* Academic Press, London.

Advances in Neurology, Vol. 46: Intensive Neurodiagnostic Monitoring, edited by R. J. Gumnit. Raven Press, New York © 1986.

Ambulatory Diagnostic Monitoring of Seizures in Adults

C. D. Binnie

Department of Clinical Neurophysiology, Instituut voor Epilepsiebestrijding, 2100 Heemstede, The Netherlands

DEVELOPMENT OF AMBULATORY MONITORING

Thirty years ago, Gastaut and Bert (20) predicted, with remarkable insight, that electroencephalography (EEG) would not be confined to recording the ongoing activity of subjects reclining on an EEG couch with their eyes closed or gazing at the ceiling, but would concern itself increasingly with electrophysiological function during a wide range of everyday activities. Indeed, the technology for such studies has been available for more than 25 years (8), but monitoring of the EEGs of active subjects was introduced only in the 1960s. At first, it was used essentially as a research technique for studying the electrophysiological correlates of various psychological activities (50).

Because of the special role of the EEG in the investigation of epilepsy, it was understandable that particular attention was directed to the effect of psychological factors on the occurrence of epileptiform discharges or epileptic seizures (23,24,47). It was then only a small step to the use of continuous EEG monitoring for clinical diagnostic purposes in epilepsy, which Stevens et al. (45), with undisguised enthusiasm, described as "unexpectedly rewarding." As a research tool, EEG monitoring has provided important new insights into the phenomena and classification of epileptic seizures (12,13,16,29,36).

The transition of EEG monitoring from a research technique to a routine clinical procedure occurred rapidly as ambulatory monitoring systems became commercially available. Epileptologists and neurologists, as well as psychiatrists and pediatricians, have enthusiastically, but in general uncritically, assimilated EEG monitoring into routine clinical practice. The potential usefulness of intensive monitoring of the ictal and interictal phenomena of epilepsy may appear so self-evident that there have been remarkably few attempts at objective evaluation of the procedure in comparison with the increasing number of reports on its application.

MONITORING TECHNIQUES

Confusion also seems to have arisen about the value of EEG monitoring, on the one hand, and the utility of the various monitoring techniques, on the other. Indeed, the introduction of EEG telemetry systems appears to have promoted the notion that it is virtually impossible to study ictal EEG phenomena without their use. All too familiar at international congresses are video presentations showing technically poor telemetric recordings of seizures, often elicited by provocation and recorded from an immobile patient seated in an armchair or confined to a small room. Under these circumstances, conventional EEG recording methods would have been entirely adequate and would have produced recordings of far higher quality. Indeed, many of the most important studies of seizure phenomena, even within the last few years, have employed hard-wired recordings from essentially static subjects (12,51).

The extent to which the patient enjoys the convenience of mobility is, for most clinical applications, not material to the usefulness of the investigation, and it may be more helpful to speak of EEG monitoring without the qualification of the term "ambulatory." Intensive EEG monitoring of epilepsy comes into its own when combined with observation of behavior aided by cine or, more recently, video recording. The requirement for close behavioral observation generally imposes such restriction on the subject's mobility and range of activities that the use of telemetric EEG recording techniques to enhance mobility is more of a luxury than a necessity. Though we have access to radiotelemetry, cassette monitoring, and telephone telemetry in our center, the com-

TABLE 1. *Main features of current EEG monitoring techniques*

Features	Hard-wired EEG machine	Cable telemetry	Radio-telemetry	Cassette: Normal tape speed	Cassette: Low tape speed
Technical quality	+++	+++	+	++	–
Mobility range	3 meters	50 meters	50 meters free field; variable in building	Unlimited	Unlimited
Cost	Nil extra	+	+++	+	+
Applications					
Intensive diagnosis	++	+++	+	+	–
Seizure frequency	+	++	++	–	+++
Precipitants	+	++	+++	++	+++
Effects of normal activity in natural environment	–	–	+	++	+++

bination of cable telemetry with video recording is the most appropriate and convenient method for studying the majority of the clinical problems that we encounter. The most important characteristics of the main EEG monitoring techniques are summarized in Table 1.

Cable Telemetry

Cable telemetry, which was pioneered by Ives et al. (27), offers the possibility of EEG recording of a quality similar to that obtainable with conventional hard-wired EEG machines, without significant restriction of channel capacity, frequency, or dynamic range, at a cost currently of about $2,000 per channel.

Radiotelemetry

The possibilities of radiotelemetry are severely limited in many countries by the prevailing regulations concerning bandwidth employed for radiotelegraphy (30), and, for instance, the most advanced radiotelemetry system commercially available cannot legally be used in Western Europe or the United States. Moreover, radiotelemetry equipment, necessarily including battery packs, is generally heavier and impedes the patient more than cable telemetry preamplifiers.

Cassette Recording

Cassette recording is regarded by some as the only true form of ambulatory monitoring and permits the study of patients actively engaged in everyday activities in their normal environment. We are, for instance, sometimes asked to assess the claim that a patient who has few seizures in hospital suffers (possibly stress-related) attacks during visits home. For this purpose, there is virtually no satisfactory alternative to ambulatory cassette recording. It is the ideal technique for determining the frequency of occurrence, under real-life conditions, of EEG phenomena, the nature and topography of which are already established. Ives (26) has described a 16-channel cassette system, but as it employs a normal tape speed, it permits only 90 min of continuous recording between cassette changes.

The diagnostic use of long-duration (low tape speed) cassette recording remains controversial. The introduction of this technique, following the report of Ives and Woods (28) and the commercial production of 3- or 4-channel EEG cassette recorders, was followed by a spate of highly uncritical reports, often originating from users with no primary interest in clinical neurophysiology and claiming an extremely high yield of diagnostically valuable information, especially in distinguishing epileptic seizures, pseudoseizures, and attacks of cardiac origin. Many reports took it for granted that epileptic seizures are invariably accompanied by spikes or spike-and-wave activity in the EEG, which is far from the case. Ictal changes in the scalp-recorded EEG are usually absent in elementary partial seizures with psychic symptoms (51) and, in some other partial seizures, may be limited to subtle and localized changes in amplitude or frequency of background activity, which are barely recognizable even in a 20-channel recording of high technical quality. Electro-decremental events, in particular, may be confined to the region of the vertex and will then be missed in 4- or 8-channel montages designed to record suspected temporal phenomena.

Simultaneous EEG Telemetry and Video Monitoring

Our findings in 100 consecutive patients investigated by EEG telemetry and video monitoring for diagnostic purposes, in whom at least two seizures were recorded, are summarized in Table 2. In 7% of the patients, the combination of elementary partial seizures (usually with psychic symptomatology) and an absence of ictal changes in the scalp-recorded EEG was considered to be compatible with an epileptic etiology, and follow-up confirmed this interpretation. Although we were able to reach a diagnostic conclusion in 89 patients, there remained 11 patients in whom we were unable to reach any conclusion. Without video documentation of clinical events, this group would necessarily have been larger.

A comparative study (17) suggested that the diagnostic yield of cassette recording is not much less than that of telemetry. However, the cable telemetry system used as a reference had only eight channels. Ambulatory monitoring of the EEG alone may resolve many diagnostic problems, particularly since the introduction of 8-channel 24-hr cassette systems, but negative ictal EEG findings often require further investigation by state-of-the-art telemetry with simultaneous video recording.

TABLE 2. *Ictal and interictal EEG activity in patients with epileptic seizures and pseudoseizures*[a]

	Ictal activity		Interictal activity[b]		
Diagnosis	Epileptiform	Nonepileptiform	Epileptiform	Nonepileptiform	Patients
Epileptic seizures	42	8	7[c]	—	57
Pseudoseizures	—	—	13	19	32
Uncertain	—	—	4	7	11

[a] 327 seizures in 100 patients.
[b] With no ictal epileptiform activity.
[c] Elementary partial seizures: 5 psychic, 2 sensorimotor.

INDICATIONS FOR MONITORING

Differential Diagnosis of Seizures

Although few detailed evaluations of intensive epilepsy monitoring have been published, several authors have reported their experience and enumerated the clinical indications for this method of investigation. Some differences in emphasis are evident from Table 3. The most important group of patients requiring intensive monitoring exhibits attacks of uncertain origin. The differential diagnosis between epileptic seizures and pseudoseizures is especially difficult in patients with undoubted epilepsy. Among the admittedly highly selected population in our institute, approximately 17.5% of the patients admitted because of diagnostic problems prove to have pseudoseizures, of whom a fourth have concomitant epilepsy. Indeed, pseudoseizures may come to the fore when the epileptic attacks are successfully treated. The underlying psychodynamics are readily understood when a patient who has adapted successfully to the handicap of epilepsy is suddenly rendered seizure-free by improved treatment, but remains socially disabled without even a claim to special consideration as a person with epilepsy.

The differential diagnosis between attacks of epileptic and cardiac origin is often cited as an important indication for diagnostic monitoring. Some studies of ambulatory cassette recording report success in determining a cardiac origin in roughly one-third of the patients with symptoms resembling syncope and an

TABLE 3. *Indications for epilepsy monitoring in nine evaluation reports*

Indication	Reference No.
Differential diagnosis	5, 7, 10, 25, 38, 40, 41, 43, 48
Subjective complaints	5, 25, 48
Pseudoseizures?	5, 10, 40, 41, 43
Enuresis	5, 10
Nocturnal restlessness/apnea	5, 10, 48
Cardiac disorder/syncope?	40, 43, 48
Diurnal sleepiness	48
Episodic behavioral disturbance	10, 25, 38, 41
Hyperventilation?	41
EEG correlates of known seizures	5, 7, 10, 40, 43, 48
Classification	5, 7, 40, 48
Focus localization	5, 48
Clinical correlates of EEG discharge	5, 10, 43
Transitory cognitive impairment	5, 10, 43
Seizure frequency	5, 10, 38, 43, 48
Seizure precipitants	5, 7, 41, 48
Reflex epilepsy	5
Self-induction	5
Situational factors	48

epileptic cause in another third (11). Whatever the reason, our experience is very different. Of about 500 annual admissions for diagnostic purposes, we identify some two patients a year with attacks of cardiac origin. In the past 8 years, all such patients known to us have been identified on the basis of the medical history, routine electrocardiography (ECG), or the single-channel ECG recording, which accompanies all our diagnostic EEGs. We have never needed to resort to intensive monitoring to establish a cardiac origin of ictal symptoms, although we have on several occasions investigated patients suspected of having cardiac dysrhythmias as epileptic ictal manifestations. A recent evaluation of 7,364 ambulatory ECG monitoring studies in cardiological practice also suggests that the yield of crucial, new diagnostic information is very modest (21).

Classification of Seizures

Diagnostic monitoring is also employed in epileptic patients in whom the classification of seizures is uncertain. In our view, the clinical importance of accurate seizure classification has been exaggerated. It is, for instance, our experience that patients who have complex partial seizures which might easily be confused with absence seizures with automatisms respond best to drugs ordinarily used for the treatment of absence seizures, such as ethosuximide and sodium valproate, and are rarely helped by agents generally more appropriate for partial seizures, such as carbamazepine. Nevertheless, whatever the therapeutic relevance, this particular differential diagnosis can be extremely difficult without ictal EEG recordings (42).

Localization of EEG Foci

A widely accepted indication for monitoring is the localization of foci in patients being considered for possible neurosurgical management. Here, there is considerable variation in approach. Some centers, following the practice of such pioneers of neurosurgical treatment of epilepsy as Falconer, make virtually no use even of ictal scalp-recorded EEGs, much less of prolonged recordings with depth electrodes (37). Stringent criteria of selection, based on the interictal EEG and the clinical and neuroradiological findings, yield excellent surgical results in these necessarily restricted cases. Others claim, probably on the basis of more varied clinical material, that ictal EEG recording with depth electrodes is usually necessary to establish reliably the site of origin of the seizures (18).

An intermediate position is adopted at the Montreal Neurological Institute, where the introduction of a sophisticated system of cable telemetry and computer-assisted data reduction (22) some 10 years ago provided the capability for very prolonged seizure monitoring, with depth electrodes if necessary.

About 3 years ago, however, the indications for depth recording had become so restricted that this method was being employed in less than 15% of neurosurgical patients. More recently, however, the indications for surgical treatment were widened by the use of prolonged monitoring of repeated seizures in patients with multiple foci (33). Excellent results were obtained in a group of patients who would have been regarded as inoperable according to the criteria previously employed in the same center (6), but it was necessary to obtain on the average 70 ictal recordings from each patient. The logistical problems of achieving this without the particular facilities existing in the Montreal Neurological Institute are, to say the least, daunting.

Seizure Frequency

Monitoring is of established value for determining the seizure frequency in types of attacks easily overlooked by the patient or observers (9). These include absence seizures, which may virtually be identified with the generalized spike-and-wave discharge, and brief complex partial seizures, which may be recognizable only by careful comparison of the EEG and video recordings. Monitoring of seizure frequency is used as an aid to adjusting medication and for evaluation of new drugs (15,35,49).

Behavioral and Psychological Correlates of EEG Discharges

The obverse of studying the ictal EEG is the use of video recording to detect possible subtle clinical correlates of known EEG discharges. Where no behavioral change is detected, continuous performance testing may, nevertheless, reveal transitory cognitive impairment accompanying the discharges. The occurrence of such psychological disturbances during generalized spike-and-wave activity is well documented (32,39), but with sufficiently sensitive tasks can also be demonstrated in some patients even during subclinical focal discharges (1).

Transitory cognitive impairment appears to be regarded more as a curiosity for psychological research than as a disability that may affect a patient's social, educational, and occupational performance. Certainly, some patients are adversely affected, and we have shown that some are benefited by drug therapy to suppress the discharges (1). Lest I should seem to advocate EEG cosmetics, however, it should be stressed that we do not yet know what proportion of patients with subclinical discharges are importantly disadvantaged, and, indeed, a study is in progress to find out. Whatever the conclusion, to engage the subject in controlled activities, the performance of which can be measured, seems a logical and desirable future extension of current monitoring procedures.

Seizure Precipitants

The study of seizure precipitants includes both investigation of general situations promoting the occurrence of seizures (19) and testing of specific triggers in possible reflex epilepsies. Our interest in the reflex epilepsies and particularly in photosensitivity led us, as a direct consequence of monitoring, to the conclusion that approximately one-fourth of photosensitive patients exhibit self-induced seizures or discharges, elicited either by hand-waving or by a particular type of slow upward deviation of the eyes (3). Therefore, intensive monitoring is indicated in all photosensitive subjects, as this phenomenon of self-induction is often associated with noncompliance or resistance to conventional antiepileptic drug therapy.

Pharmacological Monitoring

Another interest in our unit is in studies combining EEG and video recording with frequent monitoring of antiepileptic drug levels in the blood, samples of which are collected via an indwelling intravenous catheter. The clinical indications are difficult to summarize briefly, since they are different for each individual patient. Nevertheless, we have found such studies to be helpful in assessing episodic symptoms where it is unclear whether or not these are ictal manifestations or related to temporary intoxication, particularly with antiepileptic drugs having short half-lives.

Such studies have also proved helpful in explaining some otherwise obscure drug interactions. For instance, some patients who were on a regimen of phenytoin and sodium valproate experienced symptoms of phenytoin intoxication at those times of the day when the total serum phenytoin level fell to a minimum. The explanation, of course, was competition between sodium valproate and phenytoin for protein binding such that the peak valproate concentration led to an increase in free phenytoin and, presumably, to displacement of phenytoin from the intra- to the extravascular compartment. In studies such as this, the role of the EEG is secondary. Nevertheless, it is helpful in some patients as evidence of intoxication or in others where the frequency of EEG discharges or seizures is clearly related to the efficacy of pharmacotherapy, most notably, of course, in patients with absence seizures.

CURRENT AND FUTURE DEVELOPMENTS

The ideal specifications for monitoring instrumentation currently exceed the capabilities of the electronics industry, but the transition of intensive monitoring from a research technique to a clinical service has led to a sudden expansion of the equipment commercially available and in development. It is hoped that this will encourage centers engaged in monitoring to acquire a range of systems for both telemetric and portable recording, so that the most appropriate technology can be selected for each different application.

The improvements in magnetic tape technology since the introduction of the first Medilog recorders a decade ago have been such that further substantial improvements in specifications of portable monitoring systems should be possible.

Nearly 10 years ago, Ives et al. (27) introduced digital buffering of EEG signals on a computer disk, writing out on paper only those sections immediately preceding and accompanying clinical events of interest. The system has been further enhanced by automatic recognition of ictal EEG changes (22) and by more convenient solid-state buffering techniques (26). Such systems have been used by some other groups (4) and seem an essential development in order to reduce operating costs and to make monitoring more widely available. The miniaturization of such systems is already feasible, and in due course cassette recording may be superceded by portable solid-state systems that will recognize and document, or store, only events of interest.

Developments in the clinical area may be expected to include increasing study, in parallel with EEG and behavior, of multiple biological variables, such as drug levels, biochemical status, hormone levels, and psychological function. Further investigation of circadian and other slow biological changes in epileptic patients (2,31,44) and healthy subjects will be required.

EVALUATION OF INTENSIVE MONITORING

Intensive EEG monitoring is a costly undertaking: In the Netherlands, the cost is approximately $800 for 24 hr of EEG telemetry with video recording and $100 for 24 hr of ambulatory cassette recording. These costs chiefly comprise salaries, as supervision during telemetry and analysis of tapes are both labor-intensive. Determining the cost effectiveness of these activities is difficult.

Stålberg (43) and other authors have suggested that approximately 60% of investigations with intensive monitoring offer answers to the questions posed by the referring physicians. Answering questions, however, is hardly cost-effective if the result is already predictable or if the findings lead to no therapeutic action that might benefit the patient. Penry and Porter (34) estimated that 5% of all persons with epilepsy require intensive monitoring. Sutula et al. (46) demonstrated that a short admission to a unit with monitoring facilities led to sustained improvement in both seizures and social function. Unrecognized seizure types were detected in 20%, and the seizure classification was revised in 47.5% of the patients. How these findings contributed to the patients' clinical improvement was not indicated.

In order to obtain some objective assessment of intensive monitoring, we carried out a prospective study in 272 patients with epilepsy or suspected epi-

TABLE 4. *Clinical problems leading to monitoring referral and yield of questions answered by EEG and video recording*[a]

Question addressed	Records (*N*)	Patients (*N*)	Questions answered Records (%)	Patients (%)
Differential diagnosis	157	141	61	65
EEG correlates of seizures	12	11	92	91
Clinical correlates of EEG	29	27	87	85
Seizure frequency	34	28	100	100
Seizure precipitants	58	54	95	95
Pharmocotherapy	76	62	96	95

[a] There were 324 records addressing 366 questions in 272 patients.

lepsy. Before the monitoring was done, the referring clinician completed a questionnaire, giving the indication for the referral, the current assessment of the clinical problem, the diagnosis, and the proposed management of the patient. A reassessment was obtained, again by questionnaire, after monitoring and during 12-months' follow-up.

Overall, some 80% of the 366 questions were answered in 324 monitoring studies (Table 4), but this depended on the indication for monitoring, the yield being highest for those applications where, short of technical failure, we could be certain of providing the information requested, and lowest in the diagnostic group where it was essential to obtain technically satisfactory EEG and video recordings of seizures.

The findings were considered to influcnce therapy in about 68% (181/266) of those patients where an answer was provided (Table 5). The group in which

TABLE 5. *Consequences of EEG and video monitoring for clinical management and outcome of patients with epileptic seizures and pseudoseizures*[a]

Consequence and outcome	Yes	No
Question answered or other relevant information provided (*N* = 324)	262	62
Consequences for management (*N* = 262)	181	81
Management changed (*N* = 181)	135	46
Follow-up (*N* = 181)		
Improvement	62	14
> 1 year	(43)	(12)
3 months–1 year	(11)	(2)
3 months	(8)	(0)
No improvement	61	27
Not applicable or lost to follow-up	12	5

[a] Total of 324 records in 272 patients.

clinical management was unchanged requires some explanation. These were chiefly patients in whom monitoring proved the diagnosis of epilepsy and led to a decision to continue antiepileptic drug therapy, which the referring physicians had intended to terminate, since the patients were supposed to have pseudoseizures only.

At follow-up, management decisions based on the results of 23% (76/324) of the monitoring studies were considered to have led to clinical improvement in 27% of the patients. The large number of instances in which this was not the case, even though the referring physician's original question was answered, chiefly reflect therapy-resistant patients in whom providing a correct diagnosis or optimizing the antiepileptic drug regimen did not necessarily lead to seizure control. However, the 27 patients whose therapy and course were unchanged included 15 in which some benefit may be claimed for the diagnosis and treatment of epilepsy, as in preventing the aforementioned withdrawal of needed medications.

The yield from this extremely costly form of investigation may appear modest but, in fact, compares very well with the therapeutic benefits resulting from other laboratory investigations in neurology, including radiodiagnostic procedures (14). Patients with a differential diagnosis between epilepsy and pseudoseizures are more than usually socially handicapped in comparison with epileptic patients of similar neurological and mental status. In the absence of a reliable diagnosis on which to base treatment, they undergo multiple and often lengthy admissions to both neurological and psychiatric institutions due to indecision about the origin of their undoubted psychosocial dysfunction: Is it primary, or is it secondary to epileptic seizures, requiring antiepileptic treatment? Breaking this vicious circle by establishing a reliable diagnosis offers the possibility of not only seizure control but also social rehabilitation (46). In these terms, if in no others, the exercise is unquestionably cost-effective.

REFERENCES

1. Aarts, J.H.P., Binnie, C.D., Smit, A.M. and Wilkins, A.J. (1984): Selective cognitive impairment during focal and generalized epileptiform EEG activity. *Brain,* 107:293–308.
2. Binnie, C.D., Aarts, J.H.P., Houtkooper, M.A., Laxminarayan, R., Martins da Silva, A., Meinardi, H., Negelkerke, N., and Overweg, J. (1984): Temporal characteristics of seizures and epileptiform discharges. *Electroencephalogr. Clin. Neurophysiol.,* 58:498–505.
3. Binnie, C.D., Darby, C.E., De Korte, R.A., and Wilkins, A.J. (1980): Self-induction of epileptic seizures by eye closure: incidence and recognition. *J. Neurol. Neurosurg. Psychiatry,* 43:386–389.
4. Binnie, C.D., Overweg, J., and Rowan, A.J. (1980): Long-term EEG and video monitoring in epilepsy. In: *Proceedings of the 2nd European Congress of EEG and Clinical Neurophysiology,* Salzburg, September 16–19, 1979, edited by H. Lechner and A. Aranibar, pp. 83–88. Excerpta Medica, Amsterdam.
5. Binnie, C.D., Rowan, A.J., Overweg, J., Meinardi, H., Wisman, T., Kamp, A., and Lopes de Silva, F. (1981): Telemetric EEG and video monitoring in epilepsy. *Neurology* (NY) 31:298–303.
6. Bloom, D., Jasper, H., and Rasmussen, T. (1959/60): Surgical therapy in patients with temporal lobe seizures and bilateral EEG abnormality. *Epilepsia,* 1:351–365.

7. Bowden, A.N., Fitch, P., Gilliatt, R.W., and Willison, R.G. (1975): The place of EEG telemetry and closed-circuit television in the diagnosis and management of epileptic patients. *Proc. R. Soc. Med.,* 68:246–248.
8. Breakell, C.C., Parker, C.S., and Christopherson, F. (1949): Radio transmission of the human electroencephalogram and other electrophysiological data. *Electroencephalogr. Clin. Neurophysiol.,* 1:243–244.
9. Browne, T.R., Penry, J.K., Porter, R.J., and Dreifuss, F.E. (1974): A comparison of clinical estimates of absence seizure frequency with estimates based on prolonged telemetered EEGs. *Neurology (Minneapolis*), 24:381–382.
10. Bruens, J.H., and Knijff, W. (1980): Ambulatory EEG monitoring with a 24-hour cassette recorder in epileptic patients. *Monogr. Neural Sci.*, 5:295–297.
11. Callaghan, N., and McCarthy, N. (1982): Ambulatory EEG monitoring in fainting attacks with normal routine and sleep EEG records. In: *Mobile Long-term EEG Monitoring*, edited by H. Stefan, and W. Burr, pp. 61–65 Fischer, Stuttgart.
12. Delgado-Escueta, A.V. (1979): Epileptogenic paroxysms: modern approaches and clinical correlations. *Neurology* (*Minneapolis*), 29:1014–1022.
13. Delgado-Escueta, A.V., Nashold, B., Freedman, M., Keplinger, C., Waddell, G., Miller, P., and Carwille, S. (1979): Videotaping epileptic attacks during stereoelectroencephalography. *Neurology* (*Minneapolis*), 29:473–489.
14. Derouesne, C., Golmard, J.L., Bilbeau, H., Asselain, B., and Salamon, R. (1979): Evaluation of the usual supplementary tests in neurological diagnosis. In: *Evaluation of Efficacy of Medical Action,* edited by A. Alperovitch, F.T. De Dombal, and F. Gremy, pp. 179–183. North-Holland, Amsterdam.
15. Dreifuss, F.E., Penry, J.K., Rose, S.W., Kupferberg, H.J., Dyken, P., and Sato, S. (1975): Serum clonazepam concentrations in children with absence seizures. *Neurology (Minneapolis)*, 25:255–258.
16. Dreyer, R., and Wehmeyer, W. (1978): Die EEG-Abflachung bei psychomotorischen Anfaellen, ihre Haeufigkeit, Dauer, Form und Bedeutung: eine Video-Band-Analyse von 78 Patienten mit 187 Anfaellen. *Arch. Psychiatr. Nervenkr.*, 225:263–274.
17. Ebersole, J.S., and Leroy, R.F. (1983): Evaluation of ambulatory cassette EEG monitoring: III. Diagnostic accuracy compared to intensive inpatient EEG monitoring. *Neurology (Cleveland)*, 33:853–860.
18. Engel, J., Rausch, R., Lieb, J.P., Kuhl, D.E., and Crandall, P.H. (1981): Correlation of criteria used for localizing epileptic foci in patients considered for surgical therapy of epilepsy. *Ann. Neurol.,* 9:215–224.
19. Fariello, R.G., Booker, H.E., Chun, R.W.M., and Orrison, W.W. (1983): Reenactment of the triggering situation for the diagnosis of epilepsy. *Neurology* (*Cleveland*), 33:878–884.
20. Gastaut, H., and Bert, J. (1954): EEG changes during cinematographic presentation. *Electroencephalogr. Clin. Neurophysiol.,* 6:433–444.
21. Gibson, T.C., and Heitzman, M.R. (1984): Diagnostic efficacy of 24-hour electrocardiographic monitoring for syncope. *Am. J. Cardiol.,* 53:1013–1017.
22. Gotman, J. (1982): Automatic recognition of epileptic seizures in the EEG. *Electroencephalogr. Clin. Neurophysiol.,* 54:530–540.
23. Guey, J., Bureau, M., Dravet, C., and Roger, J. (1969): A study of the rhythm of petit mal absences in children in relation to prevailing situations: the use of EEG telemetry during psychological examinations, school exercises and periods of inactivity. *Epilepsia,* 10:441–451.
24. Harrison-Covello, A., and De Barros-Ferreira, M. (1975): Modulation des foyers de pointes chez l'enfant étudies par biotelemetrie. *Rev. Electroencephalogr. Neurophysiol. Clin.,* 5:82–85.
25. Holmes, G.L., McKeever, M., and Russman, B.S. (1982): Prolonged EEG and videotape monitoring in children *Am. J. Dis. Child.*, 136:608–611.
26. Ives, J.R. (1982): A completely ambulatory 16-channel cassette recording system. In: *Mobile Long-term EEG Monitoring*, edited by H. Stefan, W. Burr, pp. 205–217. Fischer, Stuttgart.
27. Ives, J.R., Thompson, C.J., and Gloor, P. (1976): Seizure monitoring: a new tool in electroencephalography. *Electroencephalogr. Clin. Neurophysol.*, 41:422–427.
28. Ives, J.R., and Woods, J.F. (1975): 4-Channel 24-hour cassette recorder for long-term

EEG monitoring of ambulatory patients. *Electroencephalogr. Clin. Neurophysiol.*, 39:88–92.

29. Lieb, J.P., Walsh, G.O., Babb, T.L., Walter, R.R., and Crandall, P.H. (1976): A comparison of EEG seizure patterns recorded with surface and depth electrodes in patients with temporal lobe epilepsy. *Epilepsia*, 17:137–160.
30. Manson, G. (1974): EEG radio telemetry. *Electroencephalogr. Clin. Neurophysiol.*, 37:411–413.
31. Martins da Silva, A., Aarts, J.H.P., Binnie, C.D., Laxminarayan, R., Lopes da Silva, F.H., Meijer, J.W.A., and Nagelkerke, N. (1984): The circadian distribution of interictal epileptiform EEG activity. *Electroencephalogr. Clin. Neurophysiol.*, 58:1–13.
32. Mirsky, A.F., and Van Buren, J.M. (1965): On the nature of the "absence" in centrencephalic epilepsy: a study of some behavioral, electroencephalographic and autonomic factors. *Electroencephalogr. Clin. Neurophysiol.*, 18:334–348.
33. Olivier, A., Gloor, P., Felipe Quesney, L., and Andermann, F. (1983): The indications for and the role of depth electrode recording in epilepsy. *Appl. Neurophysiol.*, 46:33–36.
34. Penry, J.K., and Porter, R.J. (1977): Intensive monitoring of patients with intractable seizures. In: *Epilepsy: The Eighth International Symposium*, edited by J.K. Penry, pp. 95–101. Raven Press, New York.
35. Penry, J.K., Porter, R.J., and Dreifuss, F.E. (1971): Quantification of paroxysmal abnormal discharge in the EEGs of patients with absence (petit mal) seizures for evaluation of antiepileptic drugs. *Epilepsia*, 12:278–279.
36. Penry, J.K., Porter, R.J., and Dreifuss, F.E. (1975): Simultaneous recording of absence seizures with video tape and electroencephalography: a study of 374 seizures in 48 patients. *Brain*, 98:427–440.
37. Polkey, C.E. (1981): Selection of patients with chronic drug-resistant epilepsy for resective surgery: 5 years' experience. *Proc. R. Soc. Med.*, 74:574–579.
38. Ramsay, R.E. (1982): Clinical usefulness of ambulatory EEG monitoring of the neurological patient. In: *ISAM-GENT-1981: Proceedings of the Fourth International Symposium on Ambulatory Monitoring and Second Gent Workshop on Blood Pressure Variability*, edited by F.D. Stott, E.B. Raftery, D.L. Clement, and S.L. Wright, pp. 234–243. Academic Press, London.
39. Schwab, R.S. (1939): A method of measuring consciousness in petit mal epilepsy. *J. Nerv. Ment. Dis.*, 89:690–691.
40. Sindrup, E. (1980): Technical contributions to the differential diagnosis in epilepsy. *Acta Neurol. Scand.* (*Suppl.*), 79:47–48.
41. Smith, E.B.O. (1982): The value of prolonged EEG monitoring to the clinician in a psychiatric liaison service. In: *ISAM-GENT-1981: Proceedings of the Fourth International Symposium on Ambulatory Monitoring and Second Gent Workshop on Blood Pressure Variability,* edited by F.D. Stott, E.B. Raftery, D.L. Clement, and S.L. Wright, pp. 162–170. Academic Press, London.
42. So, E.L., King, D.W., and Murvin, A.J. (1984): Misdiagnosis of complex absence seizures. *Arch. Neurol.*, 41:640–641.
43. Stålberg, E. (1976): Experiences with long-term telemetry in routine diagnostic work. In: *Quantitative Analytic Studies in Epilepsy,* edited by P. Kellaway, and I. Petersen, pp. 269–277. Raven Press, New York.
44. Stevens, J.R., Kodama, H., Lonsbury, B., and Mills, L. (1971): Ultradian characteristics of spontaneous seizure discharges recorded by radio telemetry in man. *Electroencephalogr. Clin. Neurophysol.*, 31:313–325.
45. Stevens, J.R., Milstein, V.M., and Dodds, S. (1969): Prolonged recording of EEG by radiotelemetry: an aid to localization and treatment of epilepsy. *Electroencephalogr. Clin. Neurophysiol.*, 27:544.
46. Sutula, T.P., Sackellares, J.C., Miller, J.Q., and Dreifuss, F.E. (1981): Intensive monitoring in refractory epilepsy. *Neurology (NY)*, 31:243–247.
47. Vidart, L., and Geier, S. (1967): Enregistrements téléencéphalographiques chez des sujets épileptiques pendant le travail. *Rev. Neurol.* (*Paris*), 117:475–480.
48. Vignaendra, V., Walsh, J., and Burrows, S. (1979): The application of prolonged EEG telemetry and videotape recording to the study of seizures and related disorders. *Clin. Exp. Neurol.*, 16:81–94.
49. Villarreal, H.J., Wilder, B.J., Willmore, L.J., Bauman, A.W., Hammond, E.J., and

Bruni, J. (1978): Effect of valproic acid on spike and wave discharges in patients with absence seizures. *Neurology (Minneapolis)*, 28:886–891.
50. Walter, D.O., Rhodes, J.M., and Adey, W.R. (1967): Discriminating among states of consciousness by EEG measurements: a study of four subjects. *Electroencephalogr. Clin. Neurophysiol.*, 22:22–29.
51. Wieser, H.G. (1979): "Psychische Anfaelle" und deren stereoelektroenzephalographisches Korrelat. *EEG EMG*, 10:197–206.

Advances in Neurology, Vol. 46: Intensive Neurodiagnostic Monitoring, edited by R. J. Gumnit. Raven Press, New York © 1986.

Ambulatory ECG and EEG Monitoring in the Differential Diagnosis of Cardiac and Cerebral Dysrhythmias

L. D. Blumhardt

Department of Neurology, Associated Unit of Neuroscience, University of Liverpool, Mersey Regional Unit of Medical and Surgical Neurology, Walton Hospital, Liverpool L91AE, United Kingdom

But oh my two troubles they reave me of rest,
The brains in my head and the heart in my breast.

A. E. Housman (1859–1936)

A complaint of a "funny turn" or a "black-out" is a common reason for the referral of a patient to a neurology or cardiology clinic in the United Kingdom. These terms cover a wide variety of nonfocal transient disturbances of consciousness which range from brief episodes of "dizziness" or short periods of amnesia perhaps unnoticed by observers, to dramatic collapses in which loss of consciousness may be complicated by injuries. Although many of these symptomatic episodes are "funny," i.e., peculiar and frightening to the patient, they are generally readily diagnosed by a physician without resort to special tests. However, there remains a significant group of patients whose symptoms may defy diagnosis despite protracted "interictal" investigations which, all too frequently, prove time-consuming, negative, and expensive. The physician needs to know how ambulatory monitoring of cardiac and cerebral activity can help in the management of these patients when other more conventional methods of diagnosis have proved inadequate.

PROBLEM AREAS

There are many possible causes for unexplained episodes of disturbed consciousness. It may be difficult, for a variety of reasons, to distinguish the symptoms of cardiac syncope from epilepsy and from other causes of "funny turns." The patient's description may be too vague or fragmentary to allow a confident diagnosis to be made. An almost daily occurrence for the neurologist is the lack of a crucial eye-witness. Even when an accurate history is available, the problem still frequently resolves into one of epilepsy versus syncope. The physician may be confounded by the absence of features considered "characteristic" of epilepsy or, for example, of Stokes-Adams syndrome ("nonspecific attacks"); or by the presence of features consistent with *both* epilepsy and syncope in the same symptomatic episode. When the sequence of events is vaguely described, the overlap in the symptomatology means that a diagnosis of epilepsy or syncope cannot be supported by the mere presence or absence of such features as loss of consciousness, increased salivation, incontinence, tongue-biting, and postictal fatigue, or even tonic or clonic elements, as all these phenomena may occur in both conditions (11). In practice the diagnosis is often complicated by the symptoms of migraine, vertebrobasilar ischemia, vasovagal syncope, depression, anxiety, or hysteria, conditions which may either prove to be the cause of the symptoms or which merely coexist to obscure the true etiology of the attacks. Even when the symptoms appear to be due to unequivocal epileptic convulsions, doubts may be raised by the demonstration of coexisting structural heart disease or a "serious," but asymptomatic, cardiac arrhythmia. Alternatively, an arrhythmia on the ECG may precipitate elaborate investigations when the cause of the unexplained nonspecific attack is epilepsy.

As the consequences of misdiagnosis and inappropriate treatment are potentially serious, we need to know the limitations of clinical methods in distinguishing patients with symptoms that are likely to be due either to cardiac or cerebral dysrhythmias from those whose symptoms have some other cause. Apart from the common difficulties outlined above, there are three areas with potential for confusion which require more detailed investigation.

Cardiogenic Attacks Which Mimic Epilepsy ("Cardiogenic Neurology")

Stokes (33) was the first person to link cerebral symptoms with cardiac abnormalities. The "premonitory aura" and other features in his original case could easily be mistaken for the aura of a complex partial seizure. A variety of visceral, sensory, and visual disturbances have been described in patients with this syndrome which may closely mimic the temporal lobe aura. Other arrhythmias may give rise to similar symptoms. Some descriptions of attacks in patients with cardiac conduction disorders could be interpreted as seizures arising from the temporal lobe, while others are vague and nonspecific. For example, one patient might develop a vacant stare with trembling and deep sighing respiration (25), while another might look anxious and pale and stand swaying with closed eyes and twitching hands (21). Episodes ushered in by the sudden cessation of activities and characterized by pallor, sweating, anxious facies, and apnea have been described in patients with the long QT syndrome (10). Possible *forme frustes* of epileptic seizures, such as "jactitations," nocturnal incontinence, apnea, amnesia, cyanosis, brief lapses of consciousness, drop-attacks, and postictal confusion, may occur in association with a variety of cardiac arrhythmias. Some descriptions of attacks confidently attributed to a cardiac cause might seem to the neurologist to be indistinguishable from focal seizures.

For example, Pearson (26) described a patient whose attacks of sinoatrial arrest were initiated by pallor and an anxious facies, followed by version of the head and eyes to the right with repetitive swallowing, movements of the hands, teeth-grinding, and deep sighing respiration. Similar attacks have been described with the long QT syndrome (8). Reports of EEGs obtained during cardiac arrhythmias are rare and the recordings are said to show only slowing and flattening (30,37).

Up to 25% of patients with tonic anoxic seizures secondary to reflex cardiac arrest may be mistakenly diagnosed and treated as having generalized motor seizures (32). Neurologists are occasionally surprised enough by these patients to publish short case reports extolling the virtue of simultaneous ECG and EEG monitoring (4,20). How often these patients may be misdiagnosed from ambulatory ECG tapes as primary rather than reflex cardiac arrests is unknown.

Even when the diagnosis of an epileptic convulsion seems clinically unequivocal, an arrhythmia cannot be excluded. As anoxia is a potent cause of convulsions, it is not surprising that tonic-clonic seizures may be associated with heart block (34) or the long QT syndrome (1,8), or that patients with seizures which are caused by an undetected cardiac arrhythmia are "treated" with anticonvulsants to no avail (8,35,40).

These case reports in the cardiological literature raise the question of how frequently seizures may be precipitated by clinically unsuspected cardiac arrhythmias. While the prevalence of such secondary "cardiogenic seizures" is not likely to be high, the number of patients who may be at risk from inappropriate anticonvulsant medication will be difficult to establish without carefully designed prospective studies. This important question may have implications for the prevention of the sudden unexplained deaths that occur in some epileptic patients. It cannot be answered by the anecdotal, uncontrolled publications which extoll the "value" of ambulatory EEG in making a "diagnosis" of epilepsy.

Cardiac Arrhythmias Triggered by Epileptic Seizures (Neurogenic Cardiology)

Hughlings Jackson regarded epileptic fits as "experiments made by disease" which demonstrated that the heart like other organs was represented in the highest centers. In 1887, he noted the slowing of the heart in "some slight seizures of le petit mal" and acknowledged the earlier observation of François Franck that: "le ralentissement du coeur est lie à la periode tonique l'accélération à la periode clonique des grandes accès."

Virtually any type of cardiac arrhythmia may occur as a secondary effect of seizures, whether induced in animals or spontaneous in man (7,38,41). As autonomic features such as sweating, flushing, pallor, palpitations, and apnea are frequent accompaniments of complex partial seizures (19), it is not uncommon for this type of attack to be confused with primary cardiogenic syncope. The fact that relatively minor complex partial seizures can have profound effects on cardiac rate and rhythm is seldom appreciated by neurologists, although occasional case reports have suggested links between cardiac arrhythmias and EEG discharges, and "normalization" of tachyarrhythmias with anticonvulsant therapy (27,28,39) has been reported. There is a curious lack of recognition of this problem even in combined ECG/EEG ambulatory monitoring studies. In one report a bigeminal rhythm coincided with an epileptic seizure, a finding that the authors could not explain (12). More alarmingly, the generation of tachycardias and arrhythmias by seizures is virtually totally ignored in the cardiological literature. These features are easily recognized in combined ambulatory ECG/EEG recordings, even during quite minor attacks (2).

A 19-year-old male was admitted for investigation of "black-outs." He was initially seen by a physician in an immediate postictal state when a pronounced tachycardia and injected conjunctivae were noted. The possibility of "inorganic solvent intoxication" was raised. Subsequent referral to a neurologist revealed a 33-month history of multiple minor episodes of disturbed consciousness which were characterized by déjà-vu, spatial disorientation, and a feeling of being "possessed from outside." These attacks were ushered in by a sinking feeling in the stomach with "butterflies." Witnesses observed a vacant facies with facial automatisms and either unresponsiveness, or slurred speech with nonsensical content. A diagnosis of temporal lobe epilepsy was made.

Ambulatory monitoring captured several attacks in which typical epileptic seizure activity began over the right hemisphere after a short period of EEG attenuation and spread to the left (Figs. 1A, 1B, and 1C). At the same time a rapid acceleration of the heart rate was followed by extrasystolic beats and sinus or supraventricular tachycardias alternating abruptly with short periods of bradycardia.

The attacks were successfully terminated with carbamazepine.

The alterations in heart rate and rhythm which so frequently accompany temporal lobe discharges may be confusing for cardiologists. The extent to which epilepsy is responsible for the minor arrhythmias and tachycardias which are recorded in ambulatory ECG studies, and often considered to be insufficient to explain the patient's symptoms, is unknown. Unless simultaneous EEG data are available to demonstrate the presence or absence of seizure activity, cardiac arrhythmias which coincide with nonspecific symptoms are very likely to be interpreted as causative.

Finally, epileptic seizures and cardiac arrhythmias may occur independently in the same patient but, until both EEG and ECG are captured in the attacks, the relationship between the cerebral and cardiac abnormalities remains speculative.

A 70-year-old female gave an 18-month history of "drop-attacks" occurring up to three times a week. There was no warning in most attacks, but a minority had been preceded by weakness in the legs, sweating, palpitations, and a feeling that "my heart is in my mouth."

Other attacks were observed in which there was sweating, flushing, palpitations, and an increased blood pressure.

There was a past history and a strong family history of ischemic heart disease. A cardiologist made a tentative diagnosis of cardiac arrhythmias and 90 hr of ECG monitoring captured several symptomatic episodes as well as several asymptomatic bursts of supraventricular tachycardia. Several minor events of giddiness and flushing occurred without a detectable abnormality and a typical "black-out" or "drop-attack" was associated only with a moderate sinus tachycardia.

Referral to a neurologist led to intensive investigations with a tentative diagnosis of cardiac arrhythmia or cryptogenic drop-attacks. A trial of antiarrhythmic medication was ineffective.

Simultaneous ECG and EEG monitoring for 9 consecutive days captured three symptomatic events. The first was associated with an unequivocal short burst of supraventricular tachycardia, possibly paroxysmal atrial fibrillation, with rates up to 250 beats/min. (Fig. 2A). The other two coincided with slight increases in heart rate and semi-rhythmic or rhythmic slow activity which was either right-sided (no drop-attack), or bilateral (associated with drop-attack) (Fig. 2B).

Phenytoin was commenced and at follow-up 38 months later no further drop-attacks have occurred.

The cerebral and cardiac dysrhythmias in these complex cases may be unrelated, or perhaps related by previous embolic or ischemic cerebral damage. The extent to which such combinations of dysrhythmias may confound diagnosis in patient populations studied by ambulatory ECG or EEG monitoring alone is again an unknown quantity. It is, nevertheless, instructive briefly to review this literature in order to recognize some of the pitfalls which may be carried over to multimodality studies.

Ambulatory ECG Monitoring

Cardiologists tend to monitor patients when symptoms are considered to be suggestive of cardiac arrhythmias (dyspnea or palpitations), or of cerebral ischemia (dizziness, light-headedness, or syncope). Early reports of Holter monitoring concentrated on arrhythmia detection and positive findings were considered diagnostic with or without symptoms. Later studies revealed a poor correlation between many arrhythmias and symptoms, and a high prevalence of "silent" arrhythmias in control groups. Although it remains true that serious arrhythmias are more likely to give rise to palpitations or syncope, it has been clearly shown that arrhythmias frequently occur without symptoms and symptoms without arrhythmias (22,36). When arrhythmias are present, symptoms are often vague and nonspecific but, conversely, the majority of such patients do not have cardiac arrhythmias at the time of their symptoms (17). It is therefore clear that we cannot rely on the presence or absence of so-called cardiac-specific symptoms as a method of selecting patients for ECG monitoring *alone*. Even more important is the discovery that where episodic symptoms are consistent with Stokes-Adams syndrome, but are accompanied only by a normal sinus rhythm, a 2-year follow-up shows either a spontaneous resolution of the symptoms or an "improvement" in the majority (83%) of patients (18).

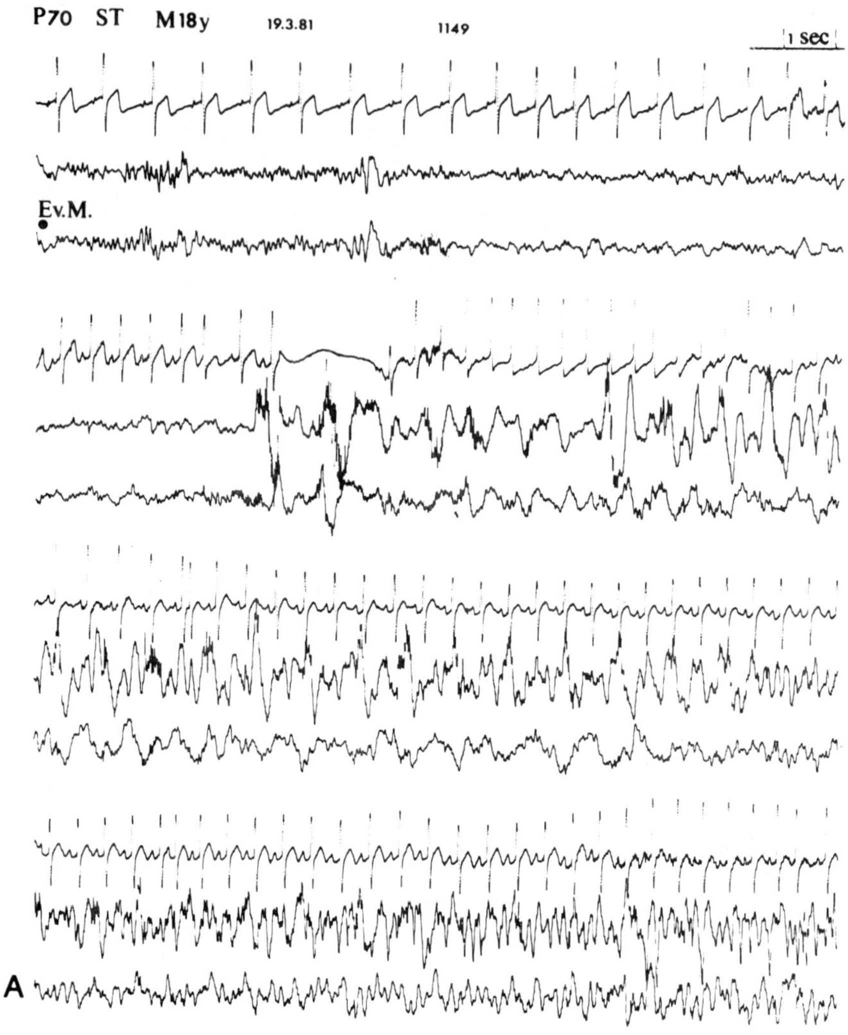

FIG. 1. **A:** The onset of a temporal lobe seizure is signaled by the event mark (Ev.M.) in the *uppermost traces*. A paroxysmal burst of high-amplitude semi-rhythmic slow activity with right-sided emphasis is accompanied by a tachycardia with abrupt onset which includes a short run of possible supraventricular arrhythmia (*second trace*). In this and all similar figures, the *upper trace* represents the electrocardiogram; the *second trace*, the right scalp leads, T4–P4; and the *third trace*, the left scalp leads, T3–P3. **B** (*facing page*): The continuation of the same attack depicted in Fig. 1a shows the rhythmic epileptic discharge lasts approximately 72 sec before it is replaced by postictal slow activity. Note the accompanying marked irregularity of the ECG. **C** (*facing page*): The same attack as in Figs. 1a and 1b is shown in compressed form. In this and all similar figures below, the *upper trace* represents EEG from scalp over the right hemisphere, the *second trace* EEG from the scalp over the left hemisphere, and the *third trace*, the ECG. The *lowest trace* is a plot of instant heart rate which shows individual R-R intervals whose height (*vertically displayed*) is proportional to the heart rate. The abrupt onset of tachycardia can be seen immediately before the event marker (▲) and the cardiac arrhythmias towards the end of the attack are clearly demonstrated. (See text for clinical details.)

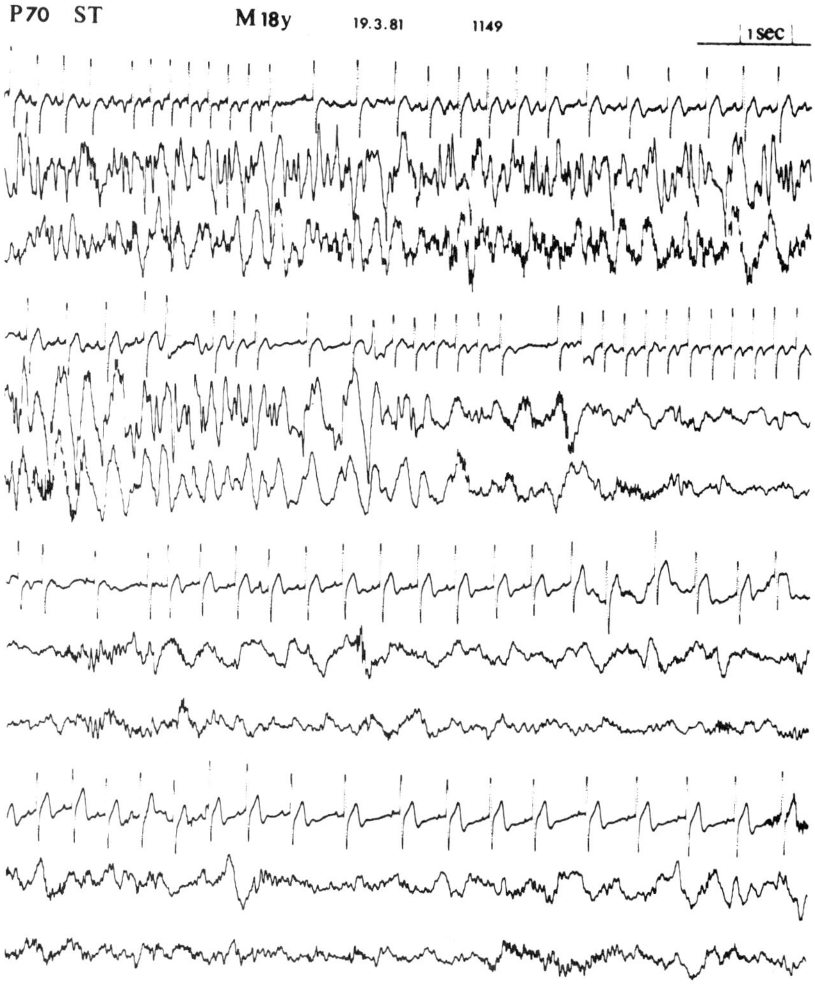
P70 ST
M 18y
19.3.81
1149
1 sec

B

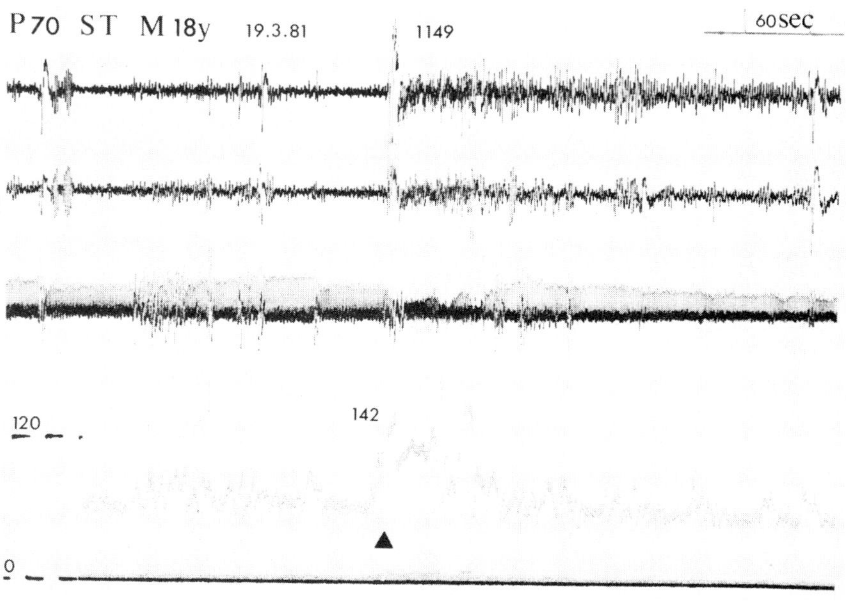
P70 ST M 18y
19.3.81
1149
60 sec
120
142
0

C

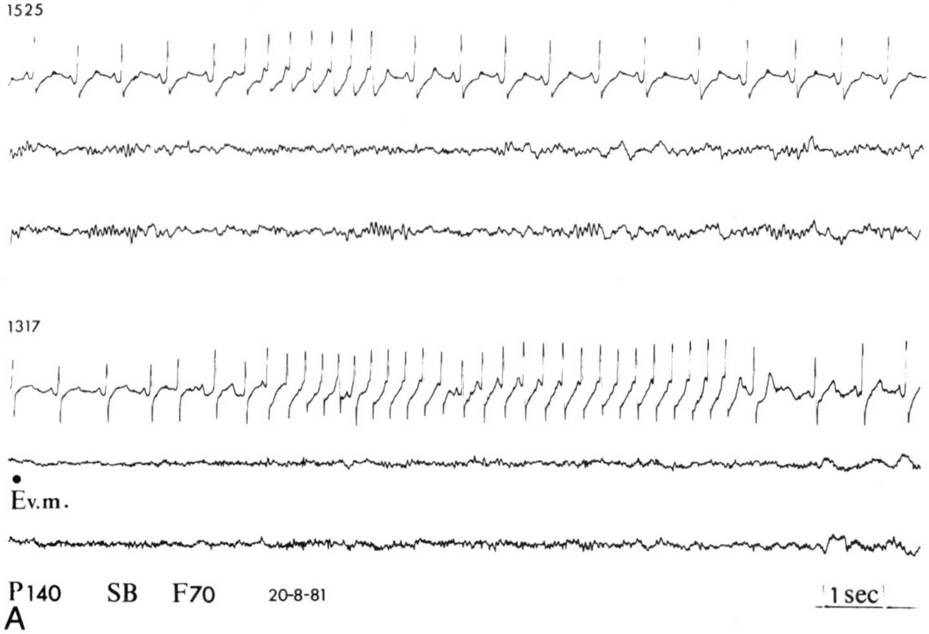

FIG. 2. **A:** *Upper traces* (15.25 hr) show asymptomatic cardiac arrhythmia while *lower trace* (15.17 hr) shows longer run of symptomatic supraventricular arrhythmia reaching rates of 250 beats/min. The EEG showed no abnormality. **B** (*facing page*): Recording obtained during the second symptomatic event (drop-attack) in the same patient as Fig. 2a. Note short burst of rhythmic bilateral slow activity at approximately 3 Hz, followed by irregular moderate- to high-amplitude slow activity which accompanies and follows the event mark (Ev.M.). Note ECG artifact at the time of the fall. (See text for clinical details.)

Furthermore, this good prognosis occurs in these patients despite a high prevalence of *asymptomatic* arrhythmias of all types. In a further small group the symptoms were subsequently shown to be due to "extracardiac" sources, but, unfortunately, no further details of these cases were provided.

The *negative* information provided by ambulatory ECG monitoring is clearly an important means for identifying patients who do *not* need anti-arrhythmia therapy, thus avoiding the potential dangers of pacemakers and drugs. The relevance of such studies to populations of patients with unexplained episodes of disturbed consciousness in *neurology* clinics (where one might expect a lower proportion of patients predisposed to cardiac arrhythmias, due to the exclusion of many cases with obvious clinical evidence of heart disease), needs to be examined.

Ambulatory ECG Studies in Neurological Patients

Neurologists involved in ambulatory ECG studies of patients attending their clinics with transient nonfocal, unexplained neurological symptoms, have also

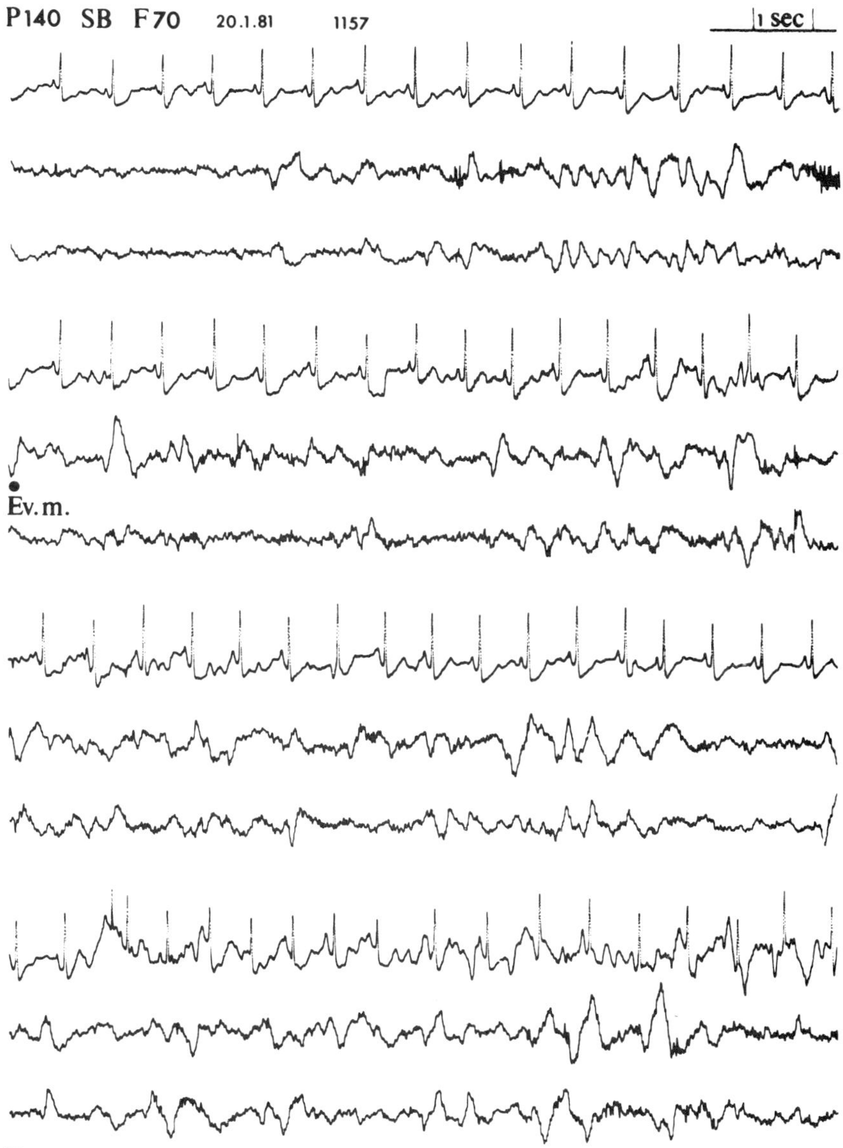

B

reported a high prevalence of cardiac arrhythmias (6,23,31). Early studies were uncontrolled and in some reports the patients were selected only on a referral diagnosis of epilepsy made by primary-care physicians, a method well known to be highly inaccurate. Extrapolations were frequently made from clinically asymptomatic arrhythmias. By this means some authors arrived at the conclusion that up to 20% of patients with a so-called diagnosis of epilepsy attending a neurological outpatient department may have a cardiac arrhythmia "significantly related to their symptoms" (31). In another study in which patients with nonfocal neurological symptoms, including light-headedness, vertigo, and "possible epilepsy or syncope," were investigated by ECG monitoring, an excess of silent arrhythmias was found compared with a control population (23). Such findings, however, are no more than suggestive, as captured symptoms were associated with an arrhythmia in only one case. Other carefully controlled studies have failed to yield such a high prevalence of abnormal results, whereas the low capture rate of symptomatic events in neurological populations precludes a positive diagnosis in more than a few percent of patients (6). In addition, despite careful preliminary neurological screening of all cases in these studies, epileptic patients were revealed by clinical follow-up. For these reasons, and in view of the very high negative correlation between symptomatic events and cardiac arrhythmias in such patients (as well as the possibility that even symptomatic arrhythmias may be generated centrally by epileptic discharges), simultaneous ECG and EEG is the investigation of choice.

Ambulatory EEG Monitoring

Reports of the diagnostic usefulness of ambulatory EEG alone, of course, provide no information on the possibility that symptoms may have a cardiac basis. Most reports have been anecdotal or primarily directed towards the problem of differentiating epilepsy from psychogenic seizures (14,24). Other studies of selected epileptic patients have not included ECG data (15). In diagnostic studies where ECG was omitted from the majority of recordings (e.g., ref. 29), an unknown number of false positives may be included due to movement artifact. Rhythmic slow activity may only be confidently attributed to a cerebral origin where coexisting movement can be excluded (i.e., by inspection of the ECG trace) (Fig. 3A).

Simultaneous Ambulatory ECG and EEG Studies

To date, publications in the field of ambulatory ECG and EEG studies have been entirely restricted to preliminary reports or feasibility studies which have been uncontrolled and lacking in follow-up data. As such, although they provide some interesting insights into the potential for solving some of the problems defined above, they allow no definitive conclusions to be reached on the overall usefulness or predictive accuracy of this technique in distinguishing cardiac from cerebral dysrhythmias in patients where either are equally possible.

A major difficulty in analyzing the results of the published studies is the variable methodology of patient selection. Some authors have merely monitored a random group of patients referred from sources of widely varying diagnostic expertise, including unknown proportions of patients who had been seen by neurologists or cardiologists (13,29). This broad approach tends to exaggerate the value of ambulatory monitoring from the inevitable inclusion of unknown numbers of patients who may have been readily diagnosed by a neurologist on clinical grounds alone. The results tell us more about the prowess of the clinicians than about the value of, or indications for, the test. Groups of patients who are difficult for a primary-care physician to diagnose, or merely because eye-witness accounts are not available, will tend to be different from those in which a diagnosis could not be reached despite full clinical histories and intensive neurological and cardiological investigations. The proportion of patients with cerebral or cardiac abnormalities on examination may also be expected to influence the likelihood of finding dysrhythmias on monitoring. Such factors have not been taken into account in any study to date. Furthermore, in some reports the results are uninterpretable as the proportions of patients who had either EEG monitoring alone, or EEG in combination with ECG, are not specified (e.g., ref. 29).

In those studies where patients were screened by neurologists prior to monitoring (details variably specified), it is often difficult to know why patients were classified as suspected epilepsy rather than syncopal attacks, and thus to what extent the test is being applied as a merely confirmatory, as opposed to a diagnostic, test. Furthermore, authors differ in their clinical terminologies. In one study the term syncope is used for any unexplained episode of loss of consciousness (12), or, idiosyncratically, in another for "attacks which do not follow the established pattern for seizures, especially . . . in patients with psychosomatic disorders" (5).

The marked variation in so-called hit rates and the proportions of positive and negative findings suggest considerable differences in patient inclusion criteria (Table 1). To some extent this may be explained by different aims of the investigators. For example, the technique has been applied to outpatient monitoring of all newly presenting patients selected only because their episodes of disturbed consciousness could not be diagnosed by neurologists (2), or to inpatients where additional information from close observation of the attacks in a hospital ward was included in the final diagnostic assessment (5). The remarkable capture rate of diagnostic events (epileptic seizures or cardiac arrhythmias in 56%) in the group of patients with "syncopal attacks" in this latter study suggests a high degree of preselection of patients. By contrast, a low capture rate of symptomatic events and a high frequency of negative findings during attacks is a common feature of most of the other studies (Table 1), paralleling the results in the ambulatory ECG literature.

In a significant number of captured attacks, a diagnosis is prevented by the occurrence of EEG artifacts. The absence of equivocal results from some studies raises the question of the EEG criteria that different authors consider sufficient for a diagnosis of epilepsy. There may be considerable differences in interpretation, but most authors have not published examples of their abnor-

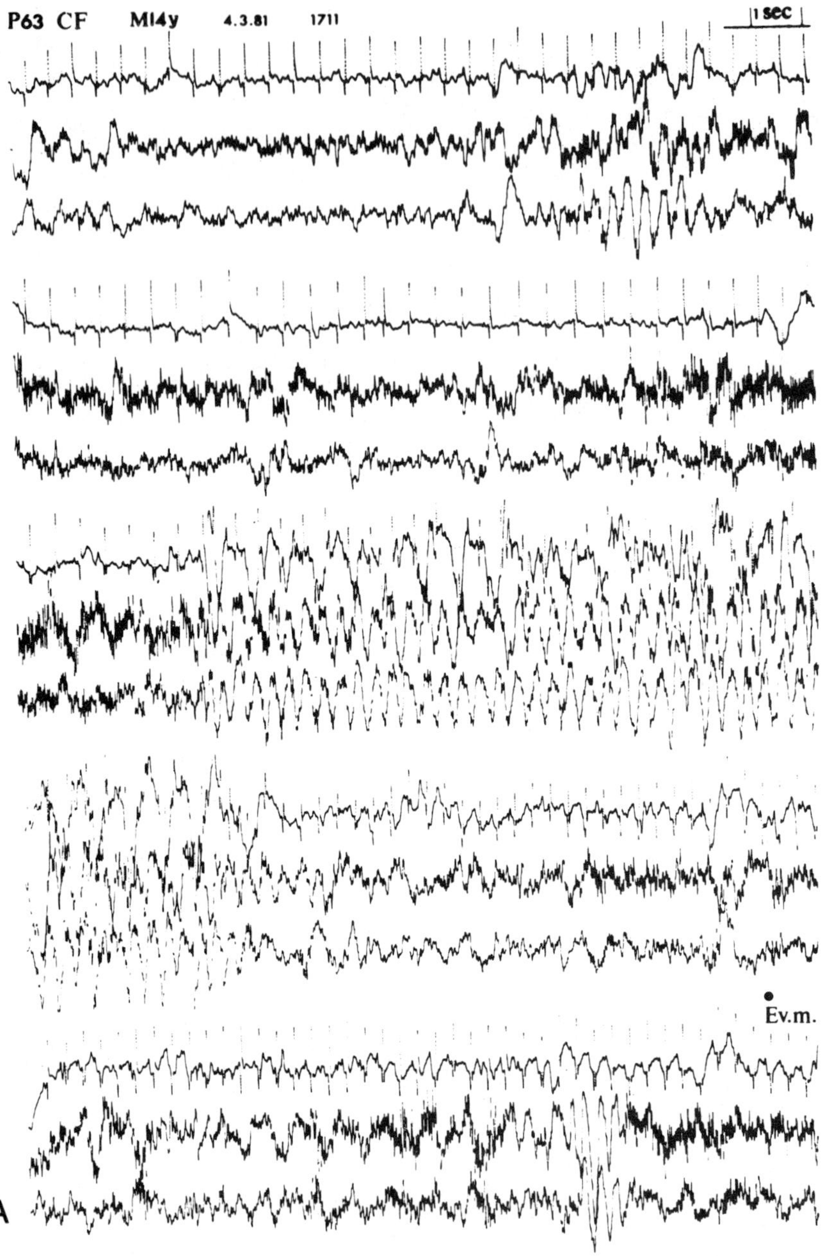

A

FIG. 3. A: Symptomatic attack in patient with minor episodes of "dizziness and weakness" (see text for clinical details). Note sinus tachycardia throughout with gradual acceleration of the heart beat, bilateral muscle and movement artifact, and high amplitude 3 HZ slow activity. The latter is intermittent, and on each occasion the rhythmic slow activity coincides with movement artifact in the ECG trace. **B** (*facing page*): The compressed instant heart rate of the same attack displayed in Fig. 3a shows a gradual step-wise increase in heart rate over several minutes (onset of tachycardia, △; event marker, ▲).

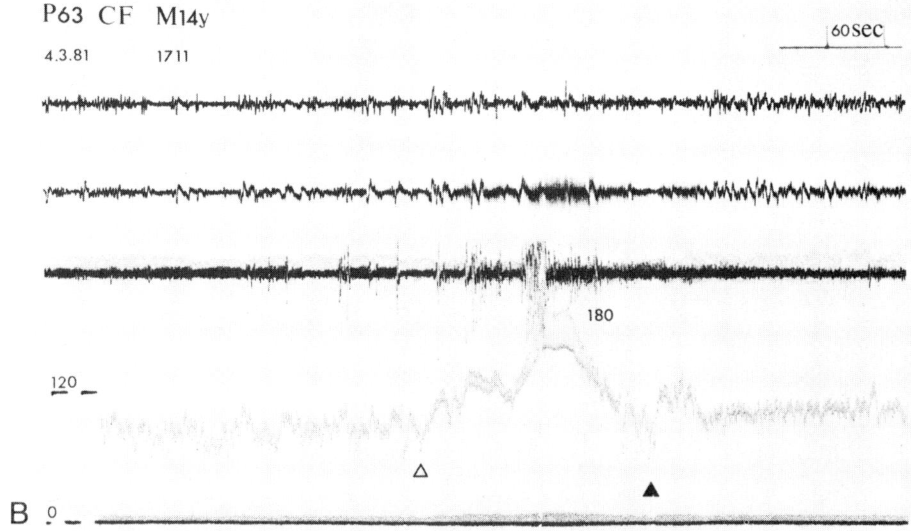

mal recordings. In some reports it is not clear whether recordings were termed inconclusive because no attacks were captured, or because the recordings obtained during symptomatic events could not be analyzed (5).

In combined studies, both ECG and EEG are likely to contain useful information, but few authors comment on changes in both parameters, merely classifying their cases as epileptic or cardiac. In most attacks where the EEG is equivocal because of associated movement or muscle artifact, very high heart

TABLE 1. *Simultaneous ECG/EEG studies of patients with "undiagnosed" episodic symptoms*

Reference	Capture rate	Epilepsy	Cardiac	Equivocal EEG	Negative
Woods and Ives (42)	12/26 (46%)	2	2	2	6
Callaghan and McCarthy (5)	32/32[c] (100%)	16	0	6[a]	10[b]
	16/16[d] (100%)	6	5	5[b]	—
Graf et al. (12)	3/22 (14%)	1	0	0	2
Blumhardt and Oozeer (2)	11/68 (16%)	1	1	2	7

[a] Defined as "pseudoseizures" by authors.
[b] "Inconclusive" results (? negative, ? equivocal).
[c] "Suspected epilepsy".
[d] "Syncope".

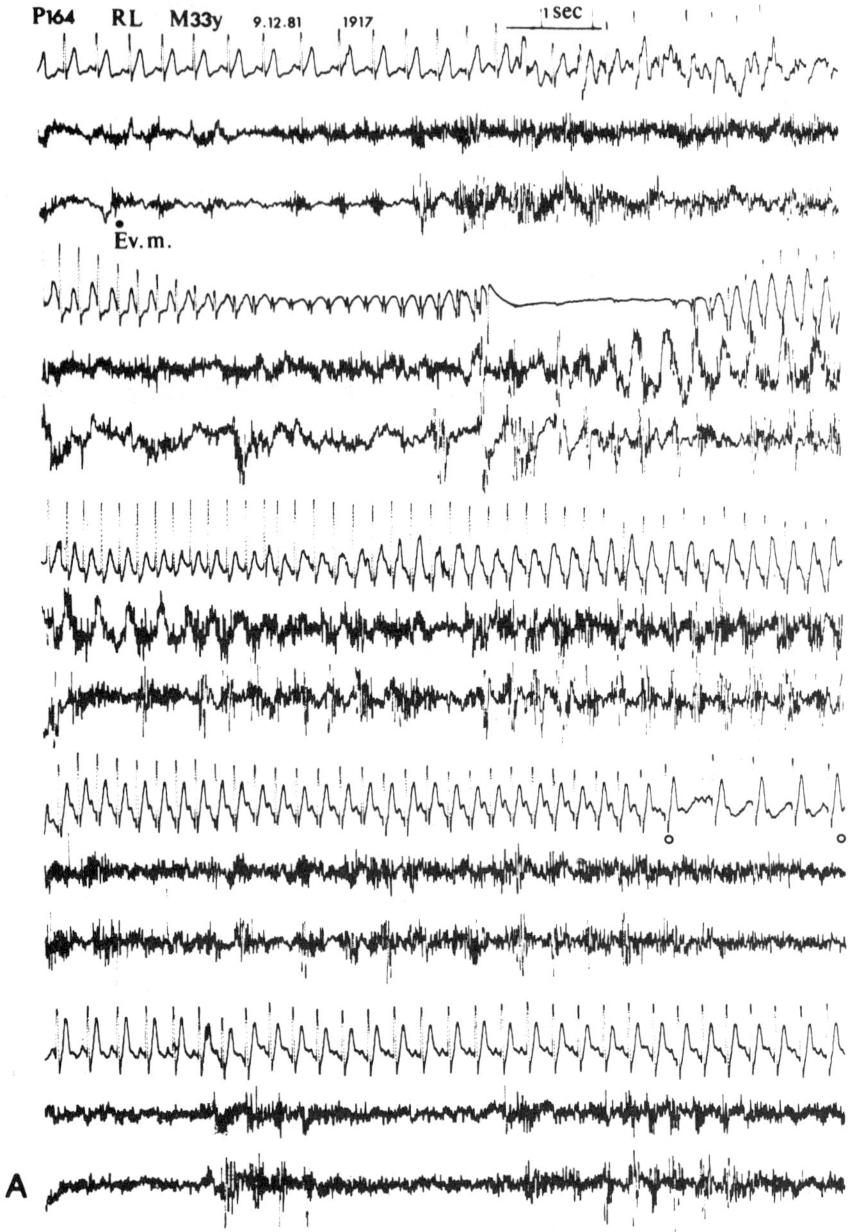

FIG. 4. A: Record of clinically definite temporal lobe seizure in epileptic control patient. Note abrupt tachycardia at onset of seizure with increased amplitude of T-waves. Note also transient decline in ECG amplitude, probably due to an associated apneic phase. The brief, irregular, high-amplitude slow activity is right-sided and there is no accompanying movement artifact in the ECG channel. Note sudden transient slowing of heart rate (marked 0–0). **B** (*facing page*): Compressed plot of the same attack shown in Fig. 4a readily reveals abrupt onset of tachycardia and several episodes of sudden slowing of heart rate (the first of which is marked 0–0) following the seizure discharge.

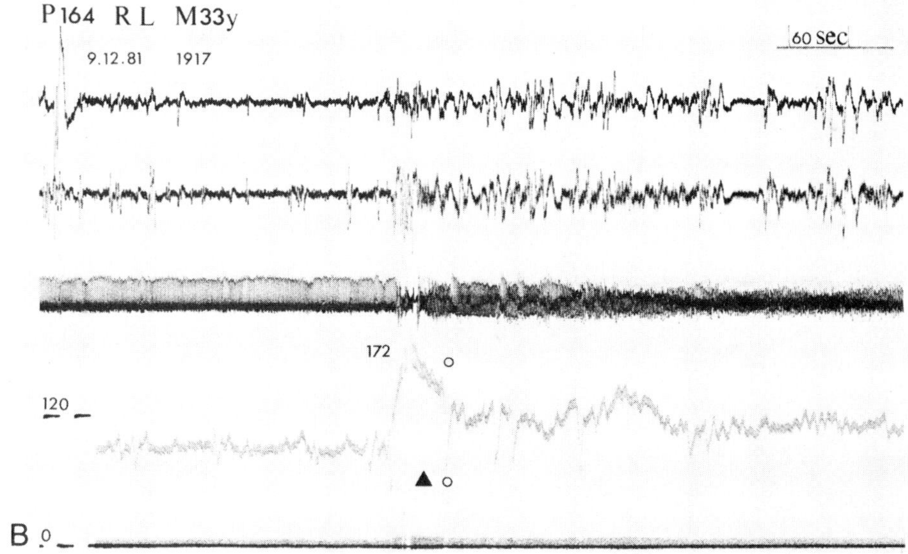

rates, often exceeding so-called normal upper limits, may occur (2). However, the *pattern* of the rate changes in some of these attacks may be quite distinct from the abrupt acceleration seen in clinically definite seizures (e.g., Figs. 1C and 4B). Further, coincidental movement artifact in the ECG tracing is a warning that apparent alterations in the EEG may also be due to movement.

A 15-year-old boy complained of episodic "tiredness and weakness" associated with dizziness, a feeling of being "not there" and of the environment closing in. Each episode could last up to 1 hr and they had been occurring for 3 years. On occasions they happened daily. Immediately prior to the recording no attacks had been experienced for 2 months. No eye witness was available, as the patient maintained there was "nothing to see." He could "control" his symptoms by going out to play. He suffered from obsessional hand-washing and gave an acceptable history of migraine headaches. His sister was said to have major convulsions. The only sign on examination was a prominent systolic ejection murmur.

Routine EEGs had shown "sharp-and-slow-wave discharges" on photic stimulation.

Several symptomatic episodes of "tiredness and weakness" were captured during 24 hr of ambulatory monitoring. The features are shown in Figs. 3A and 3B.

Following the recordings, which were judged to be equivocal on EEG criteria, no specific treatment was given. The patient later admitted to deliberate headshaking in the recorded episodes. Psychiatric counseling and behavioral therapy were administered intermittently over the following 3 years and a 39-month follow-up revealed that no further symptomatic attacks had occurred.

In our own study, follow-up data on most patients in whom recordings during attacks had shown equivocal EEG changes *and* an associated *gradual* acceleration of the heart rate (as in the example above) have revealed that attacks have ceased spontaneously without treatment in the majority. These features may be taken to suggest a nonorganic basis for the symptoms. By contrast, the abrupt ECG changes and cardiac arrhythmias which may accompany complex partial seizures in epileptic control populations can be useful in identifying symptomatic seizure activity, even when the EEG abnormalities are minimal (Figs. 4A and 4B).

No published study to date has addressed the problem of false positives or false negatives by clinical follow-up. In my own experience a mere label of "cardiac arrhythmia, refer to cardiologist" is seldom the end of the matter. Patients who remain a diagnostic problem after intensive testing often remain so even when symptomatic attacks have been captured. These complex cases are conspicuous by their absence in studies which blandly classify patients into cardiac or epileptic categories on the basis of ECG or EEG evidence alone. In our own prospective study the diagnosis remained obscure in a number of cases *despite* the capture of symptomatic arrhythmias and EEG "abnormalities." In some patients the cause of troublesome symptoms only became clear after prolonged follow-up.

A 43-year-old-female was referred in 1978 with episodes characterized by fear, a sensation of falling, hallucinations, "difficulty communicating," sweating, and tachycardia. These symptoms could last for several hours and she thought they might be precipitated by eating meat.

In the past she had suffered from "eclampsia" during a pregnancy in 1958 which was complicated by high blood pressure and a single seizure. Ever since she has been treated with a beta-blocker and barbiturates. During each pregnancy she had experienced involuntary (? myoclonic) jerks. In 1964, a diagnosis of epilepsy was made following a further episode of loss of consciousness. Mysoline was then introduced.

In 1977, somewhat similar episodic attacks of unexplained fear and palpitations had been investigated by a cardiologist but tests, including a 24-hr ECG tape, were inconclusive. In 1978, a neurologist considered that these attacks were epileptic and prescribed phenytoin. However, the attacks continued and she was subsequently referred back to the cardiologist. Extensive biochemical investigations were performed with negative results and a repeat 24-hr ECG tape showed only asymptomatic minor arrhythmias.

Ambulatory monitoring of ECG and EEG in 1980 captured three symptomatic events. Two episodes in which the patient complained of giddiness, popping ears, a "bursting head," and palpitations were clearly associated with a ventricular bigeminal rhythm with coupled beats (Fig. 5, upper traces). The third, which occurred in the early morning, was associated with a feeling of fear, misery, "pressure in the head," and "jerking of the limbs." The EEG and ECG were normal throughout this period, apart from brief (2–3 sec) bursts of 5 to 6 Hz activity over the right hemisphere (Fig. 5, lower traces).

Sometime after this inconclusive result, it was decided empirically that the beta-blocker should be stopped. There was an immediate cessation of symptoms. Despite the history and the slight EEG abnormalities, the anticonvulsant regimen was markedly reduced, and 37 months later no further symptomatic events have occurred apart from minor episodes of exercise-related palpitations.

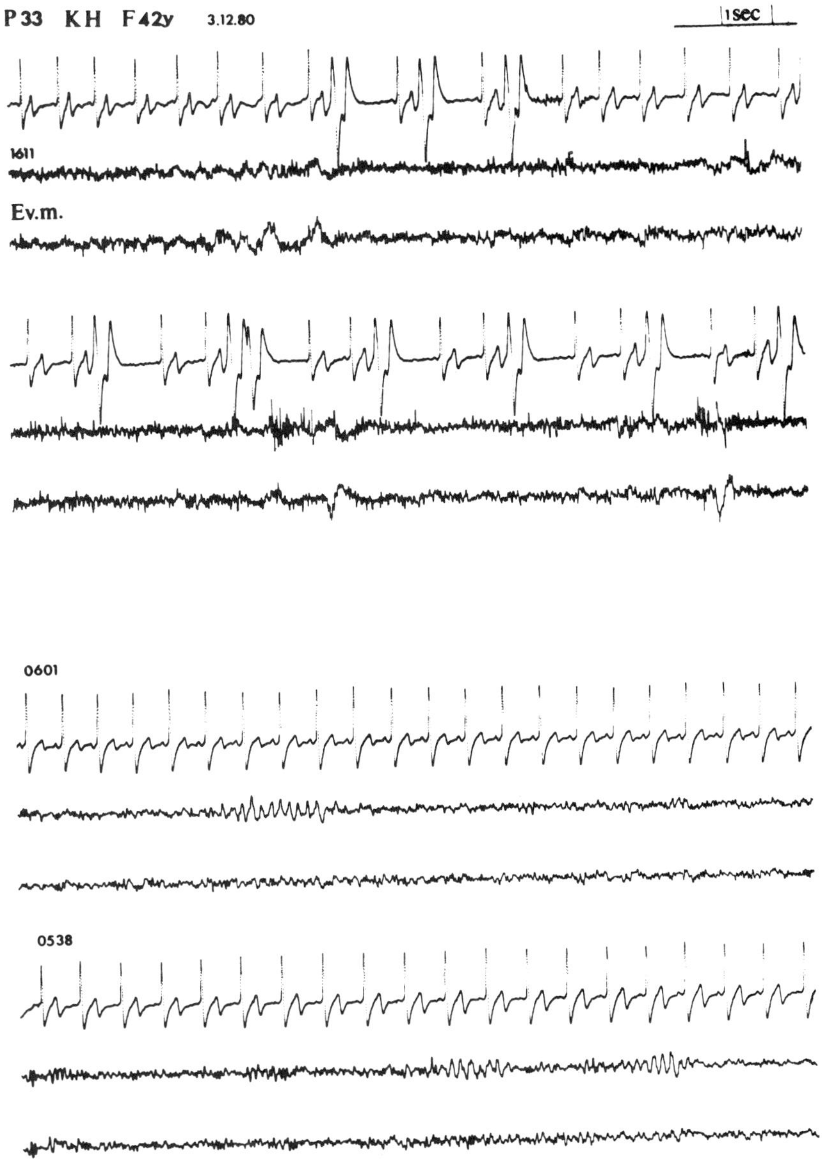

FIG. 5. Abrupt onset of ventricular ectopics with trigeminal rhythm and occasional coupled beats during symptomatic episode (*upper two traces*). *Lower traces* show episodic bursts of right-sided theta activity which was the only "abnormality" detected during a second symptomatic episode on the same tape that lasted for almost 2 hr. (See text for clinical details.)

The value of clinically silent abnormalities remains to be established. The listing of asymptomatic cardiac arrhythmias as significant results in uncontrolled studies merely repeats the errors of the early ambulatory ECG literature. Their significance can only be determined by long-term follow-up studies to determine subsequent developments and treatment outcome. Similarly, the occurrence of "silent" EEG abnormalities, for example, rhythmic slow activity, is of dubious significance, considering the difficulties in the interpretation of EEG recorded from mobile unobserved patients (3,9). Their inclusion as significant results in reports where an unknown proportion of patients had neurological deficits is even more dubious (e.g., ref. 12). In our own study, the occurrence of clinically silent asymmetric spikes-and-sharp-waves during sleep in patients with nonspecific black-outs has proved to be a reliable confirmatory sign of epilepsy, or at least a good predictor of a satisfactory response of symptoms to anticonvulsants. The predictive significance of other silent EEG abnormalities remains to be established.

CONCLUSION

There is a clear need for controlled, long-term, prospective follow-up studies in patients in whom the indications for simultaneous ambulatory EEG and ECG monitoring (or either alone) are clearly defined. These studies should be able to determine which patients will benefit from monitoring as well as the cost-efficiency and predictive accuracy of the tests. Investigators must define their criteria for inclusion and diagnosis, as well as the final results of treatment after follow-up. Merely confirmatory results should be distinguished from results of diagnostic significance. The final outcome in patients in whom ambulatory monitoring was *negative* must also be established in order to assess the overall value of the technique.

The recent advances which have made ambulatory EEG a practical everyday possibility, offer enormous potential for solving the gray diagnostic areas that lie between cardiology and neurology, and between these specialties and psychiatry. It would be a great pity if the uncritical, unscientific aspects of laboratory EEG are reproduced in the field of ambulatory monitoring.

REFERENCES

1. Ballardie, F. W., Murphy, R. P., and Davis, J. (1983): Epilepsy: a presentation of the Romano-Ward syndrome. *Br. Med. J.*, 287:896–897.
2. Blumhardt, L. D., and Oozeer, R. (1982): Simultaneous ambulatory monitoring of the EEG and ECG in patients with transient disturbances of consciousness. In: *ISAM-GENT-1981 Proceedings of the Fourth International Symposium of Ambulatory Monitoring*, edited by F. D. Stott et al., pp. 171–182. Associated Press, London.
3. Blumhardt, L. D., and Oozeer, R. (1982): Problems encountered in the interpretation of ambulatory E.E.G. recordings. In: *Mobile Long-term Recording*, edited by H. Stefan and W. Burr, pp. 37–53. Fischer, Stuttgart.

4. Braham, J., Hertzeanu, H., Yahini, J. H., and Neufeld, H. N. (1981): Reflex cardiac arrest presenting as epilepsy. *Ann. Neurol.,* 10:277–278.
5. Callaghan, N., and McCarthy, N. (1982): Ambulatory EEG monitoring in fainting attacks with normal routine and sleep EEG records. In: *Mobile Long-term Recording,* edited by H. Stefan and W. Burr, pp. 61–65. Fischer, Stuttgart.
6. De Bono, D. P., Warlow, C., and Hyman, N. (1982): Cardiac rhythm abnormalities in patients presenting with transient non-focal neurological symptoms—a diagnostic grey area? *Br. Med. J.,* 284:1437–1439.
7. Delgado, J. M. R., Mihailovic, L., and Sevillano, M. (1960): Cardiovascular phenomena during seizure activity. *J. Nerv. Ment. Dis.,* 130:477–487.
8. Driver, M. V., and Selby, P. J. (1977): Apparent epilepsy due to the intermittent tachyarrhythmia (Romano-Ward syndrome). *Electroencephalogr. Clin. Neurophysiol.,* 43: 289.
9. Ebersole, G. S., Bridges, S. L., and Silva, C. G. (1983): Differentiation of epileptiform abnormalities from normal transients and artifacts on ambulatory cassette E. E. G. *Am. J. EEG Technol.,* 23:113–125.
10. Fraser, G. R., Froggatt, P., and Gawes, T. N. (1964): Congenital deafness associated with electrocardiographic abnormalities, fainting attacks and sudden deaths. *Q. J. Med.,* 33:361–385.
11. Gastaut, H. (1974): Syncopes: generalised anoxic cerebral seizures. In: *Handbook of Clinical Neurology, Vol. 15,* edited by P. J. Vinken and G. W. Bruyn, pp. 815–835. North-Holland, Amsterdam.
12. Graf, M., Brunnei, G., Weber, H., Auinger, C., and Joskowicz, G. (1982): Simultaneous long-term recording of E.E.G. and E.C.G. in "syncope" patients. In: *Mobile Long-term Recording,* edited by H. Stefan and W. Burr, pp. 67–76. Fischer, Stuttgart.
13. Green, J., Scales, D., Nealis, D., Schott, G., and Drisler, T. (1980): Clinical utility of ambulatory E.E.G. monitoring. *Clin. Electroencephalogr.,* 11:173–179.
14. Ives, J. R., Hausser, C., Woods, J. F., and Andermann, F. (1981): Contribution of 4-channel cassette EEG monitoring to differential diagnosis of paroxysmal attacks. In: *Advances in Epileptology: XIIth Epilepsy International Symposium,* edited by M. Dam et al., pp. 329–336. Raven Press, New York.
15. Ives, J. R., and Woods, J. F. (1980): A study of 100 patients with focal epilepsy using a 4-channel ambulatory cassette recorder. In: *ISAM-1979, International Symposium on Ambulatory Monitoring,* edited by F. D. Stott et al., pp. 383–392. Academic Press, London.
16. Jackson, H. (1887): Remarks on evolution and dissolution of the nervous system. In: *Selected Writings of John Hughlings Jackson,* edited by J. Taylor, pp. 106–108. Hodder and Stoughton, London, 1932.
17. Johannson, B. W. (1977): Long-term E.C.G. in ambulatory clinical practice. *Eur. J. Cardiol.,* 5:39–48.
18. Johansson, B. W. (1981): Evaluation of alteration of consciousness and palpitations. In: *Ambulatory Electrocardiographic Recording,* edited by N. K. Wenger, M. B. Mock, and I. Ringquist, pp. 321–330. Chicago.
19. Johnson, L. C., and Davidoff, R. A. (1964): Autonomic changes during paroxysmal E.E.G. activity. *Electroencephalogr. Clin. Neurophysiol.,* 17:25–35.
20. Lai, C. W., and Ziegler, D.K. (1981): Syncope problems solved by continuous ambulatory simultaneous E.E.G./E.C.G. recording. *Neurology,* 31:1152–1154.
21. Laslett, E.E. (1909): Syncopal attacks associated with prolonged arrest of the whole heart. *Q. J. Med.,* 2:347–355.
22. Levine, B. J., Zeldis, S. M., Morganroth, J., et al. (1978): Lack of correlation between symptoms and significant arrhythmias on long-term electrocardiographic analysis. *Clin. Res,* 26:247a.
23. Luxon, L. M., Crowther, A., Harrison, M. J. G., and Coltact, J. (1980): Controlled study of 24-hour ambulatory electrocardiographic monitoring in patients with transient neurological symptoms. *J. Neurol. Neurosurg. Psychiatry,* 43:37–41.
24. Oxley, J., and Roberts, M. (1982): The role of prolonged ambulatory monitoring in the diagnosis of non-epileptic fits in a population of patients with epilepsy. In: *ISAM GENT 1981, Proceedings of the Fourth International Symposium on Ambulatory Monitoring,* edited by F. D. Stott et al., pp. 195–202. Associated Press, London.

25. Parkinson, J., Papp, C., and Evans, W. (1941): The electrocardiogram of the Stokes-Adams attack, *Br. Heart J.,* 3:171–199.
26. Pearson, R. S. B. (1945): Sinus tachycardia with cardiac asystole. *Br. Heart J.,* 7:85–90.
27. Phyzackerley, P. J. R., Poole, E. W., and Whitty, C. W. M. (1954): Sino-auricular heart block as an epileptic manifestation. *Epilepsia,* 3:89–96.
28. Poggiali, I. (1971): Considerazioni su di un caso di tachicardia parossistica sopraventriculare e giounzionale con alterazioni elettroencefalografiche. *Clin. Pediatrica,* 53:260–270.
29. Ramsay, R. E. (1982): Clinical usefulness of ambulatory E.E.G. monitoring of the neurological patient. In: *ISAM-GENT, 1981, Proceedings of the Fourth International Symposium on Ambulatory Monitoring,* edited by F. D. Stott et al., pp. 171–182. Associated Press, London.
30. Regis, H., Toga, M., and Righini, C. (1961): Clinical electroencephalographic and pathological study of a case of Adams-Stokes syndrome. In: *Cerebral Anoxia and the Electroencephalogram,* edited by H. Gastaut and J. S. Meyer, pp. 295–303. Springfield, Illinois.
31. Schott, G. D., McLeod, A. A., and Jewitt, D. E. (1977): Cardiac arrhythmias that masquerade as epilepsy. *Br. Med. J.,* 1:1454–1457.
32. Stephenson, J. B. P. (1978): Reflex anoxic seizures ("white breathholding"): non-epileptic vagal attacks. *Arch. Dis. Childhood,* 53:193–200.
33. Stokes, W. (1846): Observations in some cases of permanently slow pulse. *Dublin Q. J. Med. Sci.,* 2:73–85.
34. Storstein, O. (1949): Adams-Stokes attacks caused by ventricular fibrillation in a man with an otherwise normal heart. *Acta Med. Scand.,* 133:437–441.
35. Sulg, I. A. (1979): Dependency between cerebral and cardiac activity in physiological as well as in abnormal conditions. In: *Cerebral Manifestations of Episodic Cardiac Arrhythmias,* edited by E. Busse, pp. 30–47. Exerpta Medica, Amsterdam.
36. Swenson, R. D., Price, J. E., Fashinell, J. R., et al. (1977): High prevalence of cardiac dysrhythmias in the etiology of syncope and dizziness: Documentation of ambulatory monitoring. *Circulation,* 56 (Suppl. 3):24.
37. Tucker, J. S., and Yoe, R. H. (1956): Simultaneous E.E.G.-E.C.G. recording: study of a case with complete heart-block and paroxysmal ventricular tachycardia. *Electroencephalogr. Clin. Neurophysiol.,* 8:129–132.
38. Van Buren, J. M. (1958): Some autonomic concomitants of ictal automatism. *Brain,* 81:505–522.
39. Walsh, G. O., Masland, W., and Goldensohn, E. S. (1972): Relationship between paroxysmal atrial tachycardia and paroxysmal cerebral discharges. *Bull. Los Angeles Neurol. Soc.,* 37:28–35.
40. Wennervold, A., Melchior, J. C., and Sandoe, E. (1965): Adams-Stokes syndrome in children without organic heart disease. *Acta Med. Scand.,* 177:557–563.
41. White, P. T., Grant, P., Mosier, J., and Craig, A. (1961): Changes in cerebral dynamics associated with seizures. *Neurology,* 11:354–361.
42. Woods, J., and Ives, J. (1977): Prolonged monitoring of the E.E.G. in ambulatory patients. In: *Epilepsy: Eighth International Symposium,* edited by J. K. Penry, pp. 109–113. Raven Press, New York.

Advances in Neurology, Vol. 46: Intensive Neurodiagnostic Monitoring, edited by R. J. Gumnit. Raven Press, New York © 1986.

Intensive Monitoring of Psychogenic Seizures, Aggression, and Dyscontrol Syndromes

Venkat Ramani

Department of Neurology and Psychiatry, Albany Medical College, Section of Epilepsy and Electroencephalography, Albany Medical Center Hospital, Albany, New York 12208

PSYCHOGENIC SEIZURES

Nomenclature

Although hysteria and epilepsy both had been recognized since ancient times, a scientific inquiry into the nature of these disorders did not emerge until a hundred years ago. Hysteroepilepsy was the subject of intense interest among the neurologists of the late nineteenth century led by such illustrious men as Charcot and Gowers. Today the problem is very much with us. Over the years the disorder has been referred to by a variety of names such as hysterical seizures, conversion hysteria, psychogenic seizures, simulated seizures, pseudoseizures, and, finally, pseudo-epileptic seizures (PES). Fenton (14) in his discussion of nomenclature cogently argues in favor of the term PES.

The nomenclature currently used at the Minnesota Comprehensive Epilepsy Program recognizes that there may be many types of events that mimic genuine epileptic seizures which can be called nonepileptic (33). Many of these are organic events such as syncope related to cardiac problems. A second major subgroup is what we choose to call psychogenic seizures. These are events which superficially resemble an epileptic seizure, but under closer scrutiny (see definition by Liske and Forster, ref. 33) "are found to be lacking in an essential epilepsy component such as a disturbance in the EEG, or possessing features not compatible with epilepsy such as being precipitated, modified, or stopped by a simple command, a hypnotic suggestion, or the withdrawal of secondary gain."

Incidence

Reliable figures concerning the incidence and prevalence of psychogenic seizures are not available. It is generally stated that gross hysterical conversion symptoms are infrequently encountered in modern psychiatric practice (38). But among patients with conversion symptoms, psychogenic seizures appear to be common. Folks et al. (17) in a study of 1,000 consecutive patients referred for psychiatric consultation at a university medical center, found that 5% had conversion symptoms. In this group 14% of patients suffered from psychogenic seizures. A number of recent reports from major epilepsy centers indicate that 8 to 20% of patients admitted with the diagnosis of "intractable seizures" have psychogenic seizures, alone or in conjunction with epilepsy (12,28,29,34, 45, 47). Although most reports emphasize their occurrence in adult females, psychogenic seizures are well recognized in children (16,25,62), in adolescents (21), and in men in the military service (48). Psychogenic seizures occur in both epileptics and nonepileptics. Whether the underlying mechanisms, natural history, and prognosis differ in the two groups is unknown and is an important subject for future research. According to the reports from various epilepsy centers, 42 to 90% of psychogenic seizure patients do not have any evidence of coexisting epilepsy (19,28,29,31,34). The wide disparity in concordance rate is probably due to differences in the populations, largely the result of referral patterns.

DIAGNOSIS OF PSYCHOGENIC SEIZURES (LEVEL I)

Clinical Aspects

The majority of psychogenic seizure patients are females between 15 and 35 years of age (29). However, psychogenic seizures can and do occur in males and in all age groups. They are encountered in all levels of socioeconomic status and educational background (33). Psychogenic seizure patients differ in their personality profiles and do not necessarily conform to the hysterical type (47). According to Roy (53), the typical psychogenic seizure patient is a female, with a personal and family history of psychiatric disorder, history of sexual maladjustment and attempted suicide, and current depression. Wilkus et al. (61) found that the Minnesota Multiphasic Personality Inventory (MMPI) scores for hypochrondriasis, hysteria, and schizophrenia were significantly higher in the psychogenic seizure group compared with controls. Also psychogenic seizure patients revealed more severe psychosocial problems in the Washington Psychosocial Seizure Inventory (61).

Frequent attacks resembling generalized convulsions, of abrupt or recent onset, occurring in a young adult who has normal examination, normal computed tomogram (CT scan) of the head, and normal random EEG, and without a history of head trauma, alcohol or drug abuse should raise the clinical suspicion of psychogenic seizure. Also, unexplained increase in seizure frequency in known epileptics, in the face of therapeutic serum levels of appropriate major anticonvulsant drugs, should alert the physician to the possibility of psychogenic seizure, particularly if the patient conforms to the psychogenic seizure psychiatric profile. Inconsistent and bizarre history such as "many grand mal seizures every day" is particularly suspicious. As Liske and Forster (33) pointed out, one should be suspicious of unusual seizures with unusual precipitants. A detailed history including a careful psychiatric assessment can provide invaluable information regarding the diagnosis of psychogenic seizures. In this context, it is important to note that in the study by King et al. (28), the referring physician was correct in 67% of cases in suspecting psychogenic seizure. The importance of obtaining a detailed history before undertaking an involved and expensive intensive neurodiagnostic monitoring cannot be overemphasized.

Routine EEG

Once the diagnosis of psychogenic seizure is strongly suspected on clinical grounds, the next step is to obtain a routine EEG with photic stimulation and hyperventilation. A normal interictal EEG does not rule out epilepsy, nor does it confirm the diagnosis of psychogenic seizure. Also, the presence of interictal epileptiform abnormalities does not rule out the possibility of psychogenic seizure, since real and psychogenic seizures may coexist. The diagnosis of psychogenic seizure is best supported by documenting the fact that the EEG obtained simultaneously during the clinical episode does not show any ictal changes. A normal EEG before, during, and after a generalized tonic clonic seizure-like episode is reasonable evidence for the diagnosis of psychogenic seizure. However, this criterion is not reliable in partial seizure-like episodes. The surface EEG may be normal in partial elementary and partial complex seizures as well as in myoclonic seizures.

The EEG recording should conform to the minimum technical requirements of the American EEG Society (3). Adequate number of recording channels, adequate recording time, and standard activation procedures are essential in order to minimize diagnostic errors. Verbal suggestion is often a very effective activation technique for psychogenic seizure. Psychogenic seizure patients in general are highly suggestible and an "ictal" event can often be provoked even during a routine outpatient EEG recording. In Krumholz and Niedermeyer's study (29) psychogenic seizure occurred during standard EEG recording in 33% of patients. Thus, in many cases, the diagnosis of psychogenic seizure can be made with reasonable certainty even on an outpatient basis (51). Why some patients readily have a psychogenic seizure attack during routine EEG recording, and others do not, is unclear.

DIAGNOSIS OF PSYCHOGENIC SEIZURES (LEVEL II)

EEG with Activation

When no ictal events occur during the standard EEG session, further diagnostic evaluation is necessary. Sleep-deprived EEG recording with nasopharyngeal or sphenoidal electrodes may be of value in activation or detection of epileptiform abnormalities. But merely demonstrating the presence of interictal abnormalities is not diagnostically helpful, and it is of fundamental importance to provoke an habitual seizure so that the ictal EEG can be studied. Cohen and Suter (7) recommend a provocative EEG test employing intravenous saline injection and suggestion for recording psychogenic seizures. In the study by Luther et al. (34), psychogenic seizures occurred spontaneously in 20% of patients, and in response to saline injection in another 27%. Suggestion alone or in combination with photic stimulation and hyperventilation was found to be the most effective, eliciting psychogenic seizures in 53% of cases.

Ambulatory Cassette-Recorded EEG

When a seizure cannot be provoked in the outpatient EEG laboratory, ambulatory cassette recording (ACR) in the patient's own living environment is a convenient alternative. The technique and usefulness of ACR is presented in J. S. Ebersole (*this volume*). ACR has several advantages: (a) the recorder is lightweight and portable, (b) prolonged recording is possible, (c) hospitalization is not required and recording can be done in the patient's own natural environment, and, finally, (d) the frequency of seizures can be ascertained (58). Given these advantages, it would seem that ACR is ideally suited for the study of psychogenic seizures, but there are a few specific drawbacks. The original 4-channel system (26) is not adequate for reliably diagnosing psychogenic seizures. The situation is worse when only two channels are available for recording EEG, the other two channels having been sacrificed for ECG and event marker, respectively. A careful montage design, although extremely important, is not a substitute for an adequate number of recording channels. The recently introduced 8-channel recorders are a significant improvement over the previous system. Here again, montage design is very important and should be guided by a careful review of the patient's symptoms (30). A complex montage design requires greater expertise on the part of the person who is scanning and interpreting the EEG. Sometimes it is too much to expect of the scanning technologist to be able to recognize subtle electrographic ictal changes which may occur in partial seizures. Psychogenic seizures in response to the perception of true epileptic aura, in particular, may cause diagnostic difficulties (47), especially when a limited number of recording channels is used. When ACR monitoring is done at the patient's home, the physician does not have the opportunity to observe the clinical events and has to depend entirely on the information provided by the patient or the family. A reasonable degree of patient cooperation is essential. Reliable electroclinical correlation is not possible if the patient does not keep an accurate diary or remember to activate the event marker appropriately. An occasional psychogenic seizure patient may deliberately disable the recorder or pull out the electrodes. One of our patients removed the cassette tape during recording and inserted it into her "Walkman" recorder so that she might listen to her "brain waves." Another patient attempted to flush the recorder down the toilet. A few patients may shower with electrodes on or dislodge the wires while attempting to hide them under a hat. Such problems are not insurmountable but an awareness of these practical difficulties is important.

Technical problems can be annoying. Instrumental malfunctioning is not an uncommon problem. Meticulous attention is required in electrode applications to the scalp. Periodic applications of electrolyte solutions to the electrode cups is essential. Generally the various commonly encountered EEG artifacts can easily be recognized. An occasional problem is 60-Hz interference from a household appliance. In summer, excess sweating may cause considerable electrode artifacts. Unfortunately, the various artifacts and instrumental malfunctioning cannot be immediately recognized and corrected during ACR recording. Despite these disadvantages, ACR has a definite place as an intermediate level monitoring technique in the diagnostic study of carefully selected psychogenic seizure suspect patients, by physicians with expertise in this area.

The one-channel Cerebral Function Monitor (42) has neither the portability of ACR nor the multichannel recording capability of a standard EEG machine and, therefore, has no place in the diagnosis of psychogenic seizures.

DIAGNOSIS OF PSYCHOGENIC SEIZURES (LEVEL III)

Intensive Monitoring

Not everyone suspected of psychogenic seizures requires intensive neurodiagnostic monitoring. In about 50% of cases the diagnosis of psychogenic seizures is reasonably certain on the basis of history and outpatient EEG recordings. In the remaining group accurate diagnosis is difficult and sometimes impossible without inpatient intensive monitoring. This is especially the case when the clinical episodes resemble partial seizures or when real and psychogenic seizures coexist. Also in many instances the clinical impression of psychogenic seizures proves erroneous when the patient is subjected to intensive monitoring (41,59). Intensive monitoring includes behavioral observation, serum anticonvulsant level monitoring, simultaneous video-EEG recording and telemetry. The inpatient monitoring unit should be staffed with personnel trained in various aspects of epilepsy diagnosis and management, in order to facilitate accurate behavioral assessment. The indications for intensive monitoring are (a) to confirm the diagnosis of psychogenic seizures, (b) to rule out real seizures, and (c) to define the relationship between real and psychogenic seizures when they coexist. The purpose of hospitalization should be explained to the patient and the family in a simple, straightforward manner. We generally tell the patient, "You say that you are having many seizures. We do not know what kind of seizures you are suffering from. We want to study these seizures or spells in more detail so that we can know how to help you better."

Behavioral Observation

Following admission to the inpatient unit, baseline serum anticonvulsant levels are determined which are then serially monitored. Anticonvulsant drug toxicity should be ruled out since it may facilitate the emergence of psychogenic seizures in certain predisposed individuals (37). In a recent monograph, Trimble (60) has thoroughly discussed the subject of anticonvulsant drugs and psychogenic seizures. The well-known clinical characteristics of psychogenic seizures have been critically reviewed in the paper by Desai et al. (12). Generally psychogenic seizures are bizarre and uncoordinated but at times they can be sophisticated and very convincing, resembling various partial and generalized epilepsies. Gates et al. (19) reviewed the ictal characteristics of psychogenic seizures in 72 videotaped episodes from 53 patients. Thirty-five of these episodes resembled generalized tonic-clonic seizures, and the rest, partial seizures. In Krumholz and Niedermeyer's study (29), 66% resembled major motor seizures, and the rest, minor motor spells. Out-of-phase arm and leg movements, vigorous side-to-side head movements, continuous prolonged vocalizations, and even articulated speech during a "seizure" are quite characteristic of psychogenic seizures (19). Pelvic thrusting and even arching of the body may be seen in both pseudo- as well as epileptic seizures and, therefore, are not reliable differentiating signs. Incontinence is not rare but self-injury is most unusual. Avoidance responses to attempted eye opening, physical threats, etc., are highly suggestive of psychogenic seizures (34), although a postictally confused patient following a genuine seizure may also exhibit such behavior. In any case it is important for the staff to accurately document the ictal sequence and the circumstances in which the seizures occur in order to facilitate differentiation of psychogenic seizures from epileptic seizures. Estimation of serum prolactin levels may be of value in differential diagnosis, since a significant rise occurs only following an epileptic generalized tonic-clonic seizure and not after psychogenic seizures (8).

Video/EEG Recording

After approximately one week of behavioral observation, prolonged video-EEG monitoring is undertaken. Each recording session may last from 4 to 6 hr.

Verbal suggestions are used to enhance the possibility of provoking an attack during the recording. In the majority of psychogenic seizure patients a positive "ictal" recording can usually be obtained during the very first video-EEG session (28,47), while repeated recordings and anticonvulsant drug withdrawal may be necessary to induce an epileptic ictal event. Once an attack is precipitated, efforts should be made to terminate it by suggestion. Even in case of obvious psychogenic seizures, it is important to review the simultaneously recorded EEG carefully for evidence of ictal changes of partial seizures. Patients may react with a psychogenic seizure to the perception of a true epileptic aura. It is also important to establish that the recorded clinical episodes represent the patient's habitual seizures.

If an "ictal" recording is not obtained during the initial video-EEG session, partial anticonvulsant drug withdrawal is undertaken. This tends to unmask latent epileptic activity and facilitates a sharper distinction between epileptic and psychogenic seizures during the monitoring period. It is our practice to proceed with drug withdrawal even after successful recording of a psychogenic seizure, in order not to overlook real seizures that may coexist. The ictal characteristics of psychogenic seizures on videotape have been described in detail by several investigators (12,19,22). Psychogenic seizures may be manifested by almost an infinite variety of individual phenomena, but as Gulick et al. (22) point out, only rarely does the complete pattern of psychogenic seizure resemble an epileptic seizure. Video-EEG recording, in our experience, is the single most valuable test for diagnosing psychogenic seizures. Although psychogenic seizure may be suspected on clinical grounds alone, in many cases video-EEG documentation is necessary to confirm the diagnosis. An erroneous clinical diagnosis of psychogenic seizures can be reliably refuted only by video-EEG evidence of true epileptic events accompanying the habitual seizures. The videotape is a permanent record of the seizures and can be used to great advantage in the clinical management of psychogenic seizures (45), as well as for research, and patient and staff education.

Telemetry

The value of telemetry in intensive monitoring of seizures has been well established (6,41). Telemetered-EEG is used less often than video monitoring for diagnosing psychogenic seizures. It is best reserved for patients who do not have "seizures" in front of the camera during video/EEG sessions but complain of many attacks in the ward when not under staff observation. These patients may represent a subgroup of psychogenic seizure patients, who are more manipulative and sociopathic and less hysterical or attention-seeking than the ones who readily have their attacks in the presence of an audience. Telemetry allows greater freedom of movement compared with video/EEG recording. The clinical episodes may easily escape staff observation when the patient is on telemetry and there is no permanent record of the seizure for electroclinical correlations. In our unit patients on radiotelemetry are kept under constant one-to-one observation by the nursing staff. Night-time observation can be a problem unless special video arrangements are available for all-night recordings. The currently available combined video-telemetered EEG system is interesting but may pose certain technical problems. It is difficult to keep the patient constantly in the range of the video camera unless he or she is confined to a small area. This system may be useful in certain special situations such as observing a patient who habitually has "seizures" during stressful group therapy sessions.

Conclusions

Psychogenic seizures, either occurring alone or in conjunction with epilepsy, are increasingly being recognized as a major clinical problem. The diagnostic investigation for psychogenic seizures may be undertaken at three levels. Although the diagnosis may be made with reasonable certainty on the basis of history, outpatient EEG recordings, and ambulatory monitoring (levels I and II), intensive monitoring (level III) is necessary in many patients. Intensive monitoring is the only reliable way to document psychogenic seizures in difficult cases, especially when the attacks resemble partial seizures and when real and psychogenic seizures coexist.

AGGRESSION AND DYSCONTROL SYNDROMES

Diagnostic assessment of episodic aggression and dyscontrol syndromes presents major conceptual and practical problems. Human aggression is a complex phenomenon which is determined by varying degrees of interaction between biological, psychosocial, and environmental factors. The neural bases of aggression and violent behavior, despite the enormous body of available information (15,20), remain incompletely understood. Reliable information regarding the incidence of episodic aggression is lacking. Aggressive behavior is commonly encountered in prisons, mental institutions, group homes for the retarded, and psychiatric emergency rooms, but only infrequently in neurological practice. The reason for referral to the neurologist, in most cases of episodic aggression, is to rule out epilepsy or some form of brain dysfunction.

Clinical Assessment of Episodic Aggression

A comprehensive clinical classification of aggression is difficult. Aggressive behavior may be seen transiently in a variety of acute toxic or metabolic encephalopathies and as a secondary symptom in chronic progressive cerebral disorders. In episodic aggression, on the other hand, aggressive outbursts are chronic and recurrent and constitute the dominant clinical symptom. For diagnostic purposes, episodic aggression can be broadly divided into three subgroups: (a) aggression as a maladaptive behavior which results from adverse psychosocial influences and traumatic life experiences, (b) episodic dyscontrol syndromes, and (c) aggression related to epilepsy. These three groups are not precisely defined, mutually exclusive categories, and some degree of overlap among them is more often the rule than the exception.

Group 1

Many aggressive, violent patients also manifest other evidence of severe psychopathology. Their backgrounds frequently reveal a number of pathological features which occur consistently enough to be reliable predictors of future violent behavior. These include childhood maternal deprivation, poor father identification, or both, nocturnal enuresis, possibly fire-setting, violence towards animals, and brutalization by one or both parents (20). Severe psychopathology and alcoholism in the family are common.

Group 2

The term episodic dyscontrol was introduced by Bach-y-Rita et al. (5) although the same concept also has been expounded by Mark and Ervin (35) and Monroe (36). These authors, while not discounting the importance of psychological and environmental influences, suggest that at least in some individuals cerebral dysfunction especially involving the temporolimbic system may be the fundamental defect which is responsible for recurrent episodes of aggression.

Group 3

The relationship between epilepsy and aggression is complicated and involves a number of questions: (a) Does epilepsy per se, rather than nonspecific brain damage, predispose to aggression?; (b) Is aggression unique to temporal lobe or limbic epilepsy?; (c) Is aggression in epilepsy ictal or interictal?; (d) If interictal, what is the nature of the interaction between the neural dysfunction and environmental factors?; and, finally, (e) Can ictal aggression lead to acts of violence? (44). The answers to these questions still remain controversial and a review of this subject is beyond the scope of this chapter. The relationship between episodic dyscontrol syndrome and epilepsy is uncertain, and often the dividing line between limbic dysfunction and limbic epilepsy is blurred. These issues make the diagnostic evaluation of episodic aggression a complicated undertaking.

In view of the complex nature of the problem, it is important in every case of episodic aggression to clearly define the clinical problem and formulate specific questions that need to be answered before undertaking intensive monitoring. Intensive monitoring should not be undertaken without a prior thorough investigation of the patient's life history including his or her premorbid personality, coping styles, past psychiatric illnesses, and current psychosocial stresses. It is crucial to obtain a detailed account of the aggressive episodes themselves and the circumstances in which they occur, in an attempt to differentiate psychologically determined behavioral outbursts from those resulting from epileptic or "epileptoid" disturbances of cerebral function. All patients should have a complete physical examination, CT scan of the head, and neuropsychological testing. A number of soft neurological signs have been described in violent criminals (13,40). But as Bach-y-Rita et al. (5) point out, the presence of abnormal neurological signs by itself does not imply that the aggressive episodes are "organically" determined, any more than the presence of severe psychopathology proves the "functional" nature of the problem.

Routine EEG

Riley and Niedermeyer (49) studied 212 patients who were referred to the EEG laboratory of the Johns Hopkins Hospital for evaluation of rage attacks and episodic violent behavior. No patient had evidence of overt seizures, known neurological diseases, or psychosis. An overwhelming majority of them (94%) had normal EEGs. In contrast, aggressive patients with epilepsy, mental retardation, and other cerebral disorders have a high incidence of EEG abnormalities in the form of diffuse background slowing and nonspecific paroxysmal activities (24,56). Thus, in episodic aggression the background EEG abnormalities merely confirm the presence of cerebral damage and do not shed any light on the nature of the aggressive episodes themselves. The routine EEG even with the usual activation procedures of photic stimulation, hyperventilation, sleep, and sleep deprivation, therefore, is of limited value in the investigation of episodic aggression (52). Photometrazol (18), alpha chloralose (36), and other chemical activation tests may induce nonspecific paroxysmal abnormalities (1), and their value in the investigation of episodic aggression has not found wide acceptance. The role of ACR in episodic aggression is not well established at the present time.

Interictal Epileptiform Abnormalities

The significance of interictal spikes in the EEGs of patients with episodic aggression should be interpreted with great caution. The so-called benign transients (14/sec and 6/sec positive spikes, 6/sec spike-wave, psychomotor variants, and small, sharp spikes), in the majority view, have no clinical significance with respect to the problem of aggression. Although spikes do not necessarily imply clinical seizures, most patients with frequent spikes in their EEGs do have seizures (2). Thus, in most cases of episodic aggression, the significance of interictal spikes essentially amounts to the issue of the relationship between epilepsy and aggression. Whether epilepsy per se, complex partial type or otherwise, predisposes to aggression remains a controversial issue (39,57). The presence of frontal, anterior, or mesial temporal spikes, although highly suggestive of complex partial seizures, does not necessarily imply a causal relationship between seizures and aggression unless such a direct link can be documented by ictal recordings

At this point one can summarize by saying that if a patient with episodic aggression has a normal neurological examination, normal CT scan of the head, and normal EEG, and, in addition, has a positive psychiatric history but no history of epilepsy or other neurological disorders, further intensive monitoring is unlikely to be rewarding.

Intensive Monitoring to Episodic Aggression

Intensive monitoring is indicated (a) when episodic aggression occurs in patients with known seizures and the relationship between seizures and aggression is uncertain, (b) in patients with no history of seizures who show explosive rage attacks with little or no provocation, and (c) in patients with episodic aggression who have no known history of epilepsy but who have significant interictal epileptiform abnormalities in their EEGs. Intensive monitoring for episodic aggression should ideally be undertaken only in special epilepsy centers with facilities for psychiatric and psychological assessments, video/EEG recordings, telemetry, and depth EEG studies. The ward personnel should be well trained in managing both seizures and aggressive behavior. There are certain practical problems in intensive monitoring of EA. Hospitalization is necessary. A highly specialized, adequately staffed monitoring unit is essential. Physical injury to the staff and damage to monitoring equipment are potential dangers when dealing with aggressive or violent patients. Often the aggressive behavior may dramatically decrease in a supportive inpatient milieu and, therefore, defeat the purpose of hospitalization (43).

Video/EEG Recording

It is difficult to obtain a spontaneous habitual episode of aggression during video-EEG sessions. Video monitoring is more useful for determining whether the spontaneous or activated habitual clinical seizure reveals aggression as a prominent ictal feature. A number of studies have shown that ictal, directed aggression is rare in epilepsy (10,27,43,50). Isolated instances of ictal aggression, however, have been reported (4,35,54). Further intensive monitoring is indicated when no ictal recordings are obtained during video-EEG session or when the recorded ictal events do not reveal significant aggressive component.

Aggression may be a manifestation of interictal psychosis in epilepsy. Ramani and Gumnit (46) studied the interictal psychosis in ten hospitalized epileptics using intensive monitoring techniques. Transient agitation, hyperactivity, and aggressive tendencies were observed in most of them at some point during the course of their psychotic illness. Only one patient showed forced normalization of EEG during the psychotic phase, and an inverse relationship between seizure frequency and psychosis. In others, no explanation could be found for the emergence of psychosis.

Telemetry

Telemetry is a convenient method to study episodic aggression and has certain advantages over video monitoring. It permits freedom of movement for the patient and, therefore, recording in more natural conditions is possible. Hospitalization is required because of the limited transmission range of the telemetry system and the need for close staff supervision. Because of the need for close supervision and the limitations of telemetry transmission range, patients have to be confined to the ward during the monitoring period and consequently excluded from many recreational activities. Some patients become bored and others irritable, but most tolerate the procedure fairly well. We have successfully used telemetry over the last few years to obtain ictal recordings in various epilepsies, especially in complex partial seizures. Only rarely do these seizures show aggression as an ictal feature and we have never observed directed aggression in any.

Role of Depth EEG

In many cases the investigator is considerably handicapped by the limitations of surface EEG. Depth electrode studies in psychiatric patients have shown that complex electrical activity may be present in the deep cerebral structures with little or no reflection in the surface EEG (9,23,55). The relevance of these studies to the problems of episodic aggression and epilepsy is questionable. Lieb et al. (32) studied the surface and depth EEGs in 34 patients with temporal lobe epilepsy. They found that although seizure onset in the depths of temporal lobe often did not produce any changes in the surface EEG, ictal changes were usually evident in the surface tracings once the patient developed clinical signs of impairment of consciousness or automatisms. Delgado-Escueta et al. (11) also noted that diffuse surface EEG changes occurred when the level of consciousness was affected during a seizure. In view of such evidence it seems improbable that recurrent episodes of aggression can result from subcortical ictal activity without any reflection in the surface EEG. Depth electrode studies, although of unquestioned importance in episodic aggression, are not justified in most instances and should not be undertaken without a serious consideration of the ethical issues involved. At the present time, epilepsy surgery is the only indication for depth EEG studies. One can only hope that future technology will provide powerful noninvasive methods to investigate some of the very difficult, aggressive, and violent patients, who may indeed have some type of limbic dysfunction.

Conclusions

Diagnostic evaluation of episodic aggression is complicated. Preliminary assessment of episodic aggression should include a detailed history and a careful psychiatric evaluation. Surface EEG is usually of limited value. Intensive monitoring of episodic aggression should be carried out in special epilepsy centers. Ictal aggression is rare and most often aggression in epilepsy is a multifactorially determined interictal phenomenon. The nature of the so-called episodic dyscontrol syndrome is unknown. Depth EEG studies are not justified in most cases of episodic aggression and dyscontrol syndromes at the present time.

REFERENCES

1. Ajmone-Marsan, C. (1984): Electroencephalographic studies in seizure disorders: Additional considerations. *J. Clin. Neurophysiol.,* 1:143–157.
2. Ajmone-Marsan, C., and Zivin, L. S. (1970): Factors related to the occurrence of typical paroxysmal abnormalities in the EEG records of epileptic patients. *Epilepsia,* 11:361–381.
3. American EEG Society (1980): Guidelines in EEG, No. 3, *Minimum Technical Requirements for Performing Clinical Electroencephalography.*
4. Ashford, J. W., Schulz, C., and Walsh, G. O. (1980): Violent automatisms in a partial complex seizure. Report of a case. *Arch. Neurol.,* 37:120–122.
5. Bach-y-Rita, G., Lion, J. R., Climent, C. E., and Ervin, F. R. (1971): Episodic dyscontrol: A study of 130 violent patients. *Am. J. Psychiatry,* 127:1473–1478.
6. Binnie, C. D., Rowan, A. J., Overweg, J., Meinardi, H., Wisman, T., Kamp, A., and Lopes da Silva, F. (1981): Telemetric EEG and video monitoring in epilepsy. *Neurology,* 31:298–303.
7. Cohen, R. J.. and Suter, C. (1982): Hysterical seizure: Suggestion as a provocative EEG test. *Ann. Neurol.,* 11:391–395.
8. Dana-Haeri, J., Trimble, M. R., and Oxley, J. (1983): Prolactin and gonadotrophin changes following generalized and partial seizures. *J. Neurol. Neurosurg. Psychiatry,* 46:331–335.
9. Delgado, J. M. R., and Hamlin, H. (1956): Surface and depth electrography of the frontal lobes in conscious patients. *Electroencephalogr. Clin. Neurophysiol.,* 8:371–384.
10. Delgado-Escueta, A. V., Mattson, R. H., King, L., Goldensohn, E. S., Spiegel, H., Madsen, J., Crandall, P., Dreifuss, F. E., and Porter, R. J. (1981): Special report. The nature of aggression during epileptic seizures. *N. Engl. J. Med.,* 305:711–716.
11. Delgado-Escueta, A. V., Nashold, B., Freeman, M., Keplinger, G., Waddell, G., Miller, P., and Carwille, S. (1979): Videotaping epileptic attacks during stereoelectroencephalography. *Neurology,* 29:473–489.

12. Desai, B. T., Porter, R. J., and Penry, J. K. (1982): Psychogenic seizures. A study of 42 attacks in six patients, with intensive monitoring. *Arch. Neurol.,* 39:202–209.
13. Elliott, F. A. (1976): Neurological factors in violent behavior (the dyscontrol syndrome). *Bull. Am. Acad. Psychiatry Law,* 4:297–305.
14. Fenton, G. W. (1982): Hysterical alteration of consciousness. In: *Hysteria,* edited by A. Roy, pp. 229–246. Wiley, New York.
15. Fields, W. S., and Sweet, W. H. (editors) (1975): *Neural Bases of Violence and Aggression.* Greene, St. Louis.
16. Finlayson, R., and Lucas, A. R. (1979): Pseudoepileptic seizures in children and adolescents. *Mayo Clin. Proc.,* 54:83–87.
17. Folks, D. G., Ford, C. V., and Regan, W. M. (1984): Conversion symptoms in a general hospital. *Psychosomatics,* 25:285–295.
18. Gastaut, H. (1947): Effets des stimulations physiques sur l'EEG de l'homme. *Electroencephalogr. Clin. Neurophysiol.* (*Suppl.*), 2:69–82.
19. Gates, J. R., Ramani, V., and Whelan, S. M. (1982): Ictal characteristics of pseudoseizures (abstract). *Presented at the Annual Epilepsy Society/American EEG Society Joint Meeting, Phoenix, Arizona.*
20. Goldstein, M. (1974): Brain research and violent behavior. *Arch. Neurol.,* 30:1–34.
21. Gross, M. (1979): Pseudoepilepsy. A study in adolescent hysteria. *Am. J. Psychiatry,* 136:210–212.
22. Gulick, T. A., Spinks, I. P., and King, D. W. (1982): Pseudoseizures: Ictal phenomena. *Neurology,* 32:24–30.
23. Heath, R. G. (1958): Correlation of electrical recordings from cortical and subcortical regions of the brain with abnormal behavior in human subjects. *Confin. Neurol.,* 18:305–315.
24. Hill, D., and Watterson, D. (1942): Electroencephalographic studies of psychopathic personalities. *J. Neurol. Psychiatry,* 5:47–65.
25. Holmes, G. L., Sackellares, J. C., McKiernan, J., Ragland, M., and Dreifuss, F. E. (1980): Evaluation of childhood pseudoseizures using EEG telemetry and videotape monitoring. *J. Pediatr.,* 97:554–558.
26. Ives, J. R., and Woods, J. F. (1975): 4-Channel 24-hour cassette recorder for long term EEG monitoring of ambulatory patients. *Electroencephalogr. Clin. Neurophysiol.,* 39:88–92.
27. King, D. W., and Ajmone-Marsan, C. (1977): Clinical features and ictal patterns in epileptic patients with EEG temporal foci. *Ann. Neurol.,* 2:138–147.
28. King, D. W., Gallagher, B. B., Murvin, A. J., Smith, D. B., Marcus, D. J., Hartlage, L. C., and Ward, C. L. (1982): Pseudoseizures: Diagnostic evaluation. *Neurology,* 32:18–23.
29. Krumholz, A., and Niedermeyer, E. (1983): Psychogenic seizures. A clinical study with follow-up data. *Neurology,* 33:498–502.
30. Leroy, R. F., and Ebersole, J. S. (1983): An evaluation of ambulatory cassette EEG monitoring: I. Montage design. *Neurology,* 33:1–7.
31. Lesser, R. P., Lueders, H., and Dinner, D. S. (1983): Evidence for epilepsy is rare in patients with psychogenic seizures. *Neurology,* 33:502–504.
32. Lieb, J. P., Walsh, G. O., Babb, T. L., Walter, R. D., and Crandall, P. H. (1976): A comparison of EEG seizure patterns recorded with surface and depth electrodes in patients with temporal lobe epilepsy. *Epilepsia,* 17:137–160.
33. Liske, E., and Forster, F. M. (1964): Pseudoseizures: A problem in the diagnosis and management of epileptic patients. *Neurology,* 14:41–49.
34. Luther, J. S., McNamara, J. O., Carwile, S., Miller, P., and Hope, V. (1982): Pseudoepileptic seizures: Methods and videotape analysis to aid diagnosis. *Ann. Neurol.,* 12:458–462.
35. Mark, V. H., and Ervin, F. R. (1970): *Violence and the Brain.* Harper & Row, Hagerstown.
36. Monroe, R. R. (1970): *Episodic Behavioral Disorders.* Harvard University Press, Cambridge.
37. Niedermeyer, E., Blumer, D., Holscher, E., and Walker, B. A. (1970): Classical hysterical seizures facilitated by anticonvulsant toxicity. *Psychiatr. Clin.* (*Basel*), 3:71–74.
38. Nemiah, J. C. (1980): Somatoform disorders. In: *Comprehensive Textbook of Psychiatry, 3rd Ed., Vol. 2,* edited by A. M. Freedman, H. I. Kaplan, and B. J. Sadock, pp. 1525–1544. Williams & Wilkins, Baltimore.

39. Pincus, J. H. (1980): Can volence be a manifestation of epilepsy? *Neurology,* 30:304–307.
40. Pincus, J. H., Lewis, D. O., Shanok, S. S., and Glaser, G. H. (1979): Neurologic abnormalities in violent delinquents. *Neurology,* 29:586.
41. Porter, R. J., Penry, J. K., and Lacy, J. R. (1977): Diagnostic and therapeutic reevaluation of patients with intractable epilepsy. *Neurology,* 27:1006–1011.
42. Prior, P. F. (1979): *Monitoring Cerebral Function.* Lippincott, Philadelphia.
43. Ramani, V., and Gumnit, R. J. (1981): Intensive monitoring of epileptic patients with a history of episodic aggression. *Arch. Neurol.,* 38:570–571.
44. Ramani, V., and Gumnit, R. J. (1982): Episodic aggression in epilepsy (reply). *Arch Neurol.,* 39:385–386.
45. Ramani, V., and Gumnit, R. J. (1982): Management of hysterical seizures in epileptic patients. *Arch. Neurol.,* 39:78–81.
46. Ramani, V., and Gumnit, R. J. (1982): Intensive monitoring of inter-ictal psychosis in epilepsy. *Ann. Neurol.,* 11:613–622.
47. Ramani, V., Quesney, L. F., Olson, D., and Gumnit, R. J. (1980): Diagnosis of hysterical seizures in epileptic patients. *Am. J. Psychiatry,* 137:705–709.
48. Riley, T. L., and Massey, W. E. (1980): Pseudoseizures in the military. *Milit. Med.,* 145:614–619.
49. Riley, T. L., and Niedermeyer, E. (1978): Rage attacks and episodic violent behavior: Electroencephalographic findings and general considerations. *Clin. Electroencephalogr.,* 9:131–139.
50. Rodin, E. A. (1973): Psychomotor epilepsy and aggressive behavior. *Arch. Gen. Psychiatry,* 28:210–213.
51. Rodin, E. A. (1981): Differential diagnosis of epileptic versus psychogenic seizures. In: *Advances in Epileptology,* edited by M. Dam, L. Gram, and J. K. Penry, pp. 337–342. Raven Press, New York.
52. Rodin, E. A. (1982): Aggression and epilepsy. In: *Pseudoseizures,* edited by T. L. Riley and A. Roy, pp. 185–212. Williams & Wilkins, Baltimore.
53. Roy, A. (1979): Hysterical seizures. *Arch. Neurol.,* 36:447.
54. Saint-Hilaire, J. M., Gilbert, M., and Bouvier, G. (1980): Epilepsy and aggression: Two cases with depth electrode studies. In: *Epilepsy Updated: Causes and Treatment,* edited by P. Robb, pp. 145–176. Year Book, Chicago.
55. Sem-Jacobsen, C. W., Petersen, M. C., Lazarte, J. A., Dodge, H. W., and Holman, C. B. (1955): Electroencephalographic rhythms from the depths of the frontal lobe in 60 psychotic patients. *Electroencephalogr. Clin. Neurophysiol.,* 7:193–210.
56. Silverman, D. (1943): Clinical and electroencephalographic studies in criminal psychopaths. *Arch. Neurol. Psychiatry,* 50:18–33.
57. Stevens, J. R., and Hermann, B. P. (1981): Temporal lobe epilepsy, psychopathology, and violence. The state of the evidence. *Neurology,* 31:1127–1132.
58. Stores, G. (1981): Differential diagnosis of seizures: Psychiatric aspects. In: *Advances in Epileptology,* edited by M. Dam, L. Gram, and J. K. Penry, pp. 259–263. Raven Press, New York.
59. Sutula, T. P., Sackellares, J. C., Miller, J. Q., and Dreifuss, F. E. (1981): Intensive monitoring in refractory epilepsy. *Neurology,* 31:243–247.
60. Trimble, M. R. (1982): Anticonvulsant drugs and hysterical seizures. In: *Pseudoseizures,* edited by T. L. Riley and A. Roy, pp. 148–158. Williams & Wilkins, Baltimore.
61. Wilkus, R. J., Dodrill, C. B., and Thompson, P. M. (1984): Intensive EEG monitoring and psychological studies in patients with pseudoepileptic seizures. *Epilepsia,* 25:100–107.
62. Williams, D. T., Spiegel, H., and Mostofsky, D. I. (1978): Neurogenic and hysterical seizures in children and adolescents. Differential diagnostic and therapeutic considerations. *Am. J. Psychiatry,* 135:82–86.

Advances in Neurology, Vol. 46: Intensive Neurodiagnostic Monitoring, edited by R. J. Gumnit. Raven Press, New York © 1986.

Intensive Monitoring of Seizures in Evaluating Efficacy of Antiepileptic Drugs

Ilo E. Leppik

Department of Neurology, University of Minnesota, and the Minnesota Comprehensive Epilepsy Program, 2701 University Ave. SE, Minneapolis, Minnesota 55414

To use antiepileptic drugs (AEDs) properly, intensive neurodiagnostic monitoring is needed for three reasons: to diagnose the seizure correctly, to quantify the number of events, and to allow the patient and physician to communicate accurately regarding seizures. In treating a person with epilepsy, the physician faces one of the most difficult challenges in medicine because, unlike most other illnesses where definite physical findings are readily observable, the presence and identity of a seizure almost always must be diagnosed from historical evidence. To further complicate matters, patients are, except during simple partial seizures, unaware of the manifestations of their seizures. People observing a seizure are often frightened and not trained to recognize the details required to classify a spell clearly. Diagnosis and treatment is thus based on much less objective information than in almost any other medical condition. Not uncommonly, a patient with peculiar paroxysmal behavior is diagnosed and treated as being epileptic on evidence which would be considered hearsay in other settings. Even if the diagnosis of epilepsy is correctly made, the problem of classifying the seizure remains. Since antiepileptic medications are specific for seizure types, one must know the correct classification of the seizure in order to treat the patient effectively.

Persons whose seizures are not controlled by AEDs may be failing to respond for a number of reasons. Seizures may be nonepileptic episodes (psychogenic seizures) which will not respond and may even be made worse by AEDs (7,10). Brief complex partial seizures may appear identical to generalized absence (petit mal) seizures (3). The reverse is true also as typical absence seizures may look like complex partial spells (8). It is also important to identify the specific seizure type or types a patient is having so that the patient and physician can communicate accurately in the clinic. Often, patients are not well trained to self-report their spells. Nevertheless, medical decisions made in the clinic are based on whether intervention with AEDs has improved the frequency or severity of events. Correct diagnosis of seizures is necessary to select the proper treatment and to monitor the outcome of treatment accurately.

DIAGNOSIS OF SEIZURES

Although routine EEG is the first step in evaluation, it is often not definitive. The initial EEG does not show epileptiform activity in more than 40% of perons with a known seizure disorder (1). Even if found, an interictal abnormality may not be completely reliable in delineating the seizure pattern. In routine EEG recordings, actual seizures are captured only in 2.5% to 7% of recordings (7,9). The only means by which seizures can be diagnosed accurately is by simultaneous recording of neurophysiological and somatic manifestations of the events in question. This can be accomplished by a variety of techniques (Table 1). Ideally, every event should be observed and properly recorded. At the Minnesota Comprehensive Epilepsy Program we have developed an approach to monitoring patients with intractable seizures. The inpatient evaluation actually begins during the screening visit (Table 2). At this

TABLE 1. *Equipment available for EEG*

Modality	Description	Advantages	Disadvantages
Inpatient			
Video EEG	Patient in observation suite, video-trained on bed or chair, patient wired to EEG machine, technician present	Most accurate method available	Expensive and time consuming
Mobile video EEG	As above, but video and EEG are mounted on mobile unit which can be placed in patient's room	More flexible than suite; less costly	May miss some events
Radio telemetry	EEG component sent by radio; monitoring by video unit or nurse observation	Patient fully mobile	Expensive; may miss some events
Ambulatory cassette	EEG recorded by portable unit	Inexpensive; mobile	May miss some events
Outpatient			
Ambulatory cassette		Patient in own environment	May break down
Home video cassette		Inexpensive	May not obtain full seizure

TABLE 2. *Program for diagnosing and treating patients with intractable epilepsy*

Screening Interview	Episodes identified and described in detail.
Inpatient	
Baseline phase	Compliance with AED determined; program of medication reduction developed; episodes reviewed.
Diagnostic phase	AEDs reduced; episodes recorded and classified.
Treatment phase	Treatment appropriate to episodes started; AEDs standard or new given or psychosocial intervention if pseudoseizures diagnosed.
Outpatient	
Follow up	Seizure frequency assessed and appropriate adjustments made.

visit, the nurse clinician takes a detailed seizure history and identifies what events are considered to be of importance. For example, a patient may describe one type of spell where there is a ringing in the head and a slight feeling of dizziness. The second event may be described as ringing in the ears and dizziness, followed by loss of consciousness and behavior which is described as wandering around. A third type might be described as a warning of ringing inside the head followed by falling to the floor and shaking all over. The nurse clinician would label these as type 1, 2, and 3 and provide this information to the staff prior to admission. The goal of the admission then is to elucidate the nature of each event by observation. The course of admission is divided into three phases: baseline, diagnostic, and treatment (Table 2).

The baseline phase begins at admission and is 4 to 7 days in duration. The dose of the AED and other medication is not altered. AED levels are obtained at the beginning and end of baseline and provide a measurement of compliance with the prescribed AED. A difference of more than 20% between the admission and end of baseline level is evidence for noncompliance (5). During the past few years, fewer than 2% of patients admitted to the Epilepsy Treatment Unit (ETU) have been noncompliant at admission by these criteria. The two levels are used to calculate apparent clearance of the AED, and these values are used to develop a programmed reduction of medication. Also during baseline, a complete medical and neurological history and physical examination are performed, neuropsychological test battery is given, and laboratory evaluation of hematological, hepatic, renal, and endocrinological assessment is completed. Seizure type and frequency are documented, and this information is used to plan strategy for the diagnostic phase.

In order to obtain enough seizures for adequate diagnosis, most patients have one or more AEDs slowly withdrawn during the diagnostic phase. Only patients having very frequent seizures during baseline remain on their original medications during this phase. Usually, AEDs with long half-lives, or those with metabolites with long half-lives, are withdrawn initially (phenobarbital, primidone, etc.). Other AEDs are then withdrawn if seizure frequency has not increased to permit adequate video/EEG or radiotelemetry monitoring. Seizure type is not altered significantly by AED withdrawal (12), and EEG patterns are often activated (6). To prevent an increase in generalized seizures, one drug [usually phenytoin (PHT)] effective for generalized seizures, is not withdrawn. We have had no episodes of convulsive status epilepticus using our methods in the last 2 years. Nevertheless, an individualized protocol for treatment of status is ordered on each patient in the diagnostic phase, with coverage by an in-house physician at all times.

After a sufficient number of seizures have been documented, the treatment phase begins. If more than one generalized tonic-clonic seizure occurs during the diagnostic phase, necessary treatment is instituted. Persons with nonepileptic seizures or those who might benefit from surgery are identified.

The video/EEG recording is the cornerstone of the diagnostic process. It is our goal to record on video/EEG every event listed during the screening interview and verified during the baseline. This provides both an electroencephalographic record of activity and a visual display of behavior. These can be reviewed many times by the professional staff and also be used as a teaching device for the patients and their families or care-givers. Information obtained through video/EEG is very important in determining whether the events described are nonepileptic or epileptic. A surprising number of times the most dramatic limb movements and shaking are the nonepileptic events, whereas very brief automatisms that often go unnoticed or unreported by care-givers are the "true" epileptic seizures. Video/EEG monitoring is done in a suite with a technician in attendance at all times. A mobile video/EEG machine (Modac) is now available. This device may be used in the patients' rooms to obtain overnight recording. However, this recording system may occasionally miss seizures either because the patient has moved out of camera range or other technical difficulties.

Radio telemetry is useful once the seizures have been clearly documented by video/EEG because a correlation between the EEG activity can be made with presumed clinical phenomena, even though clinical phenomena are not observed.

Prolonged recording with cassette recorders in the recent past had the disadvantage of being able to record only four channels. Because of this limitation, this method was most useful for detecting generalized epileptiform events or determining the frequency of previously diagnosed seizures (4). A cassette recording using an 8-channel recorder is now available. This is best used when a clear diagnosis has been made with video-EEG. A number of technical problems may complicate the use of these cassette recorders, however. The most severe limiting factor is that the quality of the recording is detected only when the tape is played back. Thus, technical problems which may occur at the beginning of the recording and may invalidate the recording are not detected until after the session.

QUANTIFICATION OF SEIZURES

Quantification of seizures is crucial in evaluating the outcome of AED use. While generalized tonic-clonic seizures are generally obvious, quantification of partial complex and absence may be more difficult. Estimates of seizure frequency obtained from 12-hr EEG telemetry recordings were consistently higher than counts obtained from patients' calendars, nurses' observations, neurological examinations, and even routine EEG recordings (2). Thus, for absence seizures, it appears that only EEG recording can give the kind of accuracy required in the evaluation of a new drug or determining the effectiveness of a standard therapy (11). For complex partial seizures, we have found that patient education is important.

Throughout the evaluation on the epilepsy treatment unit, information regarding patients' seizures is continually made available to them. A record is kept of a patient's ability to self-report seizures. Usually by the end of the diagnostic phase, the patient is able to accurately self-report at least 80% of his seizures. Some patients with complex partial seizures, however, because of involvement of memory, can never reliably self-report seizures. Identification of these persons is important, as other means must be developed to quantify seizures correctly.

COMMUNICATION BETWEEN PATIENT AND PHYSICIAN

All of the information obtained during inpatient monitoring is extremely useful for outpatient drug therapy. Patients are instructed to keep strict calendars listing the seizures by type. At every clinic visit, a nurse clinician carefully reviews the seizure types and their numbers. These are entered onto a computerized data base utilizing the CLINFO program (Fig. 1). Also, drug doses and the corresponding blood levels are entered so that a computerized record of response to drug therapy over time can be maintained. The data entered into the system is of little use if it is not corroborated by inpatient video/EEG correlations.

SUMMARY

Intensive neurodiagnostic monitoring is needed in the proper use of AEDs for three reasons: to diagnose the seizure correctly, to quantify the number of seizures accurately, and to allow the patient and physician to communicate accurately. The means currently available include video/EEG, radiotelemetry, ambulatory cassette recording, and various permutations of the above. In general, video/EEG is the most accurate for diagnosis but the most costly, and ambulatory cassette recording the least costly and thus most useful for quantifying the number of seizures. An organized approach starting with screening inter-

```
NAME ___________________     CEP ID ________    MD/RN ________________

LAST VISIT ___/___/___ Studies in: ______        DATE TODAY ___-___-___  Clinic__
(___________)                      ______                                Phone__
Weight ___ kgs                                 WEIGHT ____ kgs       Discharge__

       SEIZURE FREQUENCY
----------------------------------------------------------------------
                                               # reported       # SINCE
code      type of seizure                      LAST VISIT       last visit
----------------------------------------------------------------------
---   -------------------------------    ---    *          --------
---   -------------------------------    ---    *          --------
---   -------------------------------    ---    *          --------
---   -------------------------------    ---    *          --------
--- ---------------------------------    ---    *          --------
                                                *
MEDICATIONS - LAST VISIT                        *          TODAY
-----------------------------                   *          -----
                                                *
AED       dose/24hr      level   new dose       *  AED       dose    level    new dose
---------------------------------------         * ----------------------------------
                                                *
-----      -----       -----    -----           *  -----    -----    -----    -----
-----      -----       -----    -----           *  -----    -----    -----    -----
-----      -----       -----    -----           *  -----    -----    -----    -----
-----      -----       -----    -----           *  -----    -----    -----    -----
                                                *  -----    -----    -----    -----
                                                *  -----    -----    -----    -----
LAB:                                            *
----                                            *
  WBC   ____     SGOT/AST  ____                 * WBC _____      AST _____
                                                *
                                                *
SIDE EFFECTS - LAST VISIT                       *   SIDE EFFECTS - TODAY
-----------------------------                   *_____________________________
code    description                             *
-----------------------------                   * ----  ----------------
                                                * ----  ----------------
---    -----  -------------------------         * ----  ----------------
---    -----  -------------------------         * ----  ----------------
                                                *
         NPSY TEST SCORES                   ************************************
Last Visit          Today                   *         NEW ORDERS (circle)      *
------------------------------------------  *__________________________________*
-----      Preferred hand    R    L         * LAB:                 PSYCHOSOCIAL: *
-----      CRT          __.___ seconds      *                                  *
--- ---    Pegboard ___ sec ___ pegs        * Drug levels        Counselor F/U *
 ---                ____ drops              *                                  *
--- ---    Digit Span R ___   AS ___        * Liver battery        49 Admit    *
--- ---    Digit Symb R ___   AS ___        *                                  *
-----      Verbal Fluency    ___            * Fibrinogen      Full NPsy Battery *
---_---    Verbal Fluency % ___-___         *                                  *
                                            *  NPSY  CBC  CT  EEG  ECG  AST    *
                                            *                                  *
                                            *   OTHER__________________________*
                                            ************************************
*******************************************COMMENTS: _________________________
                                               *  ______________________________
Routine Follow-up in ___wks  ___mos  ___yrs *  ______________________________
                                               *  ______________________________
Approximate date of next visit ___________  *  ______________________________
```

FIG. 1. CLINFO program data sheet.

view and continuing after discharge is recommended as being, in the long-term, the most cost-effective and satisfactory approach.

REFERENCES

1. Ajmone-Marsan, C., and Zivin, L. S. (1970): Factors related to the occurrence of typical paroxysmal abnormalities in the EEG records of epileptic patients. *Epilepsia,* 11:361–381.
2. Browne, T. R., Dreifuss, F. E., Penry, J. K., Porter, R. J., and White, B. G. (1983): Clinical and EEG estimates of absence seizure frequency. *Arch. Neurol.,* 40:469–472.
3. Delgado-Escueta, A. V., Enrile Bascal, F., and Treiman, D. M. (1982): Complex partial seizures on closed circuit television and EEG: a study of 691 attacks in 79 patients. *Ann. Neurol.,* 11:292–300.
4. Ives, J. R. (1982): Long-term monitoring in epileptic patients. *EEG Clin. Neurophysiol.,* 36(Suppl.):612–622.
5. Leppik, I. E., Cloyd, J. C., Sawchuk, R. J., and Pepin, S. M. (1979): Compliance and variability of plasma phenytoin levels in epileptic patients. *Ther. Drug. Monit.,* 1:475–483.
6. Ludwig, B. I., and Ajmone-Marsan, C. (1975): EEG changes after withdrawal of medication in epileptic patients. *EEG Clin. Neurophysiol.,* 39:173–181.
7. Mattson, R. H. (1980): Value of intensive monitoring. In: *Advances in Epileptology: The Xth Epilepsy International Symposium,* edited by J. A. Wada and J. K. Penry, pp. 43–51. Raven Press, New York.
8. Penry, J. K., Porter, R. J., and Dreifuss, F. E. (1975): Simultaneous recording of absence seizures with video tape and electroencephalography: a study of 374 seizures in 48 patients. *Brain,* 98:427–440.
9. Perry, T. R., Gumnit, R. J., Gates, J. R., and Leppik, I. E. (1983): Routine EEG vs. intensive monitoring in the evaluation of intractable epilepsy. *Public Health Rep.,* 98:384–389.
10. Ramani, V., Quesney, L. F., Olson, D., and Gumnit, R. J. (1980): Diagnosis of hysterical seizures in epileptic patients. *Am. J. Psychiatry,* 137(6):705–709.
11. Sato, S., White, B. G., Penry, J. D., Dreifuss, F. E., Sackellares, J. C., and Kupferberg, H. J. (1982): Valproic acid versus ethosuximide in the treatment of absence seizures. *Neurology (Cleveland),* 32:157–163.
12. Spencer, S. S., Spencer, D. D., Williamson, P. D., and Mattson, R. H. (1981): Ictal effects of anticonvulsant medication withdrawal in epileptic patients. *Epilepsia,* 22:297–307.

Advances in Neurology, Vol. 46: Intensive Neurodiagnostic Monitoring, edited by R. J. Gumnit. Raven Press, New York © 1986.

Epilepsy Presurgical Evaluation in the Era of Intensive Neurodiagnostic Monitoring

John R. Gates

Clinical Neurophysiology Laboratory, Comprehensive Epilepsy Program of Minnesota, 2701 University Ave. SE, Minneapolis, Minnesota 55414

The surgical treatment of epilepsy has traditionally been the last court of appeal for patients with intractable seizures. It assumes all medical therapies have been exhausted, the patient is still experiencing frequent seizures, and/or he is toxic on the medications. Fortunately, the technology available for surgical assessment and treatment has evolved and improved dramatically, especially in the last decade. Consequently, techniques now exist (e.g., corpus callostomy) that allow a surgical treatment for patients who never would have been considered candidates for a surgical approach at many epilepsy centers just 5 years ago. Similarly, a reevaluation of the point in time for a surgical assessment is also actively ongoing, with many centers considering the surgical option much earlier than before, thereby potentially sparing the patient months or even years of unsuccessful medication manipulations and/or toxicity.

This chapter presents a rational approach to the evaluation of patients for epilepsy surgery, as currently followed at the Epilepsy Treatment Unit (ETU) of the Minnesota Comprehensive Epilepsy Program. The techniques and philosophies employed must be viewed as only one approach that changes with improved technology and as an increasing follow-up experience with patients treated with surgery is gained. Controversial aspects are identified and some potentially exciting new developments are described.

Any surgical work-up in the era of intensive monitoring has one invariant component, the recording on EEG with or without concomitant videotape of spontaneously occurring ictal events (33). Although interictal epileptiform activity is considered in the overall decision about surgical candidacy, there is general agreement that it is insufficient in and of itself for presurgical localization (35).

This ictal recording requirement has become even more important now that we have recognized that many of the patients referred to the ETU at Minnesota (25% of admissions) have nonepileptic (psychogenic) seizures accounting for their intractable paroxysmal episodes. Over 50% (15) of these patients also have active epileptiform interictal EEGs (Fig. 1). Therefore, without recording the characteristic ictal events identified from the preadmission history as ac-

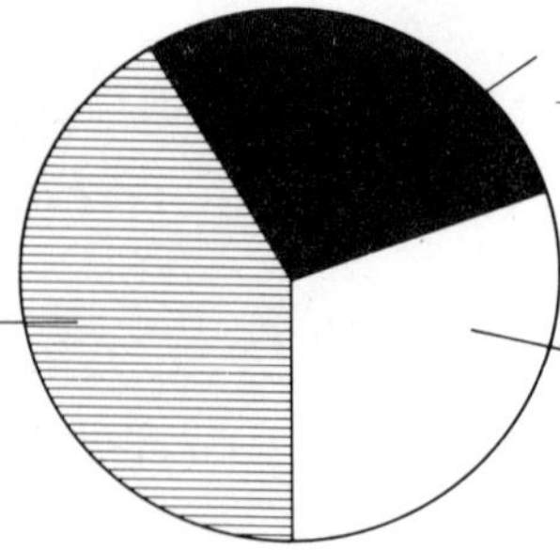

FIG. 1. Summary classification diagram for patients with psychogenic seizures (pseudoseizures). Percentages refer to patients in a series of 52 with video-recorded psychogenic seizures (pseudoseizures). (From ref. 15.) *Video-recorded epileptic and pseudoseizures. * Video-recorded pseudoseizures and highly suggestive interictal epileptiform EEG and/or history.

counting for the medical intractability, a serious therapeutic error could result by relying on interictal data, no matter how convincing.

Very often the rate of spontaneous seizures demonstrated by the patient while attempts are being made to record him in the intensive monitoring environment is not sufficiently frequent to allow the recording of any events. The "ictal yield" can be enhanced by reducing the dosage or number of anticonvulsants the patient is taking (44), though this must be done with considerable caution and only in an environment capable of immediately treating the potentially resultant status epilepticus.

With the use of a judicious reduction of medications on the ETU at Minnesota, 85 of 100 patients had seizures recorded on EEG within 2 weeks (33), 100% of presurgical candidates within 1 month. Only the occasional patient has experienced tonic-clonic status epilepticus with this approach. This complication has always been readily treatable without any long-term morbidity or a mortality in over 8 years and the treatment of over 750 intractable epilepsy patients. Pharmacological induction of seizures is not performed at the Minnesota ETU because of the potential unreliability of the localization of the induced ictal event, and the risk of inducing a nonlocalizable tonic-clonic event (18).

EQUIPMENT

A variety of recording systems now in existence for recording ictal events are described in detail by other authors in this volume. For the purposes of the presurgical evaluation, the current long-term monitoring systems can be divided into four basic categories:

1. "Hard wire" or cable telemetry with continuous paper write-out, usually also employing time-locked video/EEG.
2. Cable or radio telemetry with analog or videotape storage (with or without video).

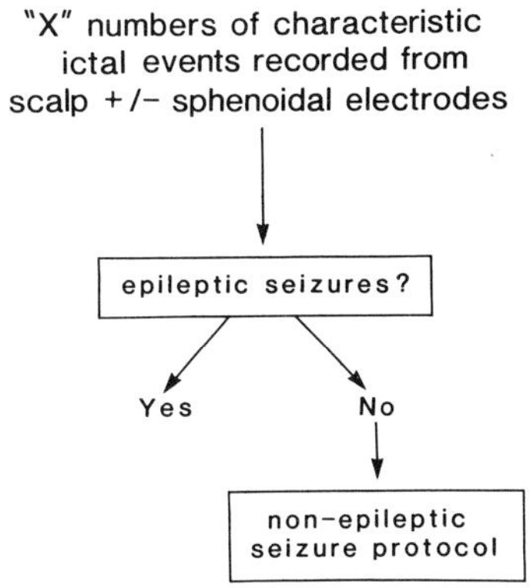

FIG. 2. Initial decision point for entry into presurgical evaluation. (See text for details.)

3. Cable or radio telemetry with digital tape/disk, computer assisted selective storage (with or without video).
4. Four-, 8-, or 16-channel ambulatory cassette with an analog cassette tape. The 16-channel system with epoch sampling only (video generally not employed).

Electrical safety is an important point when considering equipment, especially when intracranial electrodes have been placed. Any laboratory performing presurgical evaluations for epilepsy must adhere to the strictest standards of electrical safety such as performing frequent laboratory outlet ground checks; checking for equipment current leakage; interfacing biopotential isolation devices as appropriate; assessing indwelling electrode integrity before, during, and after placement; and keeping all equipment and supplies in top form (50). All technical personnel should be CPR-certified and resuscitation capability should be immediately available.

Decision Point 1

For the clarification of nonepileptic (psychogenic) from epileptic seizures, any of the above systems may be appropriate. But for definitive surgical localization at least 12, preferably 16 or more, channels of synchronized (time-locked) video monitoring are required (4). Fewer than this number of channels for surface/sphenoidal recording or with indwelling electrodes significantly increases the likelihood of missing possible multifocal epileptogenic foci.

The number of recorded ictal events required in order to decide whether a seizure type in a given patient is epileptic is quite variable. Generally, "x" at this point is usually one to two of each characteristic event of concern (Fig. 2). Once the characteristic event or events have been identified as clearly stereotyped, further ictal recording may dispense with video and rely on experienced observers' documentations of the events combined with continuous cable or radio telemetry, possibly with computer-assisted storage of the events. Definitive evaluation must include review of information from a comprehensive history, postictal prolactin levels (1,11,25,49), staff observation and interaction during the events, and a comprehensive neuropsychological evaluation.

There is clear import, both diagnostically and therapeutically, to showing the video-recorded events to family or institutional personnel caring for the patient to confirm that the documented episodes are those which precipitated the evaluation for intractable seizures. With the proliferation of portable home video recording systems, many families and institutions have the capability to record the events of concern on videotape even before admission. A side-by-side review of these events with those recorded by video-EEG can precisely document that the events recorded by the long-term monitoring system are the episodes responsible for the intractable epilepsy, regardless of type. Similarly, nursing staff and EEG technicians from the long-term monitoring facility can review the outside videotape beforehand to more precisely document behavioral changes and interact more effectively with the patient when the events are recorded.

For psychogenic episodes resembling generalized tonic-clonic epileptic seizures, video-EEG and clinical observation or review can usually readily answer the question or organicity (16). For partial seizures, a more intensive review of the comprehensive evaluation and multiple recordings of ictal events off of all medications may be required. A useful rule of thumb at the Minnesota ETU is that no patient advances to invasive intensive monitoring without recording at least one surface/sphenoidal true epileptiform ictal event, even if only a secondarily generalized seizure, no matter how convincing the clinical partial seizure is. Adhering to such a rule often requires patience combined with medication reductions to effect a wider spread or frank secondary generalization of the ictal EEG.

Decision Point 2

Having excluded nonepileptic seizures from the diagnostic options, the primary question in the presurgical evaluation is: Are the epileptic seizures of concern of unifocal origin as determined by the surface and/or sphenoidal electrode recording of "x" number of seizures (Fig. 3)? What "x" should be for this purpose is quite difficult to say. We have arbitrarily chosen eight to ten as the minimum number of characteristic seizures, as has the group at the University of California at Los Angeles (8). In our experience, this number of events is sufficient to avoid a false unifocal localization in cases of multifocal origin or to decide if invasive recording techniques (depth electrodes or subdural electrodes) are required. We have kept to this quantitative standard of ictal events, but are reviewing whether recording fewer seizures would actually sacrifice localization accuracy.

A comparison of ictal with interictal localization should also be performed. A persistently active interictal focus that does not localize to the ictal site of onset dictates a careful review of whether the seizures being recorded are but one of two or more seizure types experienced by the patient, with the frequency

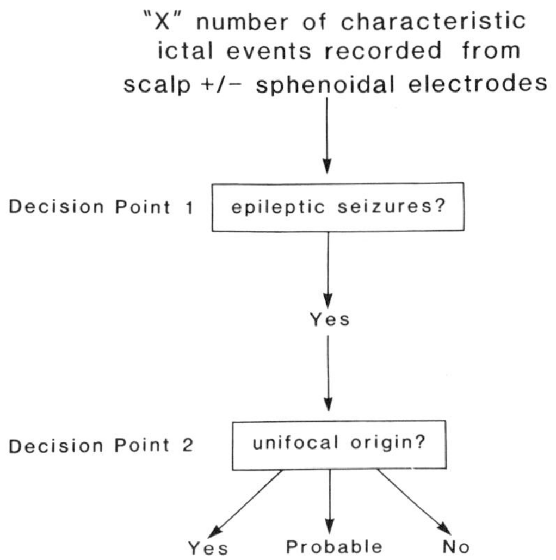

FIG. 3. Once epileptic seizures have been identified the question of unifocal origin needs to be answered. (See text for details.)

of the different episodes possibly a function of medication levels. Such false localization by medication reduction is generally not a problem, but must always be considered.

The application of computer-assisted identification, field characterization and storage of interictal activity is an exciting new development (21,22,34,41). Certainly these techniques hold the promise of expediting the presurgical evaluation as well as increasing the confidence of the epileptogenic localization. To date, however, as clearly stated by Gotman (22), the computer-assisted techniques are just that, computer-assisted, and still require the application of electroencephalographer verification of the reliability of the data analyzed.

Once the necessary number of seizures are recorded by twelve or more EEG channels using the surface/sphenoidal electrode technique, with at least five on video-EEG, there are three potential answers to the unifocal origin question.

UNIFOCAL ORIGIN IS CLEARLY ESTABLISHED

The acceptance of surface/sphenoidal EEG ictal and interictal localization as adequate for the complete presurgical evaluation is currently controversial (Fig. 4). A general agreement among the various epilepsy centers is that surface EEG recorded ictal events, even when supplemented by interictal localization, can be falsely localizing. Delgado-Escueta has suggested a false localization rate of as low as 10% from surface/sphenoidal (8), while Spencer doubts there is any utility to scalp localization (45). Quesney and Gloor (35) define a middle-of-the-road perspective with a clear electrographic localization of seizure onset by extracranial electrodes of 22 to 40% of patients with the lower yield in those with frontal lobe origin, the higher in temporal lobe onset.

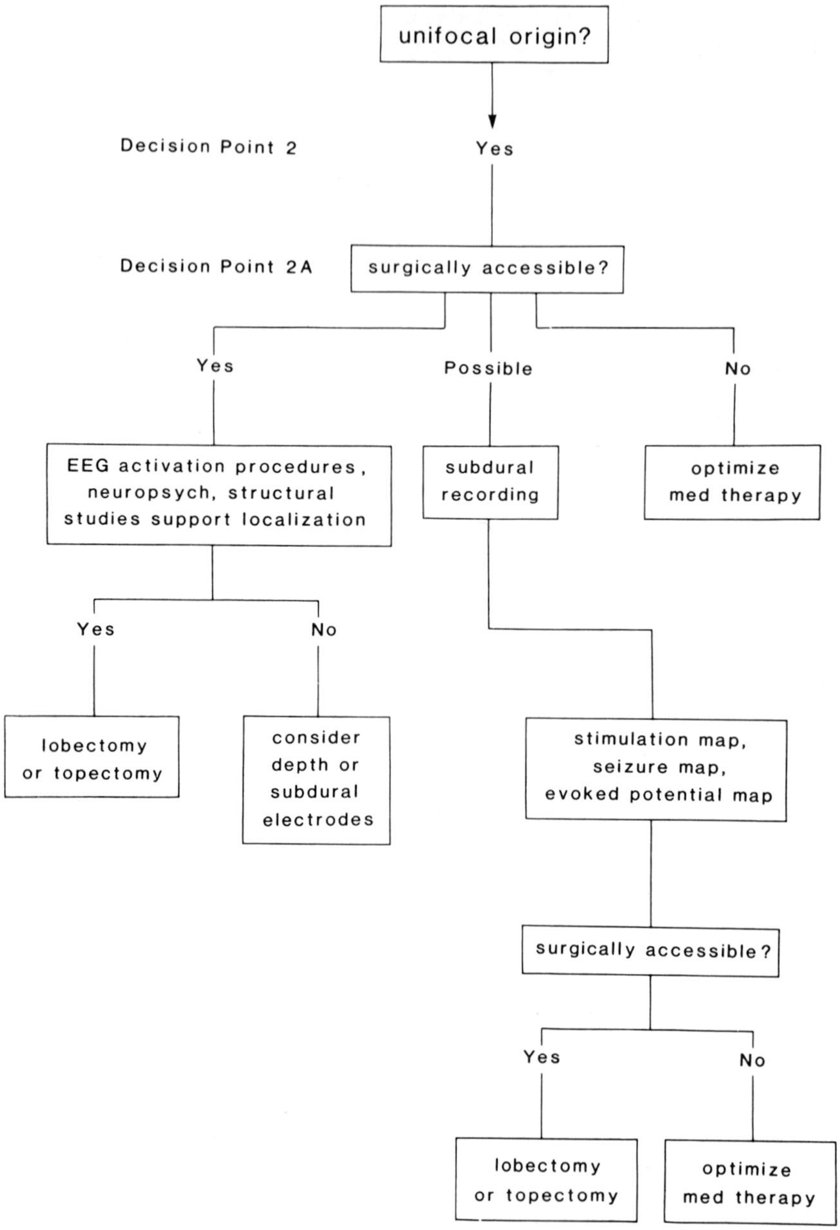

FIG. 4. Having established unifocal origin, the question of surgical accessibility then becomes paramount. (See text for details.)

The conflict can be resolved somewhat by recognizing that the EEG recording is only part of the presurgical assessment (9,10). Having established unifocal origin from surface/sphenoidal recording, the next questions are: What corroborative evidence exists for the EEG localization? Is the focus surgically accessible or is the risk of focal deficit from the proposed resection unacceptable?

The answers to these questions obviously must involve a detailed consideration of the location of the focus as it compares to the functional anatomy of the patient's cortex. The assessment of functional anatomy is difficult and crude at best, but tools do exist. Data can be assembled from a detailed neurological exam, a comprehensive neurospsychological battery, and a full complement of structural studies including CT scanning, magnetic resonance imaging, positron emission tomography, and cerebral angiography (9,31).

Further characterization and localization of the epileptogenic focus can be done with sodium pentothal injection IV (Lombroso-Erba test) (28) or diazepam (27), as well as with the Wada test (12,39) for selected patients. Magnetoencephalography may eventually be of value for a further characterization of the ictal and/or interictal epileptogenic focus because of its potential to localize more precisely in three dimensions than the EEG, however, this technology is still very much in the developmental stages (5).

With all this information in hand, the decision for lobectomy or topectomy can be made. In patients with striking inconsistencies in the localization from the neurological exam, neuropsychological studies, structural assessments, or activation studies, the possibility of a false localization from surface/sphenoidal ictal/interictal recording should be considered. Depth electrode or subdural electrode recording for a more precise epileptogenic localization may be appropriate. For those patients with a corroborative localization of dysfunction to the same cortical locus as the ictal/interictal recordings, the need for invasive ictal recording is questionable, and a successful lobectomy or topectomy is still a reasonable expectation.

A recent review (26) of 15 temporal lobectomy patients without malignant neoplasms (all selected by surface/sphenoidal recording) from the Minnesota ETU, with a mean follow-up of 32 months, demonstrated that 10 (67%) are seizure-free, and 13 (87%) were having seizures no more frequently than one per month. Preoperatively, all patients were having at least weekly seizures. The surface/sphenoidal EEG ictal/interictal criteria had been appropriately corroborated by the comprehensive presurgical studies outlined above.

UNIFOCAL ORIGIN IS PROBABLE BUT NOT CLEARLY ESTABLISHED, AND/OR THE SUPERIMPOSITION OF VITAL FUNCTIONAL CORTEX IS OF CONCERN

For the unifocal epileptogenic lesion where surgical accessibility is in question because of the presumed proximity of the focus to vital functional cortex, or where unifocal origin of the epileptogenesis is likely but not clearly established, invasive intracerebral recording electrodes should be considered (Fig. 5). Two basic techniques are available: depth electrodes and subdural electrodes.

Depth Electrodes

The utilization of invasive intracranial EEG recording was popularized by Talairach in 1962 (46–48,51). The technology has evolved considerably in the ensuing 23 years with several centers now participating in invasive EEG recording. A variety of different electrodes are in use and are interfaced with an equally varied number of long-term monitoring systems (2,9,18,30,42). Most commonly, a video system and at least 12 channels of time-locked EEG are used with careful attention to electrical safety issues (4).

We have chosen to use a flexible multicontact electrode system (30) that is stereotactically introduced in patients in whom the surface/sphenoidal EEG ictal and interictal recordings suggest a mesial temporal and/or inferofrontal focus. Because of the flexibility of the electrodes once inserted, complications from tonic-clonic seizures have not occurred in 16 patients to date. Therefore, a rather aggressive reduction of medications to increase ictal yield can be attempted. Eight to ten characteristic seizures are recorded in a 1- to 3-week period with the electrodes in place (Fig. 6). Arbitrarily, an ictal unifocality of at least 70% is required for topectomy or lobectomy. After the recorded seizures are reviewed and a therapeutic decision is made, the electrodes are removed. The patient's medications are adjusted to optimize seizure control, and he is sent home for the electrode introduction sites to heal. If surgery is indicated, the patient returns in 1 month for the procedure, at which time confirmatory and postresection corticography is employed.

Indwelling Cortical Convexity Recording Technique

The introduction of indwelling cortical recording techniques has certainly been one of the more exciting developments in epilepsy surgery in the last several years. Two schools have apparently evolved since its introduction: (a) those who utilize the established technique of Penfield and Jasper (32), involving cortical stimulation and resection under local anesthetic with electrocorticographic guidance; and (b) those who view the new indwelling cortical electrode technique as a potential significant advance over the older technology, with applicability to an expanded patient population who could not cooperate for cortical resection and stimulation while awake.

Sidney Goldring reported a 61% success rate in 29 patients (with 1- to 10-year follow-up) utilizing an epidural recording array to assist in the resection of convexity epileptogenic foci (19). This series included 17 children (ages 2–14 years) with a 70% "seizure improvement" rate for this subset.

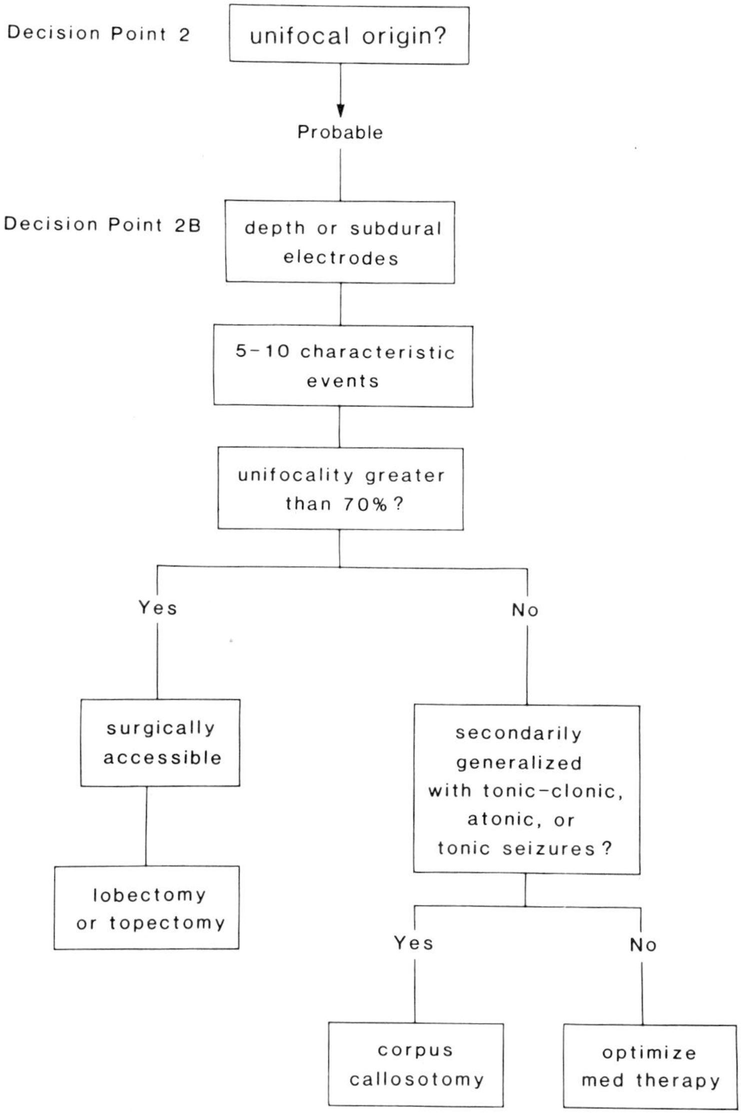

FIG. 5. If unifocal origin is only probable, invasive recording techniques are required.

Joseph Hahn from the Cleveland Clinic group indicates a 76% seizure improvement rate for his 45 patients subjected to cortical resection of an epileptogenic focus identified by a subdural array technique (23). Temporal lobectomy was the most common procedure; but the series included six patients with frontal lesions, five of whom have "had a successful result." The duration of postsurgical follow-up is not specified for the series. Nonetheless, these preliminary results for a new technology are quite encouraging, and cer-

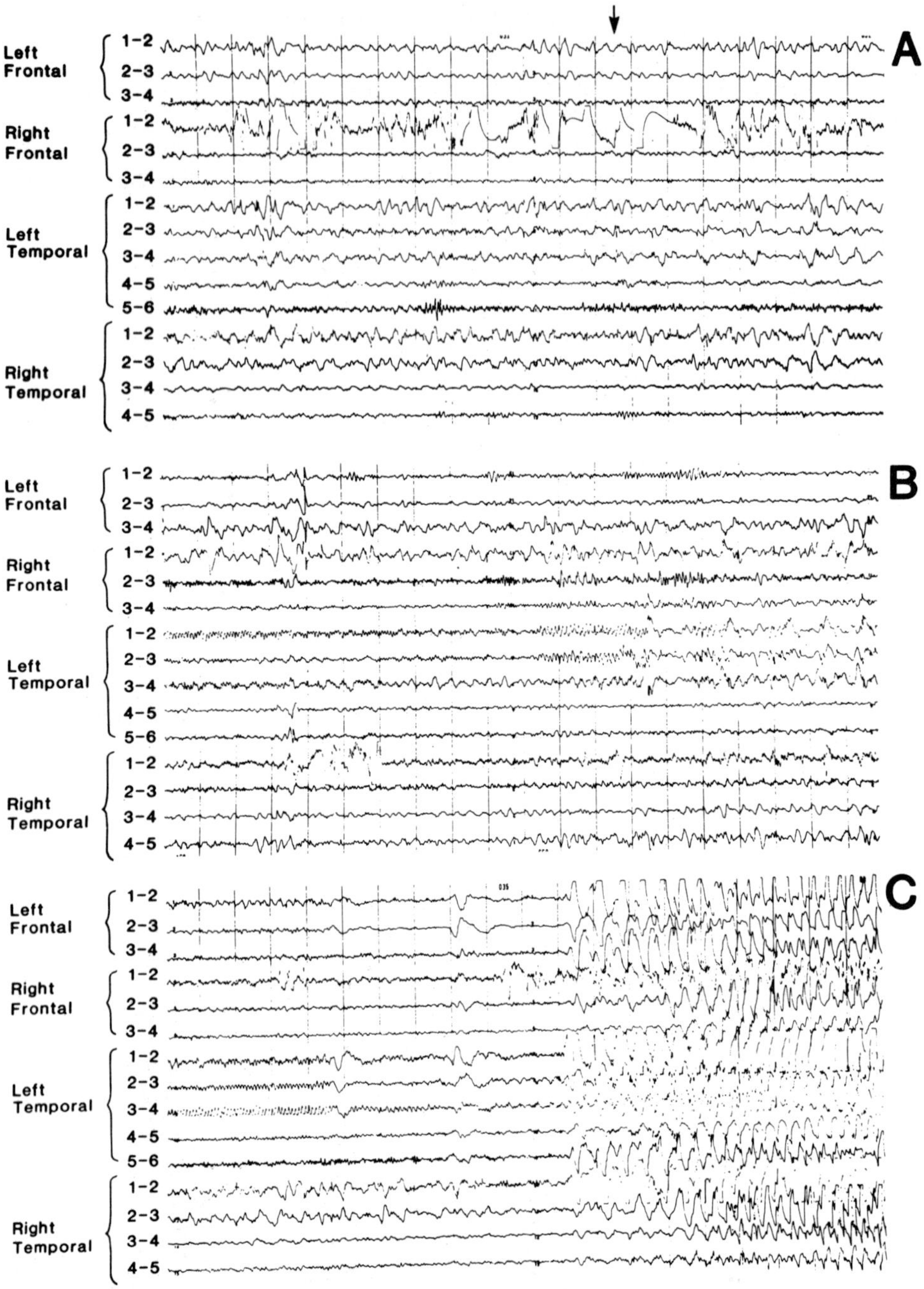

FIG. 6. Depth electrode recording from a young man who subsequently underwent temporal lobectomy. Frontal electrodes: 1, orbital frontal; 2, white matter adjacent to cingulate gyrus inferiorly; 3, white matter adjacent to cingulate gyrus superiorly; 4, superficial medial frontal region. Temporal electrodes: 1, temporal tip; 2, amygdala; 3, hippocampus; 4, white matter adjacent to superior temporal gyrus posteriorally; 5, centrum semiovale; 6, parieto-occipital junction. The *arrow* indicates onset of repetitive spikes in the left hippocampus evolving to epileptiform fast with subsequent generalization.

tainly comparable, if not an improvement, over the local anesthetic approach (36).

For various reasons, we have modelled our indwelling cortical convexity recording technique most closely after the Cleveland Clinic approach. Unlike the Cleveland group, however, as indicated above, surface/sphenoidal or depth electrode recording techniques have been utilized to date to identify potential standard anterior temporal lobectomy patients at the Minnesota ETU. Consequently, the indications for subdural array recording at our institution are more restricted, applicable to only those patients for whom surface EEG recording of interictal/ictal activity indicates the likelihood of a convexity epileptogenic focus that requires precise delineation of the coincidence of vital functional cortex with epileptogenic tissue. Such patients have included those with significant posterior penetration of the epileptogenic area into the dominant temporal lobe, and who will likely require a more aggressive temporal lobectomy than the standard four and one-half centimeters from the temporal tip.

The technique requires the identification of the area to be studied by the grid after placement to be as clearly defined as possible from surface EEG recording. The grid placement need not be precisely over the maximal area of epileptogenesis, but may better serve its purpose by being placed over the interface of a large area of epileptogenesis and adjacent vital cortical structures. "Sentinel" 4-electrode strips are slipped in medially for the temporal lobectomy cases for mesial recording purposes.

Three maps are potentially available after placement of the grid (Figs. 7–9):

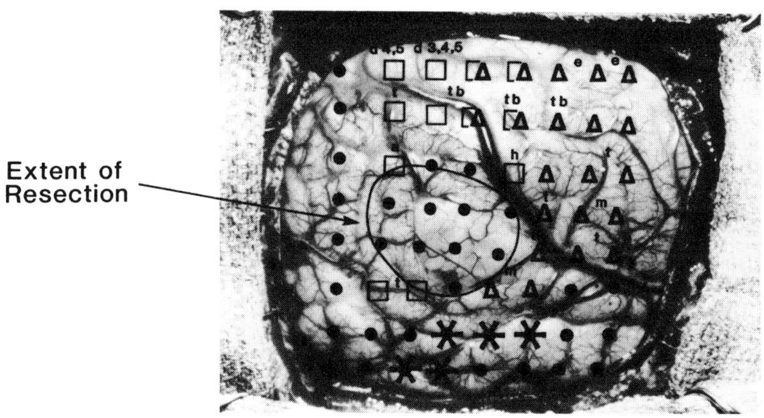

FIG. 7. The diagram shows the superimposition of the data gathered from simulation studies from a patient implanted with a 64-contact subdural grid. The grid is over the right hemisphere with the anterior to the right, posterior to the left, the temporal inferiorally, and the frontal and parietal regions represented in the *superior* portion of the photograph. The □ identifies somatosensory function. The △ refers to motor function, d identifies hand digits as numbered, t refers to tongue, tb to thumb, e to eyes, a to arm, m to mouth, and the ** refer to a sensation of hearing.

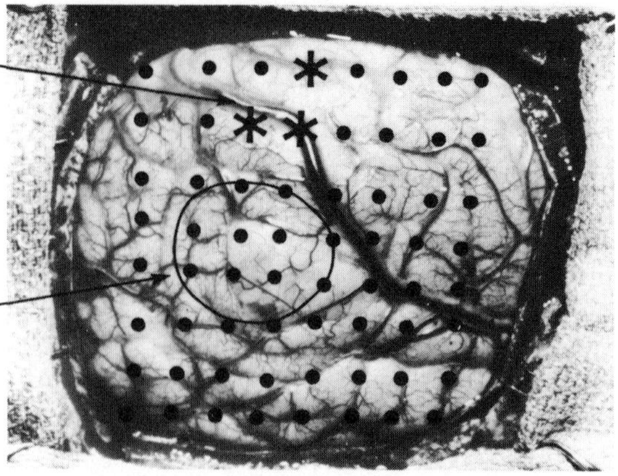

FIG. 8. Identical photograph to Fig. 7, this time showing the electrodes with maximal amplitude of the somatosensory evoked response stimulated from the left median nerve at the wrist. The extent of the ultimate resection is also identified. This evoked potential mapping was a verification technique for the stimulation studies.

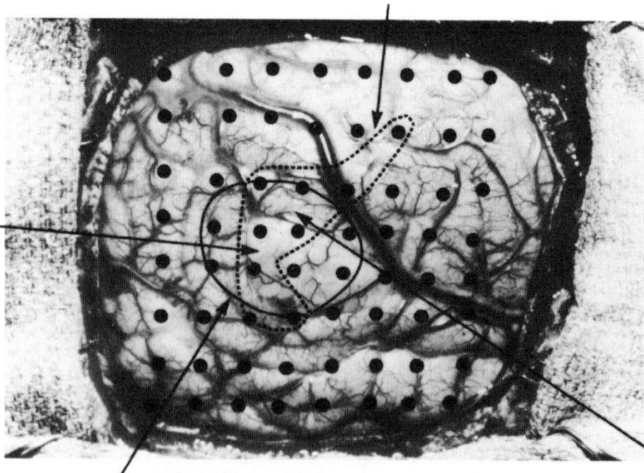

FIG. 9. Identical photograph to Figs. 7 and 8. The *stippled line* identifies the area of epileptogenesis recorded from the grid. The early and late aura regions are identified. The extent of resection is identified by the solid line.

1. A cortical stimulation map of underlying functional cortex obtained by judicious repeated stimulation of the electrodes in the array. Stimulation voltages and durations are dictated by continuous EEG monitoring after the establishment of after-discharge threshold for each electrode in the array, while the patient is on a stable anticonvulsant medication regimen.
2. A cortical-evoked somatosensory potential map generated from the array if it overlays the primary sensory cortex as a cross-check on the stimulation map. We perform this study in a separate laboratory and generate the somatosensory map from stimulation of the median nerve at the wrist without knowledge of the direct cortical stimulation map.
3. A spontaneous epileptogenesis map, generally obtained after reduction of medications after the stimulation and somatosensory maps are generated.

These maps are then superimposed and the risk of compromise of cortical function by resection is weighed against the likelihood of resecting the complete area of apparent epileptogenesis. As in the temporal lobectomy cases, confirmatory electrocorticography is used at the time of the removal of the array, before and after the cortical resection.

We regard this technology as quite promising, and the likely heir to intraoperative stimulation and resection under local anesthetic. Children can be assessed at leisure by this technique (three of our patients were 15-year-old boys), as the array can be left in up to 3 weeks with repeated stimulation studies and recording of the preferred spontaneous seizures.

It takes approximately 20 to 30 hr of physician time devoted directly to the stimulation studies alone for each 64-contact array to delineate a map of the functional cortex that is quite detailed. Whether this assessment is superior to the mapping performed by the surgeon during the brief time allowed in the high-pressure intraoperative stimulation session remains to be seen. Our experience is encouraging to date, but must be regarded as preliminary.

Again, the application of computer-assisted data reduction and analysis is exciting to contemplate for intracranial electrode recording. Gotman's lateralizing technique for rapid secondary generalization (20) could potentially dramatically expedite the preoperative recording time by salvaging those apparently nonlocalizable ictal events that so often must be excluded from consideration in the preoperative evaluation. Similarly, the application of this technique to apparently synchronous bilateral or diffuse hemispheral epileptiform discharges may identify patients for focal resection who previously would have been dismissed from consideration.

With the availability of surface/sphenoidal, depth electrodes, and subdural arrays a comprehensive approach to the patient with a potential unifocal area of epileptogenesis becomes available. Nonetheless, there remains a significant percentage of patients with medically intractable epilepsy for whom these techniques do not provide a surgical answer.

MULTIFOCAL ORIGIN OR A PRIMARY GENERALIZED PATTERN IS DOCUMENTED

For a significant subgroup of the medical failure population, yet another surgical option is available (Fig. 9). In 1940, Van Wagenen and Herren at Rochester, New York (52), introduced the concept of corpus collosotomy "in an effort to limit the spread of a convulsive wave to one-half of the cerebrum." By so doing, they believed consciousness would not be lost and the falls caused by generalized seizures could be avoided. Over the years, various combinations of sections of interhemispheric fiber tracts (corpus callosum, fornix, massa intermedia, anterior commissure, and hippocampal commissure) have been performed with mixed results, both in terms of increased seizure control and complications of surgery (3,6,7,24,29,54–56). Nonetheless, despite the more than 40 years since the introduction of the procedure, the experience of Van Wagenen and Herren with 26 patients still constitutes almost one-fourth of the published cases. This limited use of an otherwise promising technique may have been due to the significant operative morbidity of the earlier series. With the development of the operative microscope and other improvements in surgical techniques, several centers have reevaluated this technique in recent years (13,14,38,40).

At the Minnesota Comprehensive Epilepsy Program, we have been utilizing the technique since 1979, and have performed 32 callosotomies specifically for the control of tonic or atonic falling seizures associated with secondarily generalized ictal EEGs (13,14,17). Our approach is outlined in the multifocal origin protocol (Figs. 10 and 11). If such secondarily generalized falling seizures of multifocal origin or unifocal origin from a surgically unapproachable epileptogenic lesion is demonstrated from multiple surface/sphenoidal ictal recorded events on video-EEG and telemetry EEG; and the comprehensive supplemental structural, activation, and neuropsychological studies support this localization, then an anterior two-third corpus callosotomy is recommended.

The results of this procedure to date are summarized in Table 1. For the drop seizures (i.e., tonic or atonic episodes), we have found the procedure to be quite successful, with an acceptable morbidity, and no mortality (13,14,17).

Other centers have utilized different selection criteria for the procedure (37, 38,40,53), and no clear consensus has evolved from discussion between these centers as to the clear indications for callosotomy. Certainly, it is our finding that the particularly devastating atonic and tonic falling seizures intractable to anticonvulsants are significantly improved by the procedure, with a dramatic decrease in broken bones (especially the skull, neck, and jaw) and scalp or facial lacerations.

We have reviewed the other seizure types also experienced by these patients to assess how control of all types have been affected. In the Dartmouth series (38), not only atonic, but generalized tonic-clonic seizures as well, appeared to be significantly reduced postcallosotomy. Our experience has been similarly

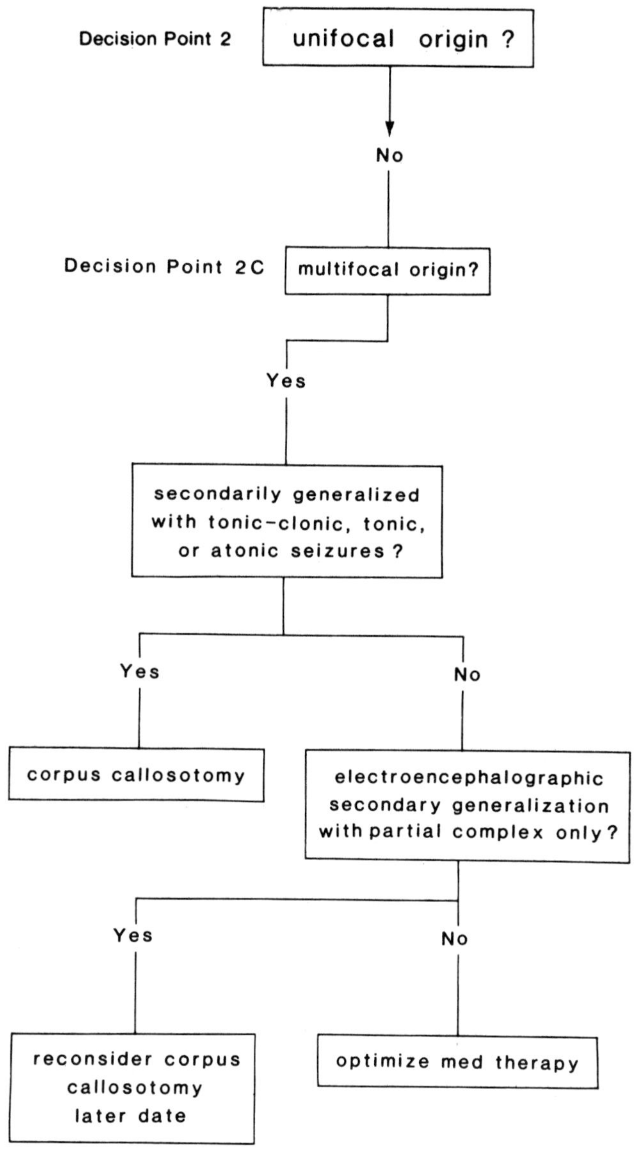

FIG. 10. When unifocality is not established, but multifocality is, the possibility of corpus callosotomy is raised. (See text for details.)

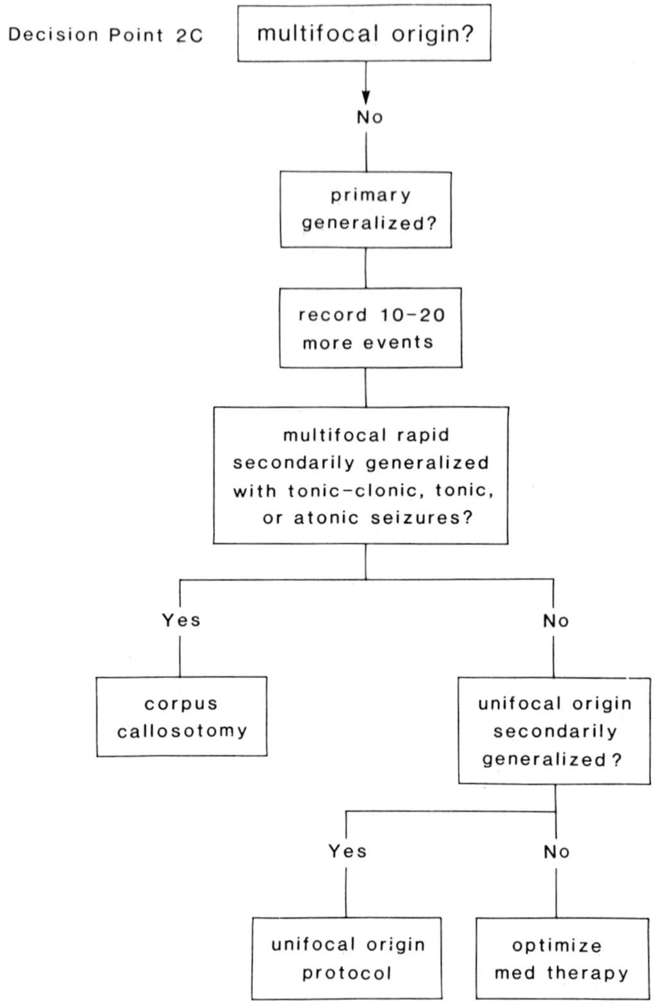

FIG. 11. Often, when a primary generalized pattern is suggested, the recording of 10 to 20 more ictal events can establish unifocal or multifocality. (See text for details.)

satisfying for postcallosotomy tonic-clonic seizure control (Table 1) (17). All 17 patients with tonic-clonic seizures as well as atonic or tonic seizures dramatically improved postoperatively.

The utility of callosotomy for partial seizures is not clear. Spencer et al. (43) observed an exacerbation of partial seizures in some patients. The Dartmouth series documents (38) a dramatic improvement in both partial complex and partial simple seizures, without describing a partial seizure exacerbation. Our experience does document an increase in the number of partial complex sei-

TABLE 1. *Response to corpus callosotomy of multiple seizure types*[a]

Patient no.	Extent of callosotomy on MRI	Months of follow-up	Partial complex Preop	Partial complex Postop	Simple Partial Preop	Simple Partial Postop	Tonic-clonic Preop	Tonic-clonic Postop	Tonic or atonic Preop	Tonic or atonic Postop
1		67	21	6	21	0	21	0	16	2
2		51	34	50[b]			17	0	56	0
3	Complete	51	40	0	0	4[b]	40	0	20	0
4	Complete	71	40	0			40	0	20	0
5	Genu intact	52	50	0	0	30[b]	4	0	4	0
6		56	80	120			80	0	56	56
7[c]	Complete	43	12	12			12	1	28	4
8	Splenium intact	48	20	30[b]			20	3	20	0.5
9	Splenium intact	39	40	16					28	2
10		37	450	50			12	0	600	60[d]
11	Complete	34	20	0	0	30[b]	12	0	14	0
12		34	30	0					11	0
13	Splenium intact	32	900	120[b]					30	1[d]
14	Complete	30	10	60[b]			30	2	60	6[d]
15		25	30	6					11	0
16	Splenium intact	23					2	1	315	120[d]
17		22	90	30[b]			2	0	70	2
18		22	4	8[b]					17	5
19	Splenium intact	21	60	10			60	0	30	3
20	Splenium intact	19							70	30
21	Splenium intact	19					20	0	50	3
22		17	60	0					12	0
23	Splenium intact	15	0	2[b]			20	0.5	12	0.5
25		15	30	30			0.5	0	10	5
	Average	35.1	20 Patients $p < 0.02$				17 Patients $p < 0.01$		24 Patients $p < 0.01$	

[a] Seizure numbers reflect average number of seizures per month for the 12 months from August 1984 to July 1985.

[b] Many of these seizures appear to be aborted tonic or atonic seizures status post-surgery

[c] This patient was operated on twice, after having been found to have an incomplete callosotomy with persistent (12 months) atonic seizures after the first surgical procedure (11/5/81). Consequently, his callosotomy was completed in a second procedure on 3/9/84.

[d] Though still technically generalized atonic or tonic seizures, thse episodes are less severe with more of a slump than an abrupt change in position of the body. Consequently, injuries are much less frequent from the resultant falls.

zures in eight patients. However, in seven of them, as well as all four of the patients with new partial simple seizures, seizure descriptions and all available ictal recordings suggest this apparent increase is the result of aborted generalized seizures. In the remaining partial complex seizure patient with more episodes postoperatively, stereotactic biopsy demonstrated bifrontal progressive radiation necrosis. Though the seizures electroencephalographically were rarely bilaterally synchronous postoperatively, the independent bifrontal discharges were so frequent that the lack of synchrony was inconsequential.

As indicated in Fig. 11, what appears to be intractable primary generalized epilepsy may prove to be secondary generalized with a more intensive recording of ictal events. If a unifocal secondary epileptogenic area can be identified in a potentially surgically approachable region, obviously a step back to the unifocal origin point in the presurgical evaluation decision tree must be made. Alternatively, a corpus callosotomy may be considered for those patients who are multifocal or unifocal, but surgically unapproachable, who secondarily generalize and experience tonic, atonic, or tonic-clonic seizures.

CONCLUSION

Dramatic advances have been made in the surgical treatment of epilepsy in the last decade. Through the improvements in intensive monitoring techniques generally and in surgical procedures and invasive intracerebral recording techniques more specifically, physicians caring for those with medically intractable epilepsy now have available to them diagnostic and therapeutic options that simply were not available or widely utilized only a few years ago.

ACKNOWLEDGMENT

This work was supported by funds from the National Institutes of Health (NINCDS), grant P50 NS 16308.

REFERENCES

1. Abbott, R. J., Browning, M. C. K., and Davison, D. L. W. (1980): Serum prolactin and cortisol concentration after grand mal seizures. *J. Neurol. Neurosurg. Psychiatry,* 43:163–167.
2. Ajmone-Marsan, C., and Van Buren, J. M. (1958): Epileptiform activity in cortical and subcortical structures in the temporal lobe of man. In: *Temporal Lobe Epilepsy,* edited by M. Baldwin and P. Bailey. Thomas, Springfield, Illinois.
3. Akelaitis, J. J. (1944): A study of gnosis, praxis and language following section of the corpus callosum and anterior commissure. *J. Neurosurg.,* 1:94–102.
4. American Electroencephalographic Society Guidelines for Long-term Neurodiagnostic Monitoring in Epilepsy (1985); *J. Clin. Neurophysiol.* 2(4):419–452.
5. Barth, D. S., Sutherling, W., Engel, J., and Beatty, J. (1982): Neuromagnetic localization of epileptiform spike activity in the human brain. *Science,* 218:891–894.

6. Bogen, J. E., Fisher, E. D., and Vogel, P. J. (1965): Cerebral commissurotomy: A second case report. *JAMA,* 194:1328–1329.
7. Bogen, J. E., and Vogel, P. J. (1962): Cerebral commissurotomy in man. *Bull. Los Angeles Neurol. Soc.,* 27:169–172.
8. Delgado-Escueta, A. V., and Walsh, G. O. (1983): The selection process for surgery of intractable complex partial seizures: surface EEG and depth electrography. In: *Epilepsy,* edited by A. A. Ward, J. K. Penry, and D. Purpura, pp. 295–325. Raven Press, New York.
9. Engel, J., Crandall, P. H., and Rausch, R. (1983): The partial epilepsies. In: *The Clinical Neurosciences,* edited by R. N. Rosenberg, R. G. Grossman, S. Schochet, E. R. Heinz, and W. D. Willis, pp. 1349–1380. Churchill Livingstone, New York.
10. Engel, J., Rausch, R., Lieb, J. P., Kuhl, D. E., and Crandall, P. H. (1980): Correlation of criteria used for localizing epileptic foci in patients considered for surgical therapy of epilepsy. *Ann. Neurol.,* 9(3):215–224.
11. Gallagher, B. B., Murvin, A., Flanigin, H. F., King, D. W., and Luney, D. (1984): Pituitary and adrenal function in epileptic patients. *Epilepsia,* 25(6):683–689.
12. Gates, J. R., Fiol, M. E., and Maxwell, M. E. (1983): Intraoperative EEG recording during complete corpus callosotomy for intractable secondarily generalized epilepsy (abstract). *Proceedings: 15th Epilepsy International Symposium and American Epilepsy Society,* Washington, D.C., September, 1983.
13. Gates, J. R., Leppik, I. E., Yap, J., and Gumnit, R. J. (1984): Corpus callosotomy: clinical and electroencephalographic effects. *Epilepsia,* 25(3):308–316.
14. Gates, J. R., Maxwell, R. E., Leppik, I. E., Fiol, M. E., and Gumnit, R. J. (1985): Electroencephalographic and clinical effects of total corpus callosotomy. In: *Epilepsy and the Corpus Callosum,* edited by A. G. Reeves, pp. 315–328. Plenum Press, New York.
15. Gates, J. R., Ramani, V., and Whalen, S. M. (1983): Ictal characteristics of pseudoseizures. *Epilepsia,* 24:246.
16. Gates, J. R., Ramani, V., Whalen, S. M., and Lowenson, R. B. (1985): Ictal characteristics of pseudoseizures. *Arch. Neurol.,* 42:1183–1187.
17. Gates, J., Rosenfeld, W., Maxwell, R. E., and Lyons, R. (1985): Response of multiple seizure types to corpus callosotomy. *Epilepsia,* 26(5):543.
18. Gloor, P. (1975): Contributions of electroencephalography and electrocorticography to the neurosurgical treatment of the epilepsies. In: *Advances in Neurology, Vol. 8, Neurosurgical Management of the Epilepsies,* edited by D. P. Purpura, J. K. Penry, and R. D. Walter, pp. 59–105. Raven Press, New York.
19. Goldring. S. (1978): A method for surgical management of focal epilepsy, especially as it relates to children. *J. Neurosurg.,* 49:344–356.
20. Gotman, J. (1983): Measurement of small time differences between EEG channels: method and application to epileptic seizure propagation. *EEG Clin. Neurophysiol.,* 56:501–514.
21. Gotman, J. (1985): Automatic recognition of interictal spikes. In: *Long-Term Monitoring in Epilepsy* (*EEG Suppl. No. 37*), edited by J. Gotman, J. R. Ives, and P. Gloor, pp. 93–114. Elsevier, Amsterdam.
22. Gotman, J. (1985): Seizure recognition and analysis. In: *Long-Term Monitoring in Epilepsy* (*EEG Suppl. No. 37*), edited by J. Gotman, J. R. Ives, and P. Gloor, pp. 133–145. Elsevier, Amsterdam.
23. Hahn, J. F., and Sellers, M. (1984): Surgical techniques for relief from seizures. *Cleveland Clin. Q.,* 51(2):307–311.
24. Huck, F. R., Radvany, J., Avila, J. O., Pires de Camargo, C. H., Marion, R., Ragazzo, P. C., Riva, D., and Arlant, P. (1980): Anterior callosotomy in epileptics with multiform seizures and bilaterial synchronous spike and wave EEG pattern. *Acta Neurochir.(Suppl.),* 30:127–135.
25. Laxer, K. D., Mullooly, J. P., and Howell, B. A. (1985): Prolactin changes after seizures classified by EEG monitoring. *Neurology,* 35(1):31–35.
26. Leppik, I. E., Cloyd, T. B., Loewenson, R., Krall, R., Cloyd, J. C., and Jacobs, M. P. (1985): Use of sequential analysis in a double-blind withdrawal of carbamazepine and phenytoin. *Epilepsia,* 26(5):544.
27. Lieb, J., Sclabassi, R., Crandall, P., and Buchness, R. (1974): Comparison of the action of

diazepam and phenobarbital using EEG-derived power spectra obtained from temporal lobe epileptics. *Neuropharmacology,* 13:769–783.

28. Lombroso, C. T., and Erba, G. (1970): Primary and secondary bilateral synchrony in epilepsy. *Arch. Neurol.,* 22:321–334.
29. Luessenhop, A. J., de la Cruz, T. C., and Fenichel, G. M. (1970): Surgical disconnection of the cerebral hemispheres for intractable seizures: Results in infancy and childhood. *JAMA,* 213:1630–1636.
30. Maxwell, R. E., Gates, J. R., Fiol, M. E., Johnson, M. J., Yap, J. C., Leppik, I. E., and Gumnit, R. J. (1983): Clinical evaluation of a depth electroencephalography electrode. *Neurosurgery,* 12(5):561–564.
31. McNaughton, F. L., and Rasmussen, T. (1975): Criteria for selection of patients for neurosurgical treatment. In: *Advances in Neurology: Vol. 8, Neurosurgical Management of the Epilepsies,* edited by D. P. Purpura, J. K. Penry, and R. D. Walter, pp. 37–48. Raven Press, New York.
32. Penfield, W., and Jasper, H. H. (1954): *Epilepsy and the Functional Anatomy of the Human Brain.* Little, Brown, Boston.
33. Perry, T. R., Gumnit, R. J., Gates, J. R., and Leppik, I. E. (1983): Routine EEG vs. intensive monitoring in the evaluation of intractable epilepsy. *Public Health Rep.,* 98(4):384–389.
34. Principe, J. C., and Smith, J. R. (1985): Automatic recognition of spike and wave bursts. In: *Long-Term Monitoring in Epilepsy* (*EEG Suppl. No. 37*), edited by J. Gotman, J. R. Ives, and P. Gloor, pp. 115–132. Elsevier, Amsterdam.
35. Quesney, L. F., and Gloor, P. (1985): Localization of epileptic foci. In: *Long-Term Monitoring in Epilepsy* (*EEG Suppl. No. 37*), edited by J. Gotman, J. R. Ives, and P. Gloor, pp. 165–200. Elsevier, Amsterdam.
36. Rasmussen, T. (1975): Cortical resection in the treatment of focal epilepsy. In: *Advances in Neurology: Vol. 8, Neurosurgical Management of the Epilepsies,* edited by D. P. Purpura, J. K. Penry, and R. D. Walter, pp. 139–154. Raven Press, New York.
37. Rayport, M., Corrie, W. S., and Ferguson, S. M. (1985): Corpus callosum section for control of clinically and electroencephalographically classified intractable seizures. In: *Epilepsy and the Corpus Callosum,* edited by A. G. Reeves, pp. 303–314. Plenum Press, New York.
38. Reeves, A. G., and O'Leary, P. M. (1985): Total corpus callosotomy for control of medically intractable epilepsy. In: *Epilepsy and the Corpus Callosum,* edited by A. G. Reeves, pp. 267–280. Plenum Press, New York.
39. Rovit, R. L., Gloor, P., and Rasmussen, T. (1961): Intracarotic amobarbital in epilepsy. *Arch. Neurol.,* 5:606–626.
40. Saint-Hilaire, J., Giard, N., Bouvier, G., and Lebrecque, R. (1985): Anterior callosotomy in frontal lobe epilepsies. In: *Epilepsy and the Corpus Callosum,* edited by A. G. Reeves, pp. 303–314. Plenum Press, New York.
41. Samson-Dollfus, D., and Senant, J. (1985): Analysis of background activity. In: *Long-Term Monitoring in Epilepsy* (*EEG Suppl. No. 37*), edited by J. Gotman, J. R. Ives, and P. Gloor, pp. 147–161. Elsevier, Amsterdam.
42. Spencer, S. S. (1981): Depth electroencephalography in selection of refractory epilepsy for surgery. *Ann. Neurol.,* 9:207–214.
43. Spencer, S. S., Spencer, D. D., Glaser, G. H., Williamson, P. D., and Mattson, R. H. (1984): More intense focal seizure types after callosal section: the role of inhibition. *Ann. Neurol.,* 16(6):686–693.
44. Spencer, S. S., Spencer, D. D., Williamson, P. D., and Mattson, R. H. (1981): Ictal effects of anticonvulsant medication withdrawal in epileptic patients. *Epilepsia,* 22(3):297–307.
45. Spencer, S. S., Williamson, P. D., Bridgers, S. L., Mattson, R. H., Cicchetti, D. V., and Spencer, D. D. (1985): Reliability and accuracy of localization by scalp ictal EEG. *Neurology,* 35(11):1567–1575.
46. Talairach, J., and Bancaud, J. (1973): Stereotaxic approach to epilepsy. *Prog. Neurol. Surg.,* 5:297–354.
47. Talairach, J., and Bancaud, J. (1974): Stereotaxic exploration and therapy in epilepsy. In: *Handbook of Clinical Neurology, Vol. 15, The Epilepsies,* edited by P. J. Vinken and C. W. Bruyn, pp. 758–782. North-Holland, Amsterdam.

48. Talairach, J., Bancaud, J., and Bonis, A. (1962): Functional stereotaxic exploration of epilepsy. *Confin. Neurol.,* 22:328–330.
49. Trimble, M.R. (1978): Serum prolactin in epilepsy and hysteria. *Br. Med. J.,* 2:1682.
50. Underwriters Laboratory, Standard for safety in medical and dental equipment, Subject 544, May 30, 1972. Melville, New York.
51. Van Buren, J. M., Ajmone-Marsan, C., and Mutsuga, N. (1975): Surgery of temporal lobe epilepsy. In: *Advances in Neurology: Vol. 8, Neurosurgical Management of the Epilepsies,* edited by D. P. Purpura, J. K. Penry, and R. D. Walter, pp. 155–196. Raven Press, New York.
52. Van Wagenen, W. P., and Herren, R. Y. (1940): Surgical division of commissural pathways in the corpus callosum: Relation to spread of an epileptic attack. *Arch. Neurol.,* 44:740–759.
53. Williamson, P. D. (1985): Corpus callosum section for intractable epilepsy: criteria for patient selection. In: *Epilepsy and the Corpus Callosum,* edited by A. G. Reeves, pp. 243–257. Plenum Press, New York.
54. Wilson, D. H., Culver, C., Waddington, M., and Gazzaniga, M. (1975): Disconnection of the cerebral hemispheres: An alternative to hemispherectomy for the control of intractable seizures. *Neurology,* 25:1149–1153.
55. Wilson, D.H., Reeves, A., and Gazzaniga, M. (1978): Division of the corpus callosum for uncontrollable epilepsy. *Neurology,* 28:649–653.
56. Wilson, D. H., Reeves, A., Gazzaniga, M., and Culver, C. (1977): Cerebral commissurotomy for control of intractable seizures. *Neurology,* 27:708–715.

Advances in Neurology, Vol. 46: Intensive Neurodiagnostic Monitoring, edited by R. J. Gumnit. Raven Press, New York © 1986.

Computer Analysis During Intensive Monitoring of Epileptic Patients

J. Gotman

Montreal Neurological Institute, and Department of Neurology and Neurosurgery, McGill University, Montreal, Quebec, Canada H3A 2B4

In long-term monitoring of the EEG in epileptic patients, the main practical problem is the large quantity of EEG that has to be recorded and reviewed. Patients are frequently monitored during several days or weeks and it is important to consider whether it is possible to reduce the requirements for EEG storage and to simplify the reviewing task of the electroencephalographer. We will see that in certain circumstances, it is possible to use computer technology to help solve both these problems. The use of such technology during monitoring brings with it the potential for additional benefits: EEGs recorded on the computer can be subjected to further analysis in order to extract information which is not directly available from traditional visual inspection.

Various methods have been developed for the analysis of the background EEG; they can be useful in the study of the influence of antiepileptic drugs on the brain and in the study of the relationships between sleep and epilepsy (see ref. 45 for a review). In this chapter we only discuss the EEG patterns which are clearly associated with epilepsy: isolated interictal spikes and sharp waves, bursts of spike-and-wave, and seizure discharges. These patterns are quite distinctive and can usually be identified easily by visual examination. Powerful modern computers should be able to identify them automatically without difficulty; but, in fact, despite the numerous attempts made in the past, there is still no computer method which can *reliably* identify epileptiform transients in the EEG of a patient subjected to long-term monitoring. (The problem is easier in a short recording during which the patient is quiet and artifacts can be eliminated.) Work is obviously necessary to improve current methods, but it is apparent that existing computer methods can be extremely useful despite their imperfection.

Methods for the computer processing of the EEG in epilepsy can be divided in two broad categories: On the one hand, detection methods aim at identifying patterns which are distinct from the background and usually also aim at quantifying their rate of occurrence; on the other hand, analysis methods take an identified epileptiform event and "dissect" it to enhance the visual analysis (these methods apply particularly to the study of seizure propagation). In the first part of this chapter *detection* methods are reviewed; in the second part, the difficult problems linked with the practical *implementation* of detection methods are discussed (artifacts, on-line analysis, integration to clinical laboratory). In the third part, *analysis* methods and their potential use in research applications are reviewed.

AUTOMATIC DETECTION OF EPILEPTIFORM PATTERNS

Interictal Spikes and Sharp Waves

Three types of methods have been used. The *mimetic* approach attempts to replicate what we believe the electroencephalographer does when reading an EEG: breaking down the EEG into waves and identifying the spikes (the term "spike" is considered here to include "sharp waves"). The detection of *nonstationarities* looks for patterns which are unexpected in a particular background. *Matched filtering* looks for recurrence of a pattern of which one sample is available.

The simplest mimetic methods attempt to detect a spike by measuring only one variable of the signal. Walter et al. (50) determined the sharpness by measuring the second derivative; they simply set a detection threshold for this variable. Smith (47) computed the first derivative (or slope) and looked for two occurrences of steep slopes of opposite direction within a few milliseconds. However, neither the slope nor the sharpness are, in isolation, sufficient for separating epileptiform transients from other EEG waveforms such as alpha waves, sleep transients, or many artifacts. Furthermore, fixed thresholds are not of general use because large changes in amplitude can take place with different types of electrodes or with varying interelectrode distance. Vera and Blume (49) propose the use of interactively adjustable thresholds in accordance with performance.

Rather than using variable thresholds, it is possible to use thresholds *relative* to the background EEG. Carrie (9, 10) measured the amplitude or the sharpness relative to average values in the preceding 128 waves. Gevins et al. (16) measured the curvature at the apex of every wave, relative to a fixed 4-sec calibration period. More complex methods involve the evaluation of several variables in order to improve discriminating power. Goldberg et al. (19) measured the amplitude and duration of each wave and set different detection thresholds according to the context (a low threshold was used in the context of slow waves and a higher one with fast activity). Guedes de Oliveira et al. (28) used discriminant analysis to decide which of several variables related to amplitude, slope, sharpness, and duration had the best discriminating power. They concluded that slope and sharpness relative to the background and total wave duration were the best features. Frost (14) also used a method based on the sequential measurements of multiple features.

In the method of Gotman and Gloor (24), the EEG was broken down into half-waves after digital filtering to remove 60-Hz activity. The amplitude of half-waves was measured relative to the average amplitude of the half-waves in the immediately preceding 5 sec (this "background" was thus constantly updated). The duration of half-waves and the sharpness at the apex of a wave were also used in a decision tree to decide if a pair of adjacent half-waves constituted a spike.

Rather than examining each wave, parametric methods represent the statistical properties of a section of EEG by a small number of parameters. These parameters can then be used to detect events which are *statistically improbable* given a certain background. Lopes da Silva et al. (35, 36) have pioneered the application of parametric methods to spike recognition. They used the autoregressive filter as parametric representation and the detected events were termed "nonstationarities." To ensure that nonstationarities have a spike-like morphology and to exclude those not likely to be related to epilepsy, the detected waves were compared to a set of predefined spike-like shapes (40).

Template matching has only rarely been used for automatic spike recognition. In this method, the computer program is provided with one sample (a template) of the spikes to be detected and searches for all occurrences of the same spike. As Barlow and Dubinsky (4) have explained, the method is too rigid given the variability in spike morphology in different patients and even for the same patient.

Some of the above methods have been used quite effectively for the detection of spikes in the EEG of patients quietly lying in an EEG laboratory when artifacts can be eliminated and when only a short section of EEG has to be analyzed. When doing long-term monitoring of epileptic patients, the problem is quite different: Artifacts are frequent and EEG analysis must proceed on-line. These practical problems are discussed later.

Bursts of Spike-and-Wave

The ideal 3/sec spike-and-wave bursts found in some patients with absence attacks is such a distinctive pattern (Fig. 1A) that many authors have attempted to develop automatic methods for its recognition. Most methods rely on the detection of spikes and the detection of slow waves as well as on some criteria for the alternation of the two patterns with an appropriate repetition rate. It must be remembered, however, that most of the bursts seen in clinical practice have a variety of morphologies which often resemble little the ideal example (Fig. 1B). This is particularly true during sleep (Fig. 1C). The detection of this latter type of burst is not simple in large part because it does not have a precise definition.

Carrie (10) used first a spike-detection method relying on the determination of the second derivative and then a slow-wave detection method based on the duration between zero-crossings; the combination of a spike and a slow wave constituted a burst. Carrie and Frost (11) describe a method which had more

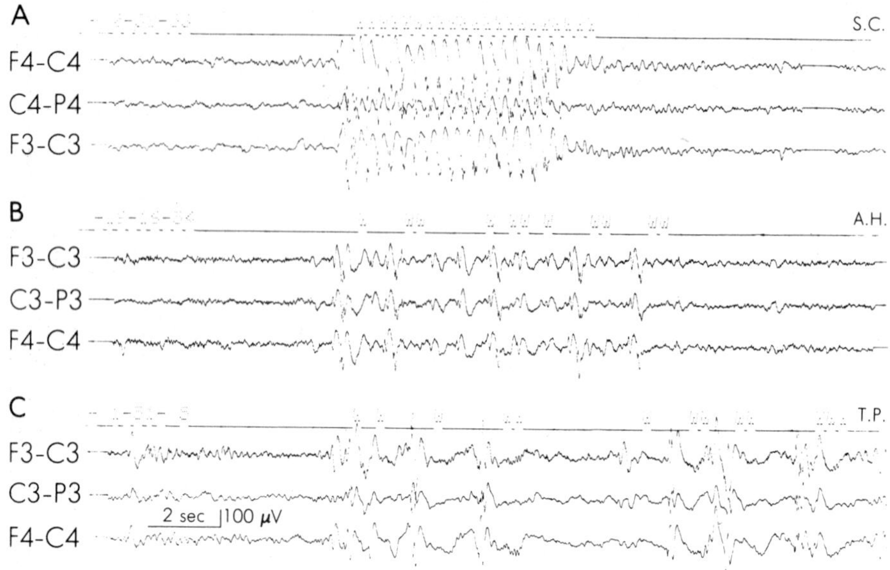

FIG. 1. Examples of the differences in morphology and duration of spike-and-wave bursts. Recordings from ambulatory cassette recorder. **A:** typical pattern; **B:** irregular and slow spike and wave; **C:** polyspike and slow wave recorded during sleep. The "W"s above each tracing indicate the bursts that were detected by the computer method (From ref. 32.)

precise criteria for the definition of slow-wave amplitude and which also incorporated a procedure for rejection of electromyographic (EMG) artifacts.

Other methods detected separately spikes and slow waves in several channels and used various criteria of spatial spread or temporal succession to perform the detection. Gevins et al. (17) analyzed four channels, detecting spikes, slow waves, and EMG waves; they required a minimum of spatial spread (appearance on several channels), synchrony between homologous channels of the two hemispheres, and a minimum duration to declare the occurrence of a generalized burst. Whisler et al. (51) developed a portable device which analyzed two channels for the recognition of spikes (by their slope, amplitude, and duration), and four channels for the detection of slow waves using filters. Decision logic required the occurrence of generalized waves and synchronous spikes to declare a burst of spike-and-wave. Principe and Smith (42) used a microprocessor to detect spikes and slow waves in one channel; before examining the time-domain characteristics of the waves, they subjected the EEG to digital filtering in order to reject activity that was not helpful in the determination of the morphology of spikes and slow waves. Burr et al. (8) used a computer to identify the EEG extrema and thus recognize spikes and slow waves; when the two patterns appeared in succession, a spike-and-wave pattern was detected.

Koffler and Gotman (32) designed a method based on the recognition of groups of spikes or sharp waves, independently of the presence of slow waves.

Analyzing three channels from ambulatory cassette recordings, they considered bursts as either spatially restricted (spikes in only one channel) but frequent in time (3 spikes in 1.3 sec) or spatially spread (spikes in all three channels) but less numerous (twice in 2 secs); intermediate criteria were used for spikes present in two channels. This method allowed to detect even extremely irregular bursts but it gave unsatisfactory results when the spike component was nonexistent (Fig. 1).

Other authors have used methods based on the filtering of the EEG into a low frequency band characteristic of the slow wave and a higher band including spike activity. We have seen above that Principe and Smith (42) used wide band filters prior to time domain analysis. Ehrenberg and Penry (13) used a modified method of amplitude integration which attenuated activity between 5 and 15 Hz, thus preserving the slow waves, below 5 Hz and the spikes, above 15 Hz. Jestico et al. (31) used a simple band-pass filter (2.2–4 Hz) to detect high-amplitude slow waves and thus quantify burst occurrence. A similar system was used by Zetterlund and Bromster (52). Quy et al. (44) improved the system of Jestico et al. (31) by adding a 12- to 18-Hz filter which allowed spike detection; in order to ensure an approximate 3-Hz rhythm, the output of this filter was rectified, filtered again between 2 and 4 Hz, and then compared to a threshold. Smith et al. (48) designed a portable device that filtered the EEG between 2.5 and 7 Hz, and then required that at least 3 waves of large amplitude be present in 1 sec.

Pinon et al. (41) used quite a different approach: They divided the EEG in 2-sec epochs which were subjected to linear discriminant analysis. Eight variables were identified for the efficient discrimination between sections with normal EEG, spike-and-wave bursts, bursts of slow wave and artifacts. The system could be made to learn automatically new detection criteria from a new set of data.

Seizures

Whereas considerable work has been done on the automatic recognition of interictal spikes and bursts of spike-and-wave, few publications have dealt with the automatic recognition of seizures not characterized by bursts of spike-and-wave. When long-term monitoring sessions are performed, automatic recognition of seizures can, however, be very helpful. Unless an EEG technologist is always present and records the EEG continuously on paper, seizures with minor or absent clinical signs can easily be missed by the patient or an observer. Automatic seizure recognition methods can detect many such seizures; all may not be detected since some may have only minimal or nonspecific EEG manifestations (1). Such a lack of EEG manifestation is due to the distance which may exist between the electrical generator of seizure activity and the recording electrodes.

Prior et al. (44) described the use of their cerebral function monitor to identify generalized tonic-clonic seizures. Such large seizures with clear motor components could also be identified in monkeys with experimental epilepsy by a characteristic pattern on low speed paper tracings (0.25 mm/sec) (33). Ives et al. (29) described a method where sixteen channels of EEG were added, band-pass filtered, and subjected to amplitude discrimination. This technique could detect large seizures but was quite insensitive. Babb et al. (2) implemented an electronic circuit for the detection of seizures in recordings from intracerebral electrodes. A seizure was recognized when a rapid succession of large-amplitude spikes, lasting at least 5 sec, was found.

Gotman (21) presented a computer method which attempted to recognize a variety of seizures. This method identified in the EEG any pattern that might represent seizure activity, for later examination by traditional visual inspection. The method was therefore designed to be as sensitive as possible. False detections, as long as they were not extremely frequent, were not detrimental. Observation of numerous seizures led to the conclusion that most seizures, at some time during their development, included activity of *paroxysmal* amplitude compared to the background, *rhythmic,* (with frequencies varying from 3–20

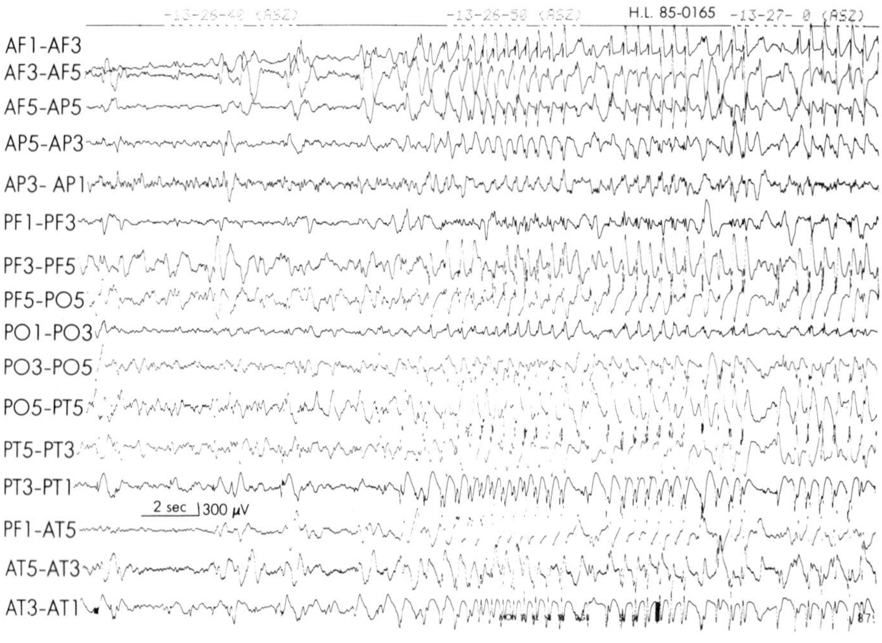

FIG. 2. Example of seizure automatically detected. Recording from subdural electrodes: six strips of five electrodes each were placed over the left hemisphere (AF, anterior frontal; AP, anterior parietal; PF, posterior frontal; PO, parieto-occipital; PT, posterior temporal; AT, anterior temporal). This seizure onset is widespread; in other seizures the onset was in the temporal region. The automatic detection program can detect seizures consisting of mostly slow activity such as this one, as well as the more frequent onsets with faster rhythms. This seizure took place during sleep and the patient was not aware of it. Subsequent examination of the video recording showed only minor motor activity.

Hz), and relatively *sustained* in duration (lasting several seconds). It was possible to obtain measurements of these characteristics by first breaking down the EEG into half-waves and then measuring, for every 2-sec epoch, the average amplitude of the half-waves relative to that of the background (indicating whether an epoch was paroxysmal), the average duration of the half-waves (indicating frequency), and the coefficient of variation of half-wave duration (indicating the regularity of duration or the rhythmicity). An example is shown on Fig. 2. A relatively small amplitude but a frequency clearly higher than that of the background also caused detections.

IMPLEMENTATION OF DETECTION METHODS IN INTENSIVE MONITORING

On-Line and Off-Line Analysis

Automatic detection methods based on computer analysis can be implemented to operate either *on-line* or *off-line.* On-line analysis means that the EEG is processed continuously as it is being recorded; at the end of the monitoring session, the analysis is also finished. Off-line analysis means that the EEG is first recorded on analog tape or even on the computer tape or disk itself, and analyzed only later after the recording is completed.

The obvious advantage of on-line analysis is that it requires no more time than that of the recording itself. It carries, however, severe limitations on the complexity of analysis methods since, for instance, only 1 min is available for the processing of 1 min of EEG. When dealing with the typical 16-channel EEG, on-line methods must be extremely streamlined or use very powerful computers.

The advantage of off-line analysis is that it allows much more freedom in the choice of the analysis method, since there is little time constraint. Cheaper computer equipment can also be used. In the context of long-term monitoring, however, it is only practical to consider on-line analysis. Consider the following example: To analyze off-line a 12-hr recording, the EEG is first recorded on analog tape; it is then played back on the computer and analyzed. This analysis may take 24 hr if the computer method requires 2 min to process 1 min of EEG. It becomes then highly impractical to subject several days of recording to computer analysis. There is room, however, for off-line computer methods which are too complex for on-line implementation: They can be used not for the detection of unpredictable epileptiform events where long hours of EEG must be processed, but for the detailed analysis of short sections of recording, such as the seizures themselves. In this case, the computer is not required to recognize a seizure; it is provided with an identified seizure pattern and asked to determine, for instance, where and when is its precise onset.

Very few of the methods for the detection of spikes and sharp waves which were reviewed above were implemented to allow the on-line analysis of eight or sixteen channels. They were mostly conceived for the analysis of a few minutes of carefully selected EEG. The methods for recognition of spike-and-wave bursts were, on the other hand, often implemented for on-line analysis. These bursts are less frequent than isolated spikes; they often correspond to absence attacks and their quantification throughout a day is often useful to assess the efficacy of drug therapy. The few seizure detection methods mentioned above were all implemented for on-line analysis since they were only used for long-term monitoring.

In the particular case of ambulatory monitoring with cassette recorders, on-line computer analysis is quite restricted since the equipment has to be carried by the patient. Automatic methods making use of analog equipment have been described (51). It is now also possible to use portable microprocessor-based equipment (41, 42, 47). The sophistication of low power consumption microprocessor will undoubtedly increase in the future and it will become possible to have quite sophisticated on-line portable analysis systems.

The Problem of Artifacts

When a monitoring session extends beyond 2 or 3 hr and when it is not under the constant supervision of an EEG technologist, a number of artifacts can be expected in scalp recordings (intracerebral recordings are usually free of artifacts because of the fixation of the electrodes and the proximity of the electrode to the neuronal generators). These artifacts are mainly due to the movements of the patient, but also to degradation of the electrode contact and to activity from scalp muscles and eye movements. The amount of artifacts is a direct function of the amount of freedom the patient is given: The worst artifacts are seen in ambulatory cassette recordings and the ensuing difficulties in interpretation have been discussed (12).

The difficulties caused by artifacts are much greater for automatic methods. Artifacts can be so varied in morphology (Fig. 3) that it is difficult to imagine an automatic method capable of identifying all of them. The human interpreters often rely on a very wide context to decide that a particular waveform is or is not an artifact; this context may be spatial (distribution and polarity of the waveform on other channels) or temporal (slow degradation of an electrode contact). Automatic methods can only rely on a very rudimentary context analysis. In some recordings, epileptiform events may be rare and false detections due to artifacts relatively more frequent, so that the results of an automatic analysis could be completely erroneous. In such a situation, one can ask whether it is possible to make clinical use of automatic detection methods without a serious risk of being misled.

It is indeed possible if the results of automatic analysis are subjected to validation by a human interpreter. In the most common approach taken in automatic analysis, the results are presented, for instance, as the number of

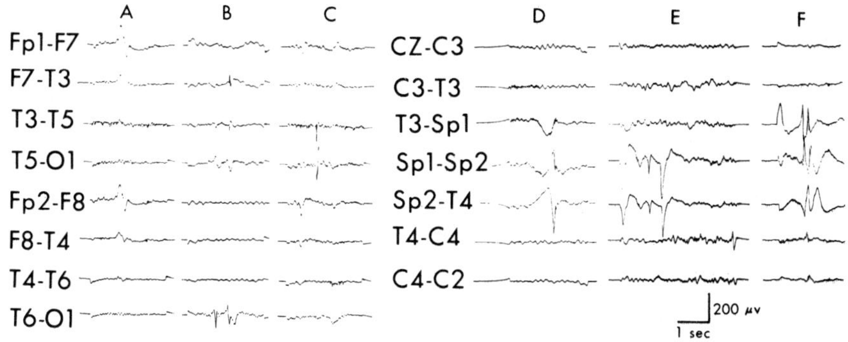

FIG. 3. Different types of artifacts which cause great difficulty to automatic spike-detection methods because they resemble spikes so much. A: unusual eyeblink; B and C: patient touches the electrodes; D, E, and F: artifacts due to movement of the sphenoidal electrodes.

spikes found in a particular channel; but this number is of little use if one does not know how many false detections it includes. An alternative approach is to have the detection method simply show the human interpreter the section of EEG where the detection took place. The computer is then used as a *selection* device, selecting from a long and largely uneventful recording the sections which are likely to be of interest (those including spikes, spike-and-wave bursts, or seizures). These sections are then subjected to human visual interpretation and artifacts can be easily identified. An implementation of this concept will be described.

Example of Implementation

The computer-assisted EEG monitoring system developed at the Montreal Neurological Institute, in use for many years, illustrates the principles discussed above. Originally implemented in 1975 on a PDP-12 computer, it has been running since 1979 on a PDP-11/60, and runs at present on the much cheaper PDP-11/73. The on-line analysis programs are aimed at recognizing seizures and interictal spikes and storing the corresponding EEG sections on the computer disk during the monitoring. At the end of the monitoring, the stored sections of EEG are played back on paper and interpreted in the traditional fashion. Events are recorded either because the program detects them or because the event button is pressed, usually because of a seizure.

The basic concept allowing the practical implementation of such a system was developed by Ives et al. (30): It is the use of the computer as a delay line for the EEG as well as a signal processor. The concept of the delay (Fig. 4) is necessary in the context of a selective recording because at the time of the event detection (by computer program or by seizure-button) a very valuable section

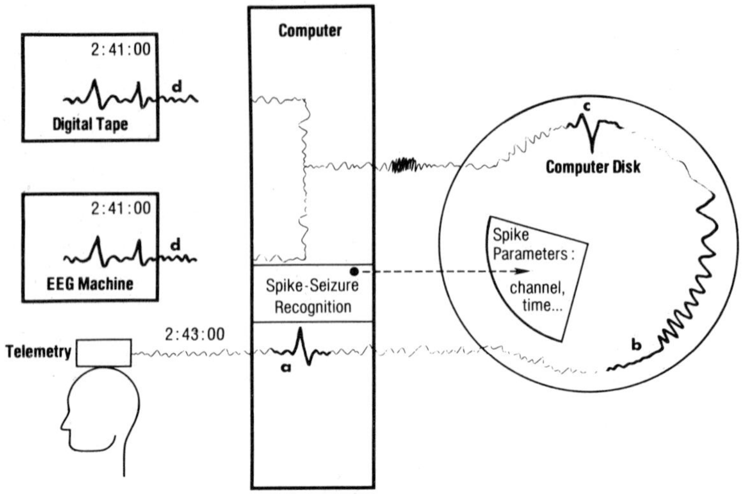

FIG. 4. Schematic representation of the use of a delay for selective EEG recordings. The diagram represents the state of the system at one instant in time. The 16-channel EEG is transmitted by cable telemetry from the patient's room to the computer laboratory. The computer processes the EEG (spike-and-seizure recognition) before writing it in a buffer memory (*large circle*) which holds at every instant the last 2 min of EEG. The computer also reads from the buffer memory the EEG which had been stored 2 min earlier and decides whether it should be written on the EEG machine and on digital disk or discarded. This decision is made according to the results of the automatic recognition programs and the push-button by the patient (the push-button is not shown on the diagram). The EEG selected for preservation is schematized in a *bold line*; the discarded segments are shown as a *thin line*. In the current EEG the computer is detecting a spike (a) and marking it for preservation; a short seizure (b) and another spike (c) were detected approximately 1 min earlier and are at present in the buffer memory; a set of two spikes (d) had been detected 2 min earlier and are now read from the buffer memory and written on disk and on paper.

of EEG, e.g., the seizure onset, may already be passed. We have found it useful to use a delay of 2 min. It is then extremely rare that a seizure onset is missed.

The computer programs are optimized so that sixteen channels can be analyzed on-line. Both the seizure and the spike-recognition programs, which run concurrently, make use of the same basic decomposition of the EEG into waves (24), thus saving processing time. The seizure recognition method (21,23) attempts to recognize EEG activity which is of paroxysmal amplitude, rhythmic (at any frequency between 3–20 Hz), lasts at least 2 sec, and is found in at least two channels simultaneously; another detection criterion involves a rapid increase in the EEG frequency, without a necessarily large amplitude. An example of a seizure automatically detected is shown in Fig. 2. The method allowed the detection of numerous seizures for which the seizure button had not been pressed for one of the following reasons: No observer was present and the patient was not aware of his or her seizure; the clinical signs were minimal and the observer did not notice them; there were no observable clinical signs (as later determined on the video recording). Small, purely "electrographic" seizures are frequent in some patients with intracerebral electrodes. It must also be stressed, however, that all seizures cannot be automatically recognized; this is due to the sometimes nonspecific EEG changes seen during a seizure (1); in some seizures only artifacts are present; in others the seizure discharge may not involve the electrodes used. The automatic seizure detection program also makes frequent mistakes, recording events which are clearly not seizures; this is not a serious problem since such events can easily be identified on visual inspection and ignored.

At the same time as the EEG is scanned for seizures, spike recognition is performed (25). When a spike is recognized in any channel, a short section of EEG (2.5 sec) is retained with the spike in its center (Fig. 5). As for the seizures, false detections can be frequent, particularly during the waking hours when scalp electrodes are used. If the electroencephalographer finds in the paper tracing that false detections are absent for a period of time (often during the night or at any time with intracranial electrodes), then a quantitative computer display can be obtained showing the actual number of spikes in each channel

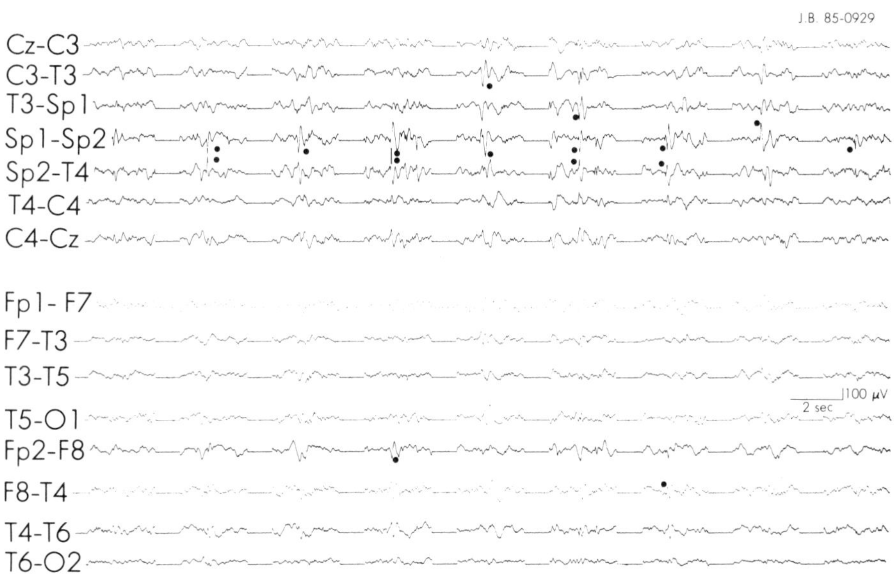

FIG. 5. Samples selected by the computer because of automatically detected spikes. Each section lasts 2.5 sec and the detected spike is approximately in its center (detected spikes are marked by a *dot*). *A flat line* marks the separation between the sections. Independent epileptiform activity is seen in the left and right temporal lobes, particularly clear at the sphenoidal electrodes (Sp1 and Sp2).

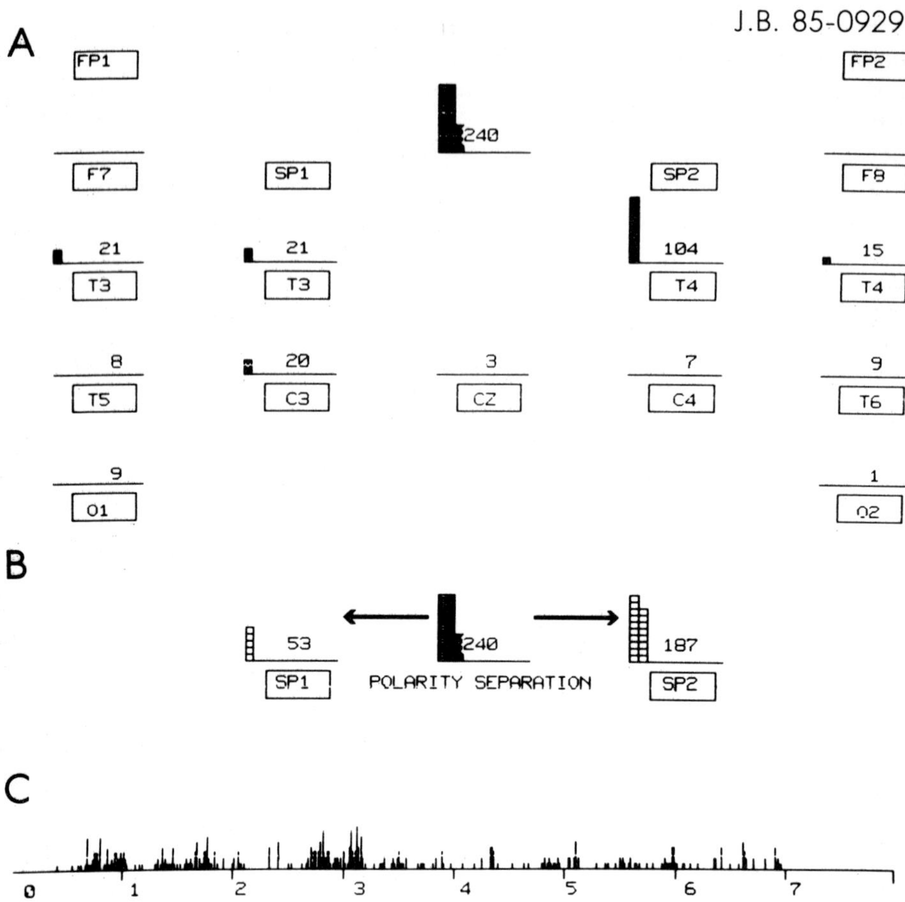

FIG. 6. **A:** Computer display representing the spatial distribution of spikes detected during a 7-hr period (midnight to 7.00 a. m.); some of the detected spikes are shown on Fig. 5. There are 21 spikes in the T3-Sp1 channel, 240 in Sp1-Sp2, 104 in Sp2-T4, and 7 in T4-C4. Each number is graphically represented to attract attention to the most active areas. **B:** In this montage there is a difficulty with the Sp1-Sp2 channel since spikes in this channel could originate from either the left or the right sphenoidal electrode. The computer therefore provides a separation according to spike polarity. **C:** Temporal distribution of spikes throughout the night. Each *vertical bar* represents the number of spikes in a 30-sec interval. Spikes were most frequent in the first half of the night, with rhythmic fluctuations probably associated with the sleep cycle.

(Fig. 6). If there are some false detections but a quantitative display is required, then false detections can be interactively edited from the record so that the quantitative display represents only genuine epileptiform activity.

Bursts of spike-and-wave can also be automatically recognized (32) and corresponding sections of EEG selectively retained. A quantitative display of their time distribution and duration can also be obtained.

Several practical aspects of the current implementation using a PDP-11/73 computer are worth noting: (a) Because the EEG is recorded on the computer disk, it is immediately available for further analysis (see below), whereas an EEG recorded on analog tape has to be first digitized in the computer before being analyzed; (b) the use of a disk as storage device makes it possible to almost instantaneously get to any part of the recording (there is no need to wait for tape movement); (c) the capacity of current disks is such that it is possible to retain the sections recorded during one day and start monitoring for a second day; the EEG from the first day can be played back on paper while monitoring is taking place so that the monitoring can, in effect, run without interruptions; (d) the cost of such a computer is very modest compared to the savings in personnel and supplies (paper in particular).

POSTMONITORING ANALYSIS

It is frequent that the purpose of the monitoring is simply to record the epileptiform events, ictal and interictal. Visual interpretation may provide all the information that is required and in this case the role of the computer is only to make the recording more efficient, using methods such as those described above. In some cases, however, the computer can also provide information which is not available, or is available with difficulty, from visual inspection. This is particularly the case when the rate of interictal spiking has to be quantified (e.g., for studying correlation with plasma levels of antiepileptic drugs, with sleep stages, or with seizure occurrence); it is also the case in the fine analysis of seizure discharges. We have seen above how, after the monitoring, it is possible to obtain quantified information on spike or spike-and-wave spatial and temporal distribution. We discuss here the methods which have been recently developed for the study of seizure propagation and for the removal of EMG artifact from seizure discharges. Unlike the on-line computer analysis which runs continuously during monitoring, these methods are used after the monitoring, when a visual examination of a seizure has indicated that additional information could be useful and might be obtained by computer analysis.

Removal of EMG Artifact

Artifacts are frequent in scalp recordings of epileptic seizures. Artifacts caused by movements of the electrode leads can be minimized by using short leads and head-worn amplifiers. EMG activity from the contraction of scalp muscles can totally obscure cerebral activity. We have described a method which can, in some cases, remove the EMG activity and reveal the underlying cerebral activity (26). The method is based on the use of a sharp digital filter which filters out practically all activity above 20 Hz, thus eliminating most of the EMG activity and preserving most of the EEG activity (Fig. 7). Unfortunately, the complete separation of EEG and EMG could not be achieved because some of the EMG activity is *below* 20 Hz and some of the EEG activity is *above* 20 Hz. Spectral analysis could be used sometimes to resolve the remaining ambiguities by identifying the presence of a *rhythmic* discharge buried in the EMG activity; if such a discharge has a frequency lower than 20 Hz it is likely to be of cerebral and not of muscular origin.

In practice we have found the method useful to assess the spatial and temporal extent of a seizure discharge which, at least at some time and in some channels, is visible in the original tracing but is largely obscured by EMG activity: In Fig. 7 the discharge is apparent in some channels before the filtering and it is revealed in others by the filtering. It is rare that the filter allows to identify with certainty a seizure discharge from a recording in which absolutely none was visible in the original tracing. Barlow (3) has presented an analog version of this filter, thus not requiring a computer. Extreme caution must be taken with such a filter because of the unavailability of concurrent spectral analysis to assess the presence of a rhythmic cerebral discharge.

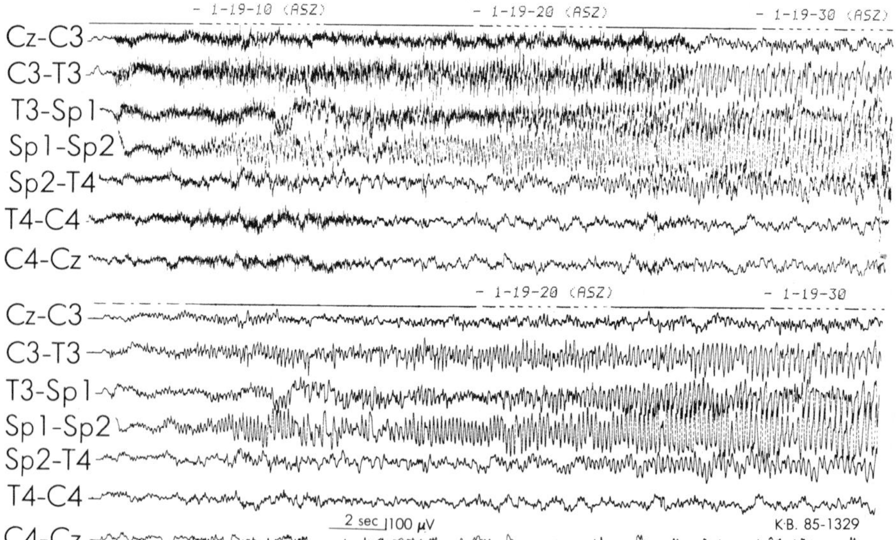

FIG. 7. Filtering of EMG artifact during an epileptic seizure. *Upper part* shows seven unfiltered channels; at the beginning of the seizure there is EMG activity in the first three channels and a visible seizure discharge in Sp1-Sp2 (left-to-right sphenoidal electrodes). The digitally filtered EEG shown on the *lower part* reveals clearly the seizure discharges in the first three channels and also a discharge in Sp1-Sp2 visible earlier than it was on the unfiltered tracing. It may also be noticed, from the "ASZ" written after the time of day, that this seizure was automatically detected and was not noticed by the patient or any observer.

Propagation of Seizure Activity

The propagation of seizure activity from one region of the brain to another can often be followed by visual examination of the EEG; seizure activity may appear in one region, a few seconds later spread to another and finally become generalized. It also happens that a seizure discharge starts simultaneously in several regions and remains synchronous in these regions. Simultaneity and synchrony are relative and in the case of EEG are limited by our visual perception of a tracing on paper. Computer methods have been developed for the measurement of small time differences between channels having apparently synchronous activity. Such small time differences may be useful in our understanding of the propagation of seizures and also in the localization of epileptic foci for clinical purposes.

Brazier (5–7) measured the phase difference between two channels at the main frequency of the seizure discharge during its first few seconds. She transformed this phase difference into a time measure and studied the propagation of several seizures recorded from intracerebral electrodes. Since seizure activity often includes mixed frequencies and a main frequency may not be apparent, the method was modified to take into consideration all frequencies which are coherent in the two channels (see the definition of coherence and the details of the method in Gotman, ref. 25). Applying this method to the measurement of interhemispheric time differences during generalized spike-and-wave activity (22), it was possible to separate the patients into two groups: (a) those having no evidence (from other EEGs or non-EEG sources) for a lateralized area of predominant epileptogenicity had no consistent interhemispheric time differences; and (b) those having evidence for a lateralized or localized epileptogenic area showed consistently an interhemispheric time difference during the generalized bursts; the most epileptogenic hemisphere was leading the other by 6 to 30 msec (Fig. 8). This procedure is used routinely in our laboratory to determine if patients with apparently synchronous bilateral spike-and-wave bursts actually have a lateralized area of predominant epileptogenicity. It serves a function similar to the intracarotid injection of amobarbital and metrazol (18) or intravenous injection of thiopental (34), but is noninvasive.

The propagation of seizure activity of morphology other than spike-and-wave can also be studied by this method (22). Figure 9A shows the example of a seizure recorded from intracerebral electrodes located in the frontal and temporal lobes. The seizure appears to start simultaneously in both regions. The measurement of small time differences indicated consistently, in this and two similar seizures, a lead from the frontal contacts over the temporal contacts. Time differences varied between 20 and 80 msec (Fig. 9B). In addition to this type of seizure, the patient had other seizures with a clear frontal onset and later a spread to the temporal region; after the spread, the discharge was similar to the one shown in Fig. 9A. An atrophic lesion was present in the frontal lobe

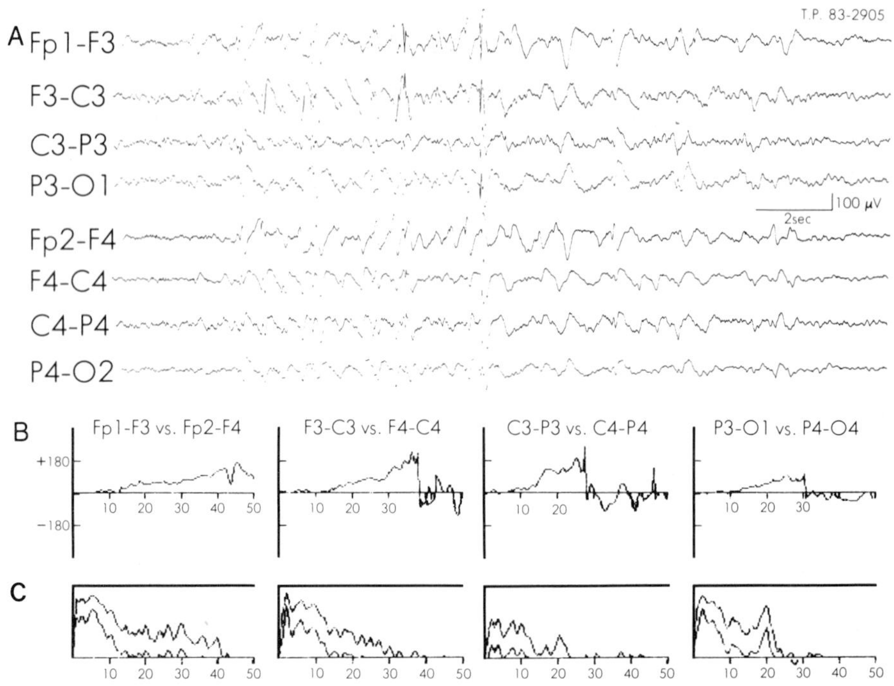

FIG. 8. Measurement of small time differences between homologous channels of the two hemispheres during apparently synchronous spike-and-wave activity. **A:** eight EEG channels with a burst of irregular spike-and-wave activity. The spikes are a little sharper in the left hemisphere. **B:** for each of the four pairs of homologous channels, the *upper curve* shows the phase of the cross-spectrum (between + 180° and − 180° from 0 to 50 Hz). A straight line is fitted to this curve, keeping only the phase values for which the coherence is significantly different from zero ($p < 0.01$). The coherence is shown on the *lower part* of the figure; it varies from 0 to 1 (1 is indicated by the *upper thick horizontal line*); the upper curve is the coherence itself and the lower one is the 99% confidence limit. If the phase is reasonably linear, a good fit is obtained and the slope of the fitted line gives the time delay between the two channels. An up-going slope indicates that the first of the two channels is leading the second and appears as a positive delay. This lead from the left side channels is present in all 4 pairs (respectively, 7, 8, 6, and 9 msec). This result can be interpreted to mean that an original discharge in the left hemisphere propagated to the right hemisphere. This interpretation is compatible with the presence of independent left frontotemporal discharges in this patient's EEG.

and all information, therefore, concurred to indicate that the frontal lobe was the most epileptogenic region.

It is important to emphasize that it is frequently impossible to make any delay measurement between two channels because the discharges are not coherent. When delay measurements can be made, however, and particularly when they are consistent in several seizures, they have, in our experience, always confirmed what was known about the patient (as in the above case). They are therefore reliable and can add an important dimension to the localization of epileptic foci.

Mars and Lopes da Silva (38) introduced another method for the measurement of small time differences: the method of average amount of mutual information. Applying this method to seizures caused by kindling in dogs, they were able to follow the different patterns of relations between several cerebral sites as the seizures evolved. Using this method, no consistent time lead was found in three patients with subdural electrodes, but higher values of mutual information were seen in the region of seizure onset (39). A somewhat different approach was used by Gersh and Goddard (15) who used the partial coherence function, trying to determine causality without making time measurements. They were able to assess that the discharge at the kindling site was causal to concurrently occurring discharges in some other brain regions.

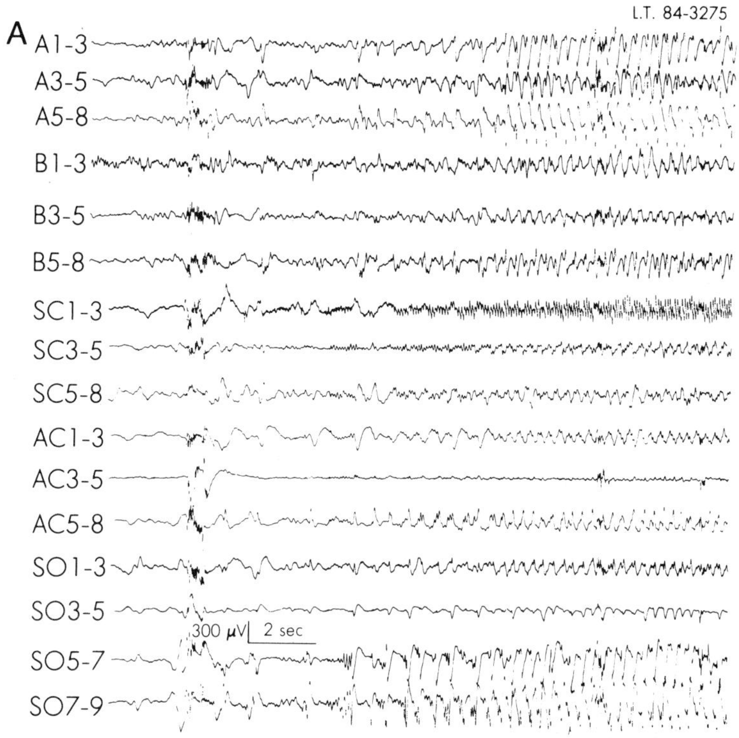

FIG. 9. Analysis of seizure propagation by measurement of small time differences. Seizure recorded from intracerebral electrodes implanted in the frontal and temporal lobes of one hemisphere; each electrode strand has nine contacts located 5 mm apart; electrodes are in a coronal plane and contact 1 is the most mesial. Recordings are bipolar between two contacts of the same electrode strand. Deepest contact of electrode A is amygdala; B is anterior hippocampus; SC in superior part of cingulate gyrus; AC in anterior part of cingulate gyrus, and SO in supra orbital region. **A:** Seizure onset simultaneous in frontal and temporal contacts.

(Continued on next page)

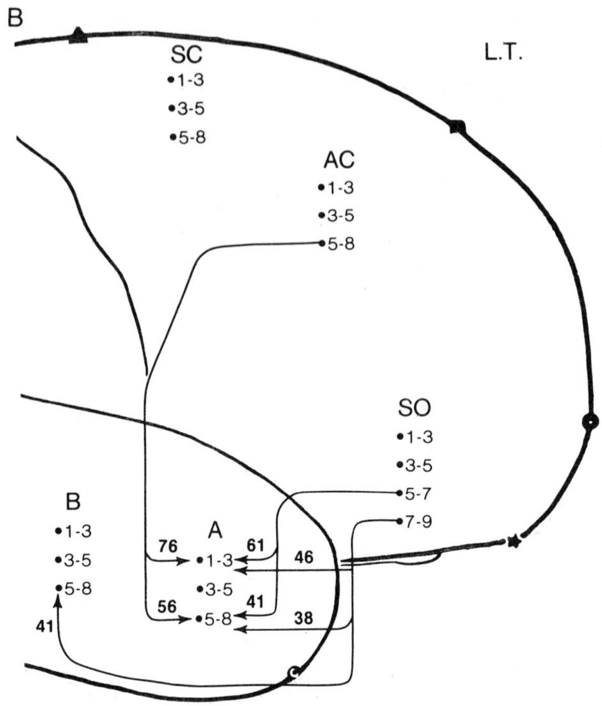

FIG. 9. (*Continued*)
B: Schematic representation of results; note that the electrodes (SC, AC, SO, A, and B) were actually in a coronal plane; *thin characters* represent contact numbers. An *arrow* between two channels indicates that a delay with consistent direction was found in the three seizures analyzed (that shown in **A** and two similar ones); the average value of time delays isgiven in *bold characters* in milliseconds. There are no arrows between many pairs of channels either because the coherence was too low to allow a time measurement or because the time measurements in the three seizures indicated inconsistent directions. Results indicate that when a delay is found consistently, the discharge in the frontal channels leads that in the temporal channels. This was corroborative evidence that the frontal lobe was the most epileptogenic region in this patient. (Several other seizures in this patient clearly started in the frontal region).

CONCLUSION

The long-term monitoring of epileptic patients is a difficult task which requires a lot of equipment and qualified personnel. Because the traditional method of EEG recording is not well adapted to such long recordings, new technologies have been developed. Commercially available equipment rely now on magnetic tapes for EEG recording, either portable cassette recorders similar to those used in cardiology or other types (standard analog tape and videotape are the most common). Such tapes can record for 12 or 24 hr unattended. The long recording still remains to be reviewed, however, and this is very time-consuming. Fast video review systems have been developed and these can be efficient when reviewing 4- or 8-channel recordings. With sixteen or more channels, the speed of replay has to be slowed down and the resolution may not be adequate. We have taken a different approach: We used a selective recording method based on computer-recognition of epileptiform events. Because the EEG is thus reduced to a small quantity, it can easily be written on paper and reviewed in the usual way. In addition to allowing easy review, the computer has allowed the pushing of limits of EEG beyond visual interpretation. For instance, the quantification of interictal activity throughout long monitoring sessions has permitted the establishment of some aspects of the relationships between plasma levels of antiepileptic drugs, spike-and-seizure occurrence (27,37). The analysis of seizures can be refined by the methods described above. When combined with video recording, the computer-assisted monitoring concepts illustrated here allow for unattended 24-hr recording and easy review. The equipment necessary cost a little more than an EEG machine; it will cost less and become easier to use in the future. The recording of thirty-two or even sixty-four channels can be envisaged without difficulty, an important improvement when dealing with recordings from multicontact intracerebral electrodes.

ACKNOWLEDGMENTS

This work was supported in part by grant MA-7204 of the Medical Research Council of Canada. The author is a "Chercheur-boursier senior" of the Fonds de la Recherche en Santé du Québec.

REFERENCES

1. Ajmone-Marsan, C. (1984): Electroencephalographic studies in seizure disorders: additional considerations. *J. Clin. Neurophysiol.*, 1(2):143–157.
2. Babb, T.L., Mariani, E., and Crandall, P.H. (1974): An electronic circuit for detection of EEG seizures recorded with implanted electrodes. *Electroencephalogr. Clin. Neurophysiol.*, 37:305–308.
3. Barlow, J.S. (1983): Muscle spike artifact minimization in the EEGs by time-domain filtering. *Electroencephalogr. Clin. Neurophysiol.*, 55:487–491.
4. Barlow, J.S., and Dubinsky, J. (1976): Some computer approaches to continuous automatic clinical EEG monitoring. In: *Quantitative Studies in Epilepsy,* edited by P. Kellaway and I. Petersen, pp. 309–327. Raven Press, New York.
5. Brazier, M.A.B. (1972): Spread of seizure discharges in epilepsy: anatomical and electrophysiological considerations. *Exp. Neurol., 36:263–272.*
6. *Brazier, M.A.B. (1972): Interactions of deep structures during seizures in man. In: Synchronization of EEG Activity in Epilepsies,* edited by H. Petsche and M.A.B. Brazier, pp. 409–427. Springer-Verlag, New York.
7. Brazier, M.A.B. (1973): Electrical seizure discharges within the human brain: the problem of spread. In: *Epilepsy: Its Phenomena in Man,* edited by M.A.B. Brazier, pp. 153–170. Academic Press, New York.
8. Burr, W., Stefan, H., and Penin, H. (1981): Spike-wave analysis in 24-hour EEG: comparison between conventional and computerized methods. In: *Advances in Epileptology: XIIth Epilepsy International Symposium,* edited by M. Dam, L. Gram, and J.K. Penry, pp. 275–285. Raven Press, New York.

9. Carrie, J.R.G. (1972): A technique for analyzing transient EEG abnormalities. *Electroencephalogr. Clin. Neurophysiol.,* 32:199–201.
10. Carrie, J.R.G. (1972): A hybrid computer technique for detecting sharp EEG transients. *Electroencephalogr. Clin. Neurophysiol.,* 32:336–338.
11. Carrie, J.R.G., and Frost, J.D. (1977): Clinical evaluation of a method for quantification of generalized spike and wave by computer. *Comput. Biomed. Res.,* 10:449–457.
12. Ebersole, J.S., and Leroy, R.F. (1983): An evaluation of ambulatory cassette EEG monitoring: II. Detection of interictal abnormalities. *Neurology (NY),* 33:8–18.
13. Ehrenberg, B.L., and Penry, J.K. (1976): Computer recognition of generalized spike-wave discharges. *Electroencephalogr. Clin. Neurophysiol.,* 41:25–36.
14. Frost, J.D. (1979): Microprocessor-based EEG spike detection and quantification. *Int. J. Biomedical Comput.,* 10:357–373.
15. Gersch, W., and Goddard, G.V. (1970): Epileptic focus location: spectral analysis method. *Science,* 169:701–702.
16. Gevins, A.S., Yeager, C.L., Diamond, S.L., Zeitlin, G.M., Spire, J.P., and Gevins, A.H. (1976): Sharp-transient analysis and thresholded linear coherence spectra of paroxysmal EEGs. In: *Quantitative Analytic Studies in Epilepsy,* edited by P. Kellaway and I. Petersen, pp. 463–482. Raven Press, New York.
17. Gevins, A., Blackburn, J., and Dedon, M. (1980): Very accurate computer recognition of three per second generalized spike-and-wave discharges. In: *Advances in Epileptology: The Xth Epilepsy International Symposium,* edited by J.A. Wada and J.K. Penry, pp. 121–128. Raven Press, New York.
18. Gloor, P., Rasmussen, T., Garretson, M., and Marown, F. (1964): Fractionized intracarotid metrazol injections. A new diagnostic method in electroencephalography. *Electroencephalogr. Clin. Neurophysiol.,* 17:322–327.
19. Goldberg, P., Samson-Dollfus, D., and Gremy, F. (1973): An approach to automatic pattern recognition of the electroencephalogram: background rhythm and paroxysmal elements. *Methods Inf. Med.,* 12(3):155–163.
20. Gotman, J. (1981): Interhemispheric relations during bilateral spike-and-wave activity. *Epilepsia,* 22:453–466.
21. Gotman, J. (1982): Automatic recognition of epileptic seizures in the EEG. *Electroencephalogr. Clin. Neurophysiol.,* 54:530–540.
22. Gotman, J. (1983): Measurement of small time differences between EEG channels: method and application to epileptic seizure propagation. *Electroencephalogr. Clin. Neurophysiol.,* 56:501–514.
23. Gotman, J. (1985): Seizure recognition and analysis. In: *Long-Term Monitoring in Epilepsy,* edited by J. Gotman, J.R. Ives, and P. Gloor, pp. 133–145. Elsevier, Amsterdam.
24. Gotman, J., and Gloor, P. (1976): Automatic recognition and quantification of interictal epileptic activity in the human scalp EEG. *Electroencephalogr. Clin. Neurophysiol.,* 41:513–529.
25. Gotman, J., Ives, J.R., and Gloor, P. (1979): Automatic recognition of interictal epileptic activity in prolonged EEG recordings. *Electroencephalogr. Clin. Neurophysiol.,* 46:510–520.
26. Gotman, J., Ives, J. R. and Gloor, P. (1981): Frequency content of EEG and EMG at seizure onset: possibility of removal of EMG artefact by digital filtering. *Electroencephalogr. Clin. Neurophysiol.,* 52:626–639.
27. Gotman, J., and Marciani, M.G. (1985): Electroencephalographic spiking activity, drug levels and seizure occurrence in epileptic patients. *Ann. Neurol.,* 17:597–603.
28. Guedes de Oliveira, P.H.H., Queiroz, C., and Lopes da Silva, F.H. (1983): Spike detection based on a pattern recognition approach using a microcomputer. *Electroencephalogr. Clin. Neurophysiol.,* 56:97–103.
29. Ives, J.R., Thompson, J.C., Gloor, P., Olivier, A., and Woods, J.F. (1974): The on-line computer detection and recording of spontaneous temporal lobe epileptic seizures from patients with implanted depth electrodes via a radio telemetry link. *Electroencephalogr. Clin. Neurophysiol.,* 37:205.
30. Ives, J.R., Thompson, C.J., and Gloor, P. (1976): Seizure monitoring: a new tool in electroencephalography. *Electroencephalogr. Clin. Neurophysiol.,* 41:422–427.
31. Jestico, J., Fitch, P., Gilliatt, R.W., and Willison, R.G. (1977): Automatic and rapid visual analysis of sleep stages and epileptic activity. A preliminary report. *Electroencephalogr. Clin. Neurophysiol.,* 43:438–441.

32. Koffler, D., and Gotman, J. (1985): Automatic detection of spike-and-wave bursts in ambulatory EEG recordings. *Electroencephalogr. Clin. Neurophysiol.* 61:165–180.
33. Lockard, J.S., Congdon, W.C., Ducharme, L.L., and Finch, C.A. (1980): Slow-speed EEG for chronic monitoring of clinical seizures in monkey model. *Epilepsia,* 21:325–334.
34. Lombroso, C.T., and Erba, G. (1970): Primary and secondary bilateral synchrony in epilepsy. *Arch. Neurol.,* 22:321–334.
35. Lopes da Silva, F.H., Dijk, A., and Smits, H. (1975): Detection of nonstationarities in EEGs using the autoregressive model—an application to EEGs of epileptics. In: *CEAN—Computerized EEG Analysis,* edited by H. Kunkel, and G. Dolce, pp. 180–199. Gustav Fischer Verlag, Stuttgart.
36. Lopes da Silva, F.H., Van Hulten, K., Lommen, J.G., Storm van Leeuwen, W., Van Veelen, C.W.M., and Vliegenthart, W. (1977): Automatic detection and localization of epileptic foci. *Electroencephalogr. Clin. Neurophysiol.,* 43:1–13.
37. Marciani, M.G., Gotman, J., Andermann, F., and Olivier, A. (1985): Patterns of seizure activation following withdrawal of antiepileptic medication. *Neurology,* 35:1537–1543.
38. Mars, N.J.I., and Lopes da Silva, F.H. (1983): Propagation of seizure activity in kindled dogs. *Electroencephalogr. Clin. Neurophysiol.,* 56:194–209.
39. Mars, N.J.I., Thompson, P.M., and Wilkus, R.J. (1985): Spread of epileptic seizure activity in humans. *Epilepsia,* 26:85–94.
40. Pfurtscheller, G., and Fischer, G. (1978): A new approach to spike detection using a combination of inverse and matched filter techniques. *Electroencephalogr. Clin. Neurophysiol.,* 44:243–247.
41. Pinon, J.M., Rubel, P., Maraval, G., Mauguière, F., and Revol, M. (1982): Analyse discriminate des grapho-éléments de l'EEG. Application à la détection des bouffées de pointes-ondes diffuses. *Int. J. Biomed. Comput.,* 13:237–261.
42. Principe, J.C., and Smith, J.R. (1982): Microcomputer-based system for the detection and quantification of petit mal epilepsy. *Comput. Biol. Med.,* 12:87–95.
43. Principe, J.C., and Smith, J.R. (1985): Automatic detection of spike-and-wave bursts. In: *Long-Term Monitoring in Epilepsy,* edited by J. Gotman, J.R. Ives and P. Gloor, pp. 115–132. Elsevier, Amsterdam.
44. Prior, P.F., Virden, R.S.M., and Maynard, D.E. (1973): An EEG device for monitoring seizure discharges. *Epilepsia,* 14:367–372.
45. Quy, R.J., Fitch, P., and Willison, R.G. (1980): High-speed automatic analysis of EEG spike and wave activity using an analogue detection and microcomputer plotting system. *Electroencephalogr. Clin. Neurophysiol.,* 49:187–189.
46. Samson-Dollfus, D., and Senant, J. (1985): Analysis of background activity. In: *Long-Term Monitoring in Epilepsy,* edited by J. Gotman, J.R. Ives, and P. Gloor, pp. 147–164. Elsevier, Amsterdam.
47. Smith, J.R. (1974): Automatic analysis and detection of EEG spikes. *IEEE Trans. Biomed. Eng.,* BME-21:1–7.
48. Smith, R.G., Houge, J.C., and Webster, J.G. (1979): Portable device for detection of petit mal epilepsy. *IEEE Trans. Biomed. Eng.,* BME-26:445–450.
49. Vera, R.S., and Blume, W.T. (1978): A clinically effective spike recognition program: its use at electrocorticography. *Electroencephalogr. Clin. Neurophysiol.,* 45:545-548.
50. Walter, D.O., Muller, H.F., and Jell, R.M. (1973): Semiautomatic quantification of sharpness of EEG phenomena. *IEEE Trans. Biomed. Eng.,* 20:53–54.
51. Whisler, J.W., ReMine, W.J., Leppik, L.E., McLain, L.W., Jr., and Gumnit, RJ. (1982): Machine detection of spike-wave activity in the EEG and its accuracy compared with visual interpretation. *Electroencephalogr. Clin. Neurophysiol.,* 54:541–551.
52. Zetterlund, B., and Bromster, O. (1981): A system for quantification of spike-and-wave episodes in 24-hour tape recordings of EEG. In: *Advances in Epileptology: XIIth Epilepsy International Symposium,* edited by M. Dam, L. Gram, and J.K. Penry, pp. 361–364. Raven Press, New York.

Advances in Neurology, Vol. 46: Intensive Neurodiagnostic Monitoring, edited by R. J. Gumnit. Raven Press, New York © 1986.

Data Reduction Methods for Intensive Neurodiagnostic Monitoring: Future Directions for Development

James D. Frost, Jr.

Section of Neurophysiology, Department of Neurology, Baylor College of Medicine, and The Methodist Hospital, Houston, Texas 77030

There is general agreement that intensive neurodiagnostic monitoring is an indispensable tool for the management of epilepsy. It has contributed significantly to improvements in both diagnosis and therapy, providing qualitative and quantitative information that is not obtainable by other means. It is, however, one of the most time-consuming of all medical procedures in terms of both data acquisition and data analysis and requires the participation of highly skilled technical and professional personnel. The application of automated data reduction techniques to monitoring offers the hope for significant improvements in overall economic efficiency, thereby making the procedure more widely available. This chapter reviews the major limitations of current methods used for computer-based analysis of EEG signals obtained during monitoring and will outline certain specific areas in which improvements are needed. The discussion will include aspects of automation as well as novel analytical approaches aimed at extension of diagnostic capability.

AUTOMATED DETECTION OF ICTAL AND INTERICTAL EPILEPTIFORM EVENTS

A typical monitoring session lasts between 8 and 24 hr and consists of simultaneously recorded multichannel EEG and video data. The approach taken to analyze the data obtained depends on the specific clinical circumstances; but in most cases, the information of primary interest is: (a) the times of occurrence and the characteristics of any ictal and interictal epileptiform EEG activity, and (b) the clinical behavior associated with any identified EEG events. The most time-consuming aspects of the analysis are the visual scanning of the EEG record and the associated tabulation of epileptiform events according to time of occurrence and type.

The various methods that have been proposed for the automatic identification and quantification of epileptiform EEG activity have been discussed previously (1,6,17) and are also reviewed by Gotman (*this volume*). In spite of the progress made in this area, it must be recognized that many problems remain unsolved and that the routine application of these methods to neurodiagnostic monitoring must await further refinements.

The most significant hindrance to the practical application of current computer-based systems to the monitoring situation is the difficulty of identifying and excluding artifactual waveforms. Several investigators have described, in detail, methods in which the automatic detection accuracy for true spikes, sharp waves, or spike-and-wave bursts can be made to approach 100% (2–4,8, 11,18,19). However, all of these approaches that have been adequately evaluated produce significant numbers of false-positive detections when required to process unselected data from prolonged monitoring sessions. The basic problem is that many nonphysiological signals, as well as certain physiological but nonepileptic events, can have waveform characteristics that are essentially identical to those of actual epileptiform EEG abnormalities. These include extraocular muscle potentials, electrode "pops," scalp muscle potentials, sharp vertex transients, lambda waves, bursts of sharp alpha activity, drug-induced fast activity, and many other waveforms that are easily recognized by the electroencephalographer.

The methods by which the human interpreter can readily exclude these similar, but nonepileptic, events have not yet been fully determined. The EEG literature, for the most part, ignores this problem. Spikes and sharp transients are defined solely in terms of their waveform characteristics, and the much more difficult concept of "context" is ignored.

The need to consider the context in EEG interpretation is easily illustrated by a simple example. Bilaterally synchronous and symmetrical sharp transient waveforms are a characteristic feature of nonrapid eye movement (NREM) sleep and, particularly in younger individuals, can have a spike-like configuration in the central regions. The experienced electroencephalographer does not, however, consider these vertex transients to be epileptiform, although the exclusion process is largely subconscious. If asked later, he would probably not even recall that such events had occurred (he would probably simply indicate that the patient fell asleep); but if an identical waveform occurred in the same region when the subject was awake, he would quickly identify it as abnormal. In this instance, the contextual clue has a purely temporal dimension. An event that is normal at a particular location and time is abnormal if it occurs in the same location at a different time. Context does, of course, also have a spatial dimension of equal importance. In the above example, an identical waveform, also occurring during NREM sleep, would be considered abnormal if it occurred only in the right frontal region rather than bilaterally in the central areas. Numerous examples of this type can be imagined, and it quickly becomes clear that strict waveform analysis, which has tended to dominate previous attempts at EEG automation, can never be successful in isolation. Stated a different way, not all "artifacts" can be distinguished by the presence of unique waveform features. They are distinguished by a combination of place of occurrence, time of occurrence, and waveform characteristics.

This problem has been a difficult one to approach, but in recent years specific attempts have been made to begin to include at least some aspects of context in computer-based spike/sharp-wave recognition systems. The 16-channel EEG analysis system developed by Gevins (8,9) incorporated specific algorithms to identify periods of EEG that were likely to be contaminated by muscle, ocular, and body movement artifacts. In this system, artifacts were identified, based on specific characteristics considered unique to artifacts; then the entire block of EEG data was excluded from consideration by other routines that searched for EEG abnormalities. The reasoning was that if certain clear-cut artifacts were present in a portion of EEG, then other events were suspect and should not be considered.

A similar, but more specific, approach was taken by Gotman (11,12). In his scheme, potential spike or sharp-wave events, detected by initial processing routines based on waveform characteristics, were rejected if a preset number of clearly artifactual events were found in the immediate vicinity. In the microprocessor-based system developed in our laboratory (4), each event detected by various waveform criteria is assigned an "artifact probability," based on the number of artifacts detected in the immediate vicinity, but rejection is delayed to permit other information to enter the decision-making process at a later stage.

These examples of the use of context-based methods for refining detection of abnormal EEG events, and similar work by other investigators, have demonstrated that significant improvement in overall reliability can be achieved. Even so, we have not yet begun to approach the level of context-based decision-making that is routine in human interpretation. This must be a major research goal of investigations in the EEG automation field, and it seems certain that entirely new methodologies will be required for a successful solution of the problem. Until this is accomplished, however, the use of computer-based technology in the monitoring area must be restricted to research situations or used as an adjunct to visual analysis, with careful confirmation of all events detected.

TECHNOLOGICAL IMPROVEMENTS

One important goal for the future is to make computer-based analysis methods more accessible to the electroencephalographer involved in the analysis of monitoring studies. In the past, systems developed for EEG analysis have generally operated off-line on tape-recorded data or, at best, on-line but at a remote location. Ideally, the computational system should be part of the monitoring laboratory environment, present as a dedicated hardware component of the overall recording system. This goal is no longer unrealistic, at least in terms of hardware cost. We are all, at least superficially, aware of the "microprocessor revolution" and the ready availability of personal and office computers. What is less well recognized, even within the computer profession, is the vast computational power now obtainable at low cost and in compact form. Most of the EEG analysis systems currently in use were developed on equipment that is now 10 to 15 years old, and although such hardware may appear quite imposing, it is functionally equivalent to modern configurations of much smaller size. For example, the 8-channel system in our laboratory was originally assembled approximately 10 years ago; it consists of a PDP 11/40 computer with standard disk drives, tapes, and input-output devices, interfaced with a large rack of special-purpose hardware, including analog filters and hybrid preprocessing apparatus. The entire system is housed in four standard 6-ft racks, exclusive of printers and terminals. We are currently reconfiguring this system, using an Apple II computer with an attached 68000 16-bit processor, together with a bank of eight parallel, single-board, Z80 microprocessors. The new configuration is considerably more powerful than the older version, permitting on-line digital filtering and other preprocessing, but it is sufficiently compact to be placed on a standard hospital cart for portable use. Whereas the original system cost more than $100,000 to assemble, the current version will cost less than $20,000 and could be duplicated for approximately $15,000.

Developers of EEG automation systems should be encouraged to make full use of the changing technology in order to bring their analytical methods into the day-to-day monitoring environment. More direct involvement of clinical personnel in the computer analysis procedures would permit current techniques, although not yet perfect, to be used as adjuncts to human analysis. This interaction would also facilitate the identification of problem areas and the acquisition of information essential for further improvement of the computer software.

IMPROVEMENT OF DIAGNOSTIC CAPABILITY

A large part of the cost of neurodiagnostic monitoring is due to the necessity for continuous recordings lasting many hours. A reasonable question is whether automated data analysis methods can contribute in any way to a reduction in the time requirements. Simple automation, or duplication of human visual analysis, although desirable for other reasons as noted above, would not, per se, alter the recording time. But the possibility exists that certain information, currently obtainable only from long-term records, might be extractable from more abbreviated sessions through unique processing of the data. It is also possible that certain clinical information, not accessible at present through human interpretation, could be made available by proper computer processing. Such capabilities have not yet been demonstrated in a convincing manner. However, some progress in this general direction seems to have been made during the past few years, and the results of some preliminary studies suggest the possibility of future practical applications to epilepsy monitoring.

One example, currently being investigated in our own laboratory, is directed toward assessing the efficacy of anticonvulsant drugs. Recent work has demonstrated that there may be consistent relationships between the degree of seizure control and the time distribution of epileptiform activity observed over 24 to 36 hr (13–15). In a group of children with partial seizures, in whom total seizure control was eventually achieved with increasing blood levels of phenobarbital, spike discharges tended to disappear first in rapid eye movement (REM) sleep, then in the awake state, and last in nocturnal slow-wave sleep. A similar pattern was observed in the response of children with 3-Hz spike-and-wave activity to ethosuximide treatment (16). This demonstrates that monitoring can provide quantitative and objective information regarding efficacy that is useful in the clinical management of the patient. It decreases reliance on subsequent reports of seizures by the patient or family, but multiple long-term monitoring studies are still required. The question we now pose is whether computer-based assessment of interictal spike characteristics can provide similar information regarding seizure probability, utilizing data based on recordings of much more limited duration. Specifically, we are using a microprocessor-based system to detect spikes and to calculate average measurements of spike amplitude, duration, and sharpness. The computer system has been described previously (4) and has undergone extensive testing to eliminate artifacts. In a pilot study, a group of seven children, 5 to 11 years of age, with benign rolandic epilepsy, were evaluated (5,7). They had C_3 or C_4 spike foci and, at the time of referral, were experiencing focal or generalized motor seizures. All patients were studied with repeated 24-hr monitoring sessions over 1 to 3 years, including a baseline session prior to initiation or modification of therapy and a session 2 to 5 weeks later, after attainment of steady-state serum drug levels. Much shorter EEG segments, typically 5 to 10 min, were selected from the first slow-wave sleep episodes of the nocturnal recording session, and from these, data samples consisting of 100 spikes were extracted by the computer system. Average values were calculated for the spike amplitude, duration, and normalized sharpness (second derivative of the voltage tracing at the spike peak divided by the peak-to-peak amplitude). Each spike selected by the computer was confirmed by visual inspection of the EEG record, and any artifactual or other false-positive event chosen by the computer was eliminated prior to determination of average parameter values.

The computer also calculated, for each 100-spike sample, a single composite spike parameter (CSP) by dividing the product of amplitude and duration by the normalized sharpness ($\mathrm{CSP} = \frac{\mathrm{AD}}{\mathrm{SA}} \times \mathrm{K}$). The CSP provides a single value that summarizes the average parameters of a spike sample, and it is reduced in value by any combination of amplitude or duration decrease or normalized sharpness increase.

The basic questions we hoped to answer were: (a) Do changes in the spike parameters occur in association with institution of drug therapy? (b) Does the nature of such changes permit the ultimate efficacy of treatment to be predicted? The results of this initial study suggest that the answer to these questions may be "yes."

In six of the seven patients, seizures were initially controlled by phenobarbital therapy, although a relapse occurred 5 weeks later in one subject and 11 months later in another. Four of the six patients continued to show frequent EEG spikes in the absence of clinical seizures, whereas spikes ceased in the other two. A consistent computer-derived pattern of changes in the spike parameters was observed in all four patients who were controlled by phenobarbital but continued to have EEG spikes: When studied shortly after institution of treatment, there was a decrease in spike amplitude (average value, −28%), a decrease in spike duration (average value, −17%) and a decrease in the CSP (average value, −57%), compared to baseline values. An increase in normalized sharpness also occurred in three of the four patients (average value, +44%). Thus, seizure control was associated with decreased amplitude and duration and increased sharpness of the spike activity. The parameter values returned to near baseline levels at the time of relapse in two patients. The single patient who was not controlled on phenobarbital had the highest baseline CSP value and showed no significant change in spike parameters when treated. These results are summarized in Fig. 1, where the CPS values from all baseline and fol-

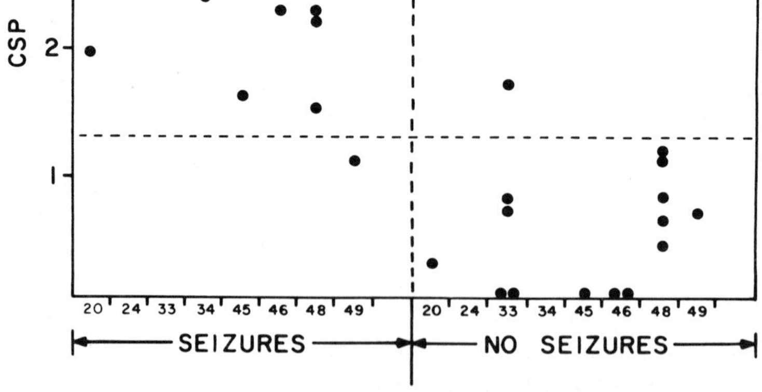

FIG. 1. Relationship between composite spike parameter (CSP) values and seizure-control status. Numbers on the horizontal axis indicate patient identification.

low-up studies are plotted versus seizure-control status. An absolute CSP value of 1.3 nearly separates the two conditions, and seizure control was always associated with a decreased CSP.

It should be emphasized that seizure-control status was determined for all patients by conventional observation and subjective reports over a period of months following institution of treatment, whereas the CSP data were obtained shortly after institution of treatment and well before the efficacy of treatment was known by the conventional approach. Consequently, this method could conceivably facilitate the achievement of an optimal therapeutic plan for an individual patient by eliminating the necessity for long subjective observation periods and/or multiple prolonged monitoring sessions prior to adjusting dosage or beginning treatment with a new drug. The reliability of the technique, and its applicability to multiple seizure types, must, of course, be determined through objective testing protocols before it can be considered for routine clinical use. We have recently started a program designed to evaluate these factors and have instituted a protocol to assess spike parameter changes in patients with seizures of temporal lobe origin.

Whether or not this particular approach proves to be advantageous, it does illustrate the potential use of computer-based analytical schemes to increase the overall efficiency of EEG monitoring studies. There are, of course, a number of other examples of analytical techniques that may eventually be valuable adjuncts to the current monitoring routines or may lead to further reduction in time requirements.

The work of Gotman and his colleagues (10) has demonstrated that computer methods can be used effectively to delineate exact interhemispheric time relationships among generalized discharges and has provided suggestive evidence that this type of information may be useful in differentiating between primarily and secondarily generalized epileptic processes. Such information is not obtainable by human analysis, at least in practical terms, and so this technique could prove to be an additional source of diagnostic information that would facilitate detection of a focal process. We have also been exploring the possibility that computer-based analysis of EEG background activity can predict the probability of future behavioral side effects of anticonvulsant medication (5). It is not unusual for behavioral problems, such as hyperactivity or poor school performance, to become manifest in individuals in whom anticonvulsant therapy has resulted in complete control of seizures. However, such problems may not become apparent for many weeks or months after institution of treatment, and when they do, a direct causal relationship to the anticonvulsant drug is sometimes difficult to establish. As with the other examples cited previously, an objective and quantitative measurement, based on EEG alterations, would allow a more timely intervention, through drug dosage alteration or replacement, with an overall increase in efficacy.

Utilization of the approaches mentioned here, as well as other recent developments in the area of EEG automation and analysis, may make it possible to decrease the complexity and time requirements of intensive neurodiagnostic monitoring while increasing its diagnostic value.

CONCLUSION

The outlook for the future of the application of computer-based methods to prolonged EEG monitoring appears optimistic, but the problems involved must not be minimized or bypassed. The successful routine application of these automated techniques will require much more work and a good deal of feedback from individuals engaged in the interpretation of monitoring studies to individuals attempting to design the computer systems. As indicated above, current systems must be used with caution, and with careful visual confirmation, to exclude false-positive detections and to validate the successful detection of actual epileptiform events. Because of the increasing availability and power of microprocessor-based systems, it is clear that such hardware will soon be a routine component of monitoring laboratories, which will facilitate the more rapid development of practical software. The ultimate goal of computer technology is not simply to automate the spike-counting and seizure-identification abilities of the human but to extend diagnostic capabilities and decrease recording-time requirements.

ACKNOWLEDGMENT

The author's work was supported by grant NS11535 from the National Institute of Neurological and Communicative Disorders and Stroke, NIH.

REFERENCES

1. Barlow, J.S. (1979): Computerized clinical electroencephalography in perspective. *IEEE Trans. Biomed. Eng.,* BME-26:377–391.
2. Carrie, J.R.G. (1972): A hybrid computer system for detecting and quantifying spike and wave EEG patterns. *Electroencephalogr. Clin. Neurophysiol.,* 33:339–341.
3. Ehrenberg, B.L., and Penry. J.K. (1976): Computer recognition of generalized spike-wave discharges. *Electroencephalogr. Clin. Neurophysiol.,* 41:25–36.
4. Frost, J.D., Jr. (1979): Microprocessor-based EEG spike detection and quantification. *Int. J. Biomed. Comput.,* 10:357–373.
5. Frost, J.D., Jr. (1981): Applications of automated EEG analysis in epilepsy. *Proceedings of the 34th Annual Conference on Engineering in Medicine and Biology,* p. 128.
6. Frost, J.D., Jr. (1985): Automatic recognition and characterization of epileptiform discharges in the human EEG. *J. Clin. Neurophysiol.,* 2:231–249.
7. Frost, J.D., Jr., and Kellaway, P. (1981): Changes in epileptic spike configuration associated with achievement of clinical seizure control. *Electroencephalogr. Clin. Neurophysiol.,* 51:20P-21P.
8. Gevins, A.S., Yeager, C.L., Diamond, S.L., Spire, J-P., Zeitlin, G.M., and Gevins, A.H. (1975): Automated analysis of the electrical activity of the human brain (EEG): A progress report. *Proc. IEEE,* 63:1382–1399.

9. Gevins, A.S., Yeager, C.L., Zeitlin, G.M., Ancoli, S., and Dedon, M.F. (1977): On-line computer rejection of EEG artifact. *Electroencephalogr. Clin. Neurophysiol.,* 42:267–274.
10. Gotman, J. (1981): Interhemispheric relations during bilateral spike-and-wave activity. *Epilepsia,* 22:453–466.
11. Gotman, J., and Gloor, P. (1976): Automatic recognition and quantification of interictal epileptic activity in the human scalp EEG. *Electroencephalogr. Clin. Neurophysiol.,* 41:513–529.
12. Gotman, J., Ives, J.R., and Gloor, P. (1979): Automatic recognition of interictal epileptic activity in prolonged EEG recordings. *Electroencephalogr. Clin. Neurophysiol.,* 46:510–520.
13. Kellaway, P., Frost, J.D., Jr., and Crawley, J.W. (1980): Influence of phenobarbital on C_3/C_4 spikes in Rolandic epilepsy of children. *Electroencephalogr. Clin. Neurophysiol.,* 50:153P.
14. Kellaway, P., Frost, J.D., Jr., and Crawley, J.W. (1980): Time modulation of spike-and-wave activity in generalized epilepsy. *Ann. Neurol.,* 8:491–500.
15. Kellaway, P., Frost, J.D., Jr., and Hrachovy, R.A. (1978): Relationship between clinical state, ictal and interictal EEG discharges, and serum drug levels: Partial seizures/phenobarbital. *Ann. Neurol.,* 4:197.
16. Kellaway, P., Saltzberg, B., Frost, J.D., Jr., and Crawley, J.W. (1979): Relationship between clinical state, ictal and interictal EEG discharges, and serum drug levels: Generalized epilepsy/ethosuximide. *Neurology,* 29:559.
17. Ktonas, P.Y. (1983): Automated analysis of abnormal electroencephalograms. *CRC Crit. Rev. Biomed. Eng.* 9:39–47.
18. Lopes da Silva, F.H., Dijk, A., and Smits, H. (1975): Detection of nonstationarities in EEGs using the autoregressive model—An application to EEGs of epileptics. In: *CEAN: Computerized EEG Analysis,* edited by G. Dolce and H. Künkel, pp. 180–199. Gustav Fischer Verlag, Stuttgart.
19. Principe, J.C., and Smith, J.R. (1982): Microcomputer-based system for the detection and quantification of petit mal epilepsy. *Comput. Biol. Med.,* 12:87–95.

Advances in Neurology, Vol. 46: Intensive Neurodiagnostic Monitoring, edited by R. J. Gumnit. Raven Press, New York © 1986.

Intensive Neurodiagnostic Monitoring: Strategy for Optimal Use

Richard H. Mattson

Department of Neurology, Yale University School of Medicine, Veterans Administration Medical Center, Neurology Service, West Haven, Connecticut 06516

Intensive neurodiagnostic monitoring (INDM) began approximately 15 years ago with simple closed circuit, reel-to-reel videotaping of clinical events and simultaneous prolonged electroencephalographic recording (video/EEG). The monitoring and immediate replay of events proved to be a major conceptual and technical advance in the evaluation and treatment of patients with seizures or seizure-like conditions. The diagnosis of epilepsy, classification of seizure type, determination of seizure frequency and severity, and localization of onset of attacks has been greatly facilitated by use of these methods (7,16,17). The value of INDM has led to its widespread acceptance and utilization in epilepsy units throughout the world. Although the complexity and technical sophistication of the procedure have increased (2,19), the principles of this approach to patient evaluation and care have not changed significantly.

Different INDM techniques are utilized in different centers for specific clinical problems. The recording may be a prolonged EEG tracing of 4 to 6 hr combined with simultaneous time-locked videotaping of the patient (18), or prolonged 24-hr EEG recording stored on magnetic tape without an audiovisual component (2,20). At the other extreme, evaluation may include up to several weeks of inpatient intensive monitoring of video/EEG recordings, as well as cardiac, pneumographic, and other physiologic measures. Display of electrographic patterns recorded directly from the surface of the cortex or from the depth of the brain using specially implanted electrodes with concomitant clinical videotape recordings are used prior to surgery for epilepsy (6,21). Signals recorded in these various clinical situations can be retained, not only on videotape and paper, but also simultaneously on magnetic tape for retrieval of information at a later time. The most elaborate units have remote control, black and white and color cameras with in-room microphones for audio pick-up connected to videotape cassette recorders (VCR). The polygraphic/EEG signal is transmitted by traditional "hard wire" cable or radiotelemetry. The signal can be written out on paper or reformatted and displayed on a video or TV monitor simultaneously with the clinical picture (19). Computer programs have been developed to recognize electrographic seizures and initiate selective video/EEG tape recordings of only the clinically important events (9,10,13). In an inpatient setting, and for combined video/EEG recording, the INDM often is attended by a professional staff member such as a physician, nurse, or EEG technician who can come to the patient during some type of clinical attack. Such interaction enhances clarification of the clinical characteristics of any type of episode that occurs or provides care during seizures (8,16).

This most highly developed INDM requires close on-site physician supervision of well trained personnel over long periods of time and is costly (11,12). Consequently, decisions must be made that direct attention to which level and type of intensive monitoring can best answer the important clinical questions relevant to each specific patient. The INDM should be simple and economical, but sufficiently detailed to provide the necessary information. For example, many problems, such as the diagnosis of absence seizures, can be answered as an outpatient with relatively simple systems, whereas complex diagnostic or treatment problems as well as presurgical evaluation require exhaustive and costly inpatient diagnostic studies. Equipment and personnel for the former indication should be available at most major medical centers. The more difficult problems require referral to highly developed INDM epilepsy centers.

TYPES OF INDM

Fifteen years of experience in intensive monitoring of more than 3,000 patients at the Veterans Administration/Yale Epilepsy Center have allowed us a special opportunity to examine retrospectively which levels of technology and personnel are required to provide the physician with information allowing for optimal care.

Our early studies provided maximal monitoring with cable ("hard wire")-recorded EEG and paper write-out, videotaping of all events, and professional interaction with the patient. These methods have been very effective in diagnosis and management (2–5,8,15,16,21). However, the cost of operating such a unit is considerable. Consequently, reevaluation of our admission process has been done to determine how much *less* intensive monitoring might have sufficed to provide comparable information for diagnosis and management. Studies of ambulatory monitoring of the EEG (1,2,4) have been the initial step in this direction. Most recently, we have completed a detailed analysis of a single representative month of admissions to the epilepsy center for inpatient evaluation. In particular, we wished to ascertain if less complex INDM might have allowed us to arrive at comparable clinical diagnoses and treatment.

OUTPATIENT INDM

INDM can be divided into a number of categories describing increasing levels of complexity (Tables 1–3). The least extensive studies, of course, are

TABLE 1. *Clinical problems suitable for evaluation by short-term outpatient INDM*

Half-day video/EEG and/or polygraphic INDM
Multiple daily events (seizures, anxiety, vertigo, syncope, sleep disorders)
Easily precipitated attacks
Intensive drug level monitoring
Prolonged EEG (polygraphic) INDM
Ambulatory cassette magnetic tape-recorded EEG
Frequent daily/nocturnal events
Events occurring or precipitated outside of hospital
Prolonged sleep EEG (polygraphic) INDM (interictal or subclinical abnormalities) for diagnosis and/or quantification

TABLE 2. *Clinical problems best evaluated by prolonged video/EEG inpatient INDM*

Tape-recorded time-locked video and EEG INDM with or without reformatting
Characterization of less frequent daytime or nocturnal events
Quantification of events
Video and paper-displayed EEG INDM
Localization of interictal EEG
Localization of ictal EEG seizure

TABLE 3. *Clinical problems best managed with attended inpatient INDM*

Characterization of subclinical or subtle events
Intracranial electrodes (depth, subdural)
Exact seizure localization
Clinical correlation
Polysomnography
Status epilepticus
Video/EEG to evaluate drug toxicity or efficacy
Recordings on patients requiring withdrawal of antiepileptic drug

usually those done on an outpatient basis. Half- or all-day video/EEG examinations may suffice to make a diagnosis, especially if attacks are frequent or reproducible. Such tests may be done in an EEG laboratory suite (18). Twenty-four hour ambulatory cassette monitoring often provides evidence of interictal epileptiform abnormality confirming a diagnosis of epilepsy and/or providing localization of onset. The EEG pattern may aid in classification of seizure or epilepsy type to assist in choice of optimal antiepileptic drug selection for treatment. Similarly, an all-day/night ambulatory monitoring EEG done as an outpatient can give evidence of an electrographic seizure that may provide a diagnosis in cases in which uncertainty exists as to whether the patient suffered from syncopy, pseudoseizures, or other types of attacks (1,2). Although the absence of a definite diagnosis may require more intensive inpatient monitoring, in may cases an answer can be found without such labor-intensive efforts.

INPATIENT INDM

Evaluation of inpatients can be divided into two broad categories. Those in which the patient is confined to an area in front of a video camera so that combined video/EEG recordings can be made, and those in which the patient is freer to move about the inpatient unit under the close scrutiny of specially trained professional personnel.

Time-Locked Video/EEG Recording

Video observation of the patient while simultaneously recording his EEG is of proven value. However, it requires close time synchronization, or time-locking, if one is to make a precise correlation between electrical events and behavioral events, as well as professional attendance and supervision. For many patients use of a video recorder at home with an EEG machine is not satisfactory, although these simple units are of advantage in the routine EEG laboratory where they make it possible for the electroencephalographer to come in at the end of the day and review what the technician saw during a routine EEG.

Tables 2 and 3 outline the types of problems that are best answered with inpatient video/EEG recording. Such recordings can be divided into two broad groups: (a) when the patient must be under constant surveillance by a technologist or nurse, and (b) when the recorded video and EEG can be reviewed later in those instances in which a clinical event has been recognized by the patient or attendant.

The initial characterization of the patient's seizures in order to make the diagnosis of specific type requires constant attention, as does the recognition of subtle clinical seizures or of those for which the patient may be amnesic. The documentation of actual ictal events may take days to achieve, and the diagnosis requires simultaneous videotape recording of a specific clinical event, especially when muscle artifact obscures the EEG, or scalp propagation of deep seizure activity does not occur.

Simultaneous ECG, respiration, and other polygraphic measures provide evidence of nonepileptic attacks simulating epileptic seizures (for example, cardiac dysrhythmias).

The most intensive neurodiagnostic monitoring is required when a precise seizure diagnosis and localization are required, whether this be for the classification of multiple types of seizures so that drug therapy may be adjusted, or during presurgical evaluations. The presence of skilled observers such as specially trained nurses or technologists to assist the physician is especially important when recording from depth electrodes or during provocation by anticonvulsant drug withdrawal with the risk of serial seizures. These personnel help protect the patient and the leads and other equipment from damage and contamination, and help to assess the patient's clinical condition.

In these cases continuous on-site supervision by a physician expert in epilepsy and electroencephalography is necessary if appropriate interventions are to be made. Careful clinical observation by the physician and his/her assistants in order to ascertain the presence or absence of motor, sensory, memory, or language problems provides especially valuable information concerning the localization of onset of the attacks.

On the other hand, once initial characterization of the seizure types has been made, there are many patients with whom video/EEG can be performed with a one-on-one observation by special technologists or nurses. These include patients in whom the characterization of easily recognized, but less frequent, daytime or nocturnal events is needed, in which the number of events must be counted, and in obtaining sufficient numbers of seizures of the same type in order to assure localization and characterization of type of interictal and ictal EEG events. This is especially useful in the diagnosis of epilepsy type and subsequent drug treatment selection.

In many centers the entire 24 hr of EEG is written out on paper. This is necessary in some cases, especially for the first 24 hr. Most interictal electroencephalographic abnormalities of importance will have become evident in that period of time (5). At present, the ambulatory cassette tape recording remains inferior to paper display for recognition and localization of interictal abnormalities and artifacts. However, many centers depend on the constant attention of a trained electroencephalographic technologist to determine which events should be written out immediately in pen and ink, and those in which the recording is marked for closer analysis and write-out later. Simultaneous magnetic tape recording can be done on a separate analog tape recorder, or the signal can be multiplexed and recorded on one of the audio channels of the videotape. This procedure assures both video and EEG are on the same tape, a safeguard against losing part of the information.

Freely Moving Patients

Many events occur only during interaction with other people, occur infrequently enough so that the patient cannot be confined to the area of focus of the video camera, or involve the patient running or making other movements that make video recording difficult or impossible. Although some of these episodes can be evaluated in cooperative patients with ambulatory cassette recordings at home, in many instances it is necessary to have the patient under the close scrutiny of specially trained personnel. For example, it is important to obtain quantification of frequency of well characterized EEG events, or record events that only occur during human interaction. Some events occur with insufficient frequency to warrant dedicating the video equipment for long periods of time to this group of patients.

These patients may be recorded on ambulatory cassette recorders while inpatients. The patient, his family, other patients on the ward, or professional personnel all can push the event button. This is particularly useful for people of limited intelligence, cooperation, or those who have no knowledge that the event is occurring.

If immediate review of the tracings is required, the ambulatory cassette recorders are not useful. Under these circumstances, either cable or radiotelemmetry recording are the devices of choice. Technologists, nurses, and physicians are then able to immediately play back an event to analyze it and determine the next course of action. Cable and radiotelemetry, coupled with tape recording of the EEG, are particularly useful in patients with well characterized seizures who are being worked up for surgery. Under these circumstances it is possible to confirm that the seizures begin in one part of the brain by recording several seizures while freeing up video equipment for other patients. The continuous EEG recording is not only essential for evaluation of attacks but also provides for analysis of interictal abnormalities to help in the diagnosis of epilepsy type. These techniques, however, are not a substitute for the initial characterization of the seizures which requires more combined video/EEG recording and come only when videoanalysis confirms that attacks are stereotyped.

RETROSPECTIVE ANALYSIS OF INDM

Retrospective analysis was done for a random month in 1984 to determine if some less extensive study would have sufficed to provide the same critical information. Thirty patients were admitted and 24 had some type of INDM (Table 4). Six patients who did not have intensive neurodiagnostic monitoring were not included in the analysis. The reason for admission and INDM for each patient was analyzed and the types of diagnostic testing were recorded, together with the ultimate diagnosis and outcome. In every case, the reasons for admission and final outcome, as well as the methods used to arrive at the decisions, were compared with possible alternative methods described in Tables 1 to 3. Six patients of the 24, if studied as outpatients, would have provided essentially the same pertinent information allowing for a diagnosis. Four of these patients required overnight or nocturnal recording of the EEG for characterization of type, extent, and severity of abnormality of the EEG. No attacks were expected in any of these individuals. Such testing could have been performed equally well using an ambulatory monitoring system with either rapid screening subsequently or, if need be, write-out onto paper. Two patients had episodes of a frequency that outpatient INDM during a half-day's time would have captured attacks and allowed the diagnosis. In one patient, multiple episodes were clearly of histrionic type and responded to encouragement to bring them on and turn them off. Such precipitation might have been equally possi-

TABLE 4. *Analysis of INDM in inpatient epilepsy patients*[a]

Group	Type INDM: Actually performed	Type INDM: Alternative
Outpatient		
Video/EEG INDM	0	2 (5)[b]
Ambulatory cassette-recorded EEG	0	4
Inpatient		
Video/EEG with selected paper write-out INDM	0	8 (5)[b]
Video/EEG with continuous paper write-out INDM	24	10
Total	24	24

[a] Analysis of INDM for 24 of 30 patients admitted to the West Haven Veterans Administration Medical Center inpatient epilepsy center over a 1-month period. All had full CCTV with professional attendance and paper-written EEG. Retrospective analysis indicated less intensive monitoring would have sufficed in all but 10 of the 24.

[b] Assignment of patient category included in parentheses was a possible alternative.

ble in an outpatient setting. The final patient had frequent afternoon episodes of dizziness and seeming confusion. On clinical video recording no concurrent electrographic abnormality was found, but transient high levels of carbamazepine were found and resulted in drug toxicity. In three other patients admitted to the hospital, seizures were captured within the first day of recording and, in retrospect, could have been successfully studied as an outpatient. In none of the individuals, however, was the frequency of attack sufficient to expect attacks could be recorded in an outpatient half-day or even all-day setting. Consequently, scheduling such a patient and recording in an outpatient setting might require repeated use of the resources and still fail to capture an attack. In view of the unlikely probability of capturing an attack, this seeming economy of using outpatient monitoring actually would be wasteful of resources by failing to make a diagnosis.

In 18 of the patients admitted, clinical attacks occurred, and replay of videotape of the attack together with write-out of tape-recorded electroencephalographic signal would have sufficed to assure the diagnosis. Continuous paper-written EEG was not necessary. Some of these attacks were nocturnal. The electrographic signal was obscured by artifact but the seizures were established by reviewing the simultaneous clinical videotape recording. In ten patients, the combined clinical and paper-written record was necessary to provide specific characterization and localization of attacks. The presence of a professional attendant was needed to interact and test the patient, manage the equipment, and provide acute care. In summary, retrospective analysis of a month's admission to the Epilepsy Center suggested that 25% of the patients could have been studied as outpatients with essentially the same information obtained.

A number of reasons can be provided to understand why most of these patients were appropriately admitted to the inpatient unit. A full range of outpatient INDM capability is not readily available in West Haven. Establishment of such a unit requires availability of space in a clinic, office, or hospital. Separate equipment is needed, as well as the availability of the necessary technical staff. Ideally, such a daytime unit might be established in the area contiguous with a monitoring facility for the inpatient center, but planning is needed early in construction to allow such an arrangement. In our center, personnel are trained and familiar with the operation of the inpatient unit, and efforts to do daytime recording often prove to conflict with the full operation of the inpatient unit.

Although ambulatory monitoring has proven useful (2), such capability requires purchase of expensive equipment or sending tapes away for "expert" review. Unfortunately, at present, there is a relative shortage of electroencephalographers who are expert and experienced in reading and interpreting these tracings. In contrast, most adequately trained electroencephalographers can accurately review a paper-written signal.

Even when outpatient INDM can give the essential diagnostic information, admission to a seizure unit also provides simultaneous care and acquisition of other information. These include the opportunity for a complete review of the patient's history, as well as a reexamination. The hospital admission provides an opportunity for multiple consultations, including psychiatrists, neurosurgeons, nurses, technicians, study assistants, etc. In approaching the problem from somewhat different vantage points, these personnel may provide valuable information or insights. A significant number of patients have other diagnostic studies while hospitalized including computerized tomographic scanning and/or magnetic resonance imaging, lumbar puncture, and angiography. The latter, in particular, is best done on an inpatient setting. In order to provoke attacks, it may be necessary to withdraw antiepileptic drugs with the attendant risk of serial seizures, or even status epilepticus. The patients being closely monitored and attended in hospital facility allows immediate treatment to terminate such attacks. Finally, after the completed evaluation has been reviewed and discussed in detail, a summary is dictated and becomes a permanent and important part of the patient's record and a foundation for future treatment and decision-making. Consequently, selection of a strategy for intensive neurodiagnostic monitoring depends on what type of approach will give the most specific answer to a problem; but the selection may be also influenced by the availability of other diagnostic or treatment approaches primarily available through admission to an inpatient intensive monitoring center. Finally, the type of INDM available at different epilepsy centers may influence the strategy more than the specific indication. The historical development of our center has led to an efficient evaluation and management in an INDM unit operating 24 hr daily, 7 days a week. A quite different inpatient approach was developed in Montreal but works well for them (13,14).

SUMMARY AND CONCLUSIONS

Intensive neurodiagnostic monitoring has proven to be a valuable approach to diagnosis and management of epilepsy and related disorders. Certain specific types of problems can be answered with fairly limited outpatient methods, whereas others require exhaustive, complex, and expensive inpatient methods. With rapid advances in technical quality of cameras, videotape recorders, and utilization of computer assistance, changes in current methods can be expected in the near future.

REFERENCES

1. Bridgers, S.L., and Ebersole, J.S. (1984): The clinical utility of ambulatory cassette EEG monitoring. *Neurology (Cleveland),* 35:166–173.
2. Ebersole, J.S. (1985): EEG telemetered and ambulatory cassette—Review of current systems and techniques. In: *Advances in Neurology, International Conference on Intensive Neurodiagnostic Monitoring.* Raven Press, New York.
3. Ebersole, J.S., and Leroy, R.F. (1983): An evaluation of ambulatory cassette EEG monitoring: II. Detection of interictal abnormalities. *Neurology (Cleveland),* 33:8–18.
4. Ebersole, J.S., and Leroy, R.F. (1983): An evaluation of ambulatory cassette EEG monitoring: III. Diagnostic accuracy compared to intensive inpatient EEG monitoring. *Neurology (Cleveland),* 33:853–860.
5. Ebersole, J.S., and Spencer, S.S. (1981): The efficacy of 24-hour EEG monitoring in the epilepsy diagnosis. *Epilepsia,* 22:235–236.
6. Engel, J. (1985): Intensive neurodiagnostic monitoring with intracranial electrodes. In: *Advances in Neurology, International Conference on Intensive Neurodiagnostic Monitoring.* Raven Press, New York.
7. Escueta, A.V., Kunze, U., Waddell, G., Boxley, J., and Nadel, A. (1977): Lapse of consciousness and automatisms in temporal lobe epilepsy: A videotape analysis. *Neurology (Minneapolis),* 27:144–155.
8. Fay M.L., and Mattson R.H. (1980): Clinical testing during intensive monitoring of ictal events. In *Advances in Epileptology: The Xth Epilepsy International Symposium,* edited by J.A. Wada and J.K. Penry, pp. 65–68. Raven Press, New York.
9. Gotman, J. (1982): Automatic recognition of the epileptic seizures in the EEG. *Electroencephalogr. Clin. Neurophysiol.,* 54:530–540.
10. Gotman, J. (1985): Current state of the art in data reduction. In: *Advances in Neurology, International Conference on Intensive Neurodiagnostic Monitoring.* Raven Press, New York.
11. Gumnit, R.J. (1985): Cost-benefit problems and information transfer to practicing physicians. In: *Advances in Neurology, International Conference on Intensive Neurodiagnostic Monitoring.* Raven Press, New York.
12. Holmes, G.L., McKeever, M., and Russman, B.S. (1981): Long term monitoring of seizure patients. *Conn. Med.,* 45:358–362.
13. Ives, J.R. (1985): Video recording during long-term monitoring. In: *Advances in Neurology, International Conference on Intensive Neurodiagnostic Monitoring.* Raven Press, New York.
14. Ives, J.R., and Gloor, P. (1978): A long term timelapse video system to document the patient's spontaneous clinical seizure synchronized with the EEG. *Electroencephalogr. Clin. Neurophysiol.,* 45:412–416.
15. Mattson, R.H. (1980): Value of intensive monitoring. In: *Advances in Epileptology. The Xth Epilepsy International Symposium,* edited by J.A. Wada and J.K. Penry, pp. 43–52. Raven Press, New York.
16. Mattson, R.H. (1983): Closed circuit televised videotape recording and electroencephalography (CCTV/EEG) in convulsive status epilepticus. In: *Advances in Neurology:*

Symposium on Status Epilepticus, edited by A.V. Escueta, C.G. Wasterlain, D.M. Treiman, and R.J. Porter, pp. 37–46. Raven Press, New York.

17. Perry, T.R., Gumnit, R.J., Gates, J.R., and Leppik, I.E. (1983): Routine EEG vs. intensive monitoring in the evaluation of intractable epilepsy. *Public Health Rep.,* 98:384–389.
18. Porter, R.J. (1980): Methodology of continuous monitoring with videotape recording and electroencephalography. In: *Advances in Epileptology: The Xth Epilepsy International Symposium,* edited by J.A. Wada and J.K. Penry, pp. 35–42. Raven Press, New York.
19. Porter, R.J., Penry, J.K., and Lacy, J.R. (1977): Diagnostic and therapeutic reevaluation of patients with intractable epilepsy. *Neurology (Minneapolis),* 27:1006–1011.
20. Sheridan, P.H., Sato, S., and Porter, R.J. (1984): Video monitoring during a single, outpatient, routine EEG recording. *Epilepsia,* 25(5):653.
21. Stores, G., Hennion, T., and Quy, R.J. (1980): EEG ambulatory monitoring system with visual play-back display. In: *Advances in Epileptology. The Xth Epilepsy International Symposium,* edited by J.A. Wada and J.K. Penry, pp. 89–94. Raven Press, New York.
22. Williamson, P.D., Spencer, D.D., Spencer, S.S., and Mattson, R.H. (1980): Presurgical intensive monitoring using depth electroencephalography in temporal lobe epilepsy. In: *Advances in Epileptology: The Xth Epilepsy International Symposium,* edited by J.A. Wada and J.K. Penry, pp. 73–81. Raven Press, New York.

Advances in Neurology, Vol. 46: Intensive Neurodiagnostic Monitoring, edited by R. J. Gumnit. Raven Press, New York © 1986.

Intensive Neurodiagnostic Monitoring: Summary and Recommendations

Robert J. Gumnit

Minnesota Comprehensive Epilepsy Program, 2701 University Avenue, SE, and Department of Neurology, University of Minnesota, Minneapolis, Minnesota 55414

INDICATIONS FOR INTENSIVE NEURODIAGNOSTIC MONITORING

In general terms, INDM is used to (a) identify the nature of the event (seizure, syncope, etc.), (b) identify the type of seizure, (c) localize the part of the brain from which a seizure begins, and (d) quantify the number of seizures. Depending on the particular clinical situation, a variety of tests may be used alone or in combination.

Precise Definition of the Event

If there is a very high probability that the event is a true seizure this step might be passed and the work-up begin with identifying the seizure type. If there is concern that the patient may be suffering from a disturbance of sleep rather than a genuine seizure, the patient might best be referred either to a sleep laboratory or to have an overnight sleep study (with concomitant measurement of ECG, respiratory effort, extraocular movements at a minimum) in the intensive monitoring suite. If it is not clear whether the patient is suffering from a seizure, syncope secondary to cardiac disturbance, or vertigo secondary to a disturbance in the vestibular/brainstem system, a 24-hr ambulatory cassette recording in which one channel of ECG, one channel of extraocular movements, and six channels of EEG are used will be found to be very helpful (20). However, since not all rhythm disturbances are symptomatic (the cardiovascular literature is full of such studies) extreme care must be taken in interpretation.

Precisely Identify the Type of Seizure

There is no substitute for intensive neurodiagnostic monitoring using time-locked video and EEG recording if one is to be certain of the type(s) of seizure the patient experiences. Some large units, in which several patients are being studied simultaneously, have developed techniques whereby constant one-on-one attention between the technologist and the patient is not always necessary. The technologist is shared among several patients with various fail-safe procedures introduced. Even in such units, however, a one-on-one relationship between the patient and technologist (with everything being recorded on tape and selected portions written out by the EEG machine) is a necessity if subtle events are to be identified. If the technologist has been properly trained in observing seizures, is known to be reliable in identifying the portion of the tape where the event occurred, and has been properly trained to test for varying degrees of disturbance of consciousness, speech, etc., then the physician need not be in constant attendance in the recording suite. However, the electroencephalographer/epileptologist must be immediately available to deal with untoward events, especially the medical problems accompanying a seizure, and to interpret what has been going on in order to make changes in the investigatory plan as changed conditions arise. This is particularly true if depth electrodes have been implanted or if anticonvulsant drugs have been withdrawn in order to increase the yield of ictal events (2,24–26,28,29,35).

Capturing a single ictal event is insufficient. Patients frequently have more than one type of seizure, and apparently similar seizures may have differing electrical correlates. Therefore, multiple events must be recorded until the epileptologist is satisfied that the diagnosis has been properly determined.

Video/EEG is particularly useful in differentiating the various forms of epileptic convulsive syndromes, in classifying nonconvulsive epilepsies, and in providing a guide to specific pharmacotherapy (1,4,5,8,9). Delgado-Escueta has pointed out that it has a practical use in uncontrolled primary generalized epilepsies. It differentiates primary or genetically determined generalized motor seizures from symptomatic or secondary generalized seizures. It also helps differentiate nonconvulsive classic absences from atypical absences and complex partial seizures, pure absence from juvenile absence, juvenile myoclonic epilepsy, myoclonus epilepsy, and myoclonic absence.

Video/EEG has provided data that has permitted the introduction of a proposed subclassification of complex partial seizures. It has provided clues to separating frontal lobe foci from mesial temporal lobe foci, and perhaps mesial from lateral cortical temporal lobe foci as well. Many bizarre episodes which, in the past, were passed off as psychogenic are in reality complex partial seizures. Similarly, some events which have been accepted as complex partial seizures are now recognizable as psychogenic. The role of video/EEG monitoring in making these distinctions is crucial, as Williamson has elegantly demonstrated (36).

Characterization and Quantification of the Types of Seizures

Once all of the types of seizures that the patient experiences have been identified, it is often necessary to know the relative frequency of the types of seizures and to come to a precise clinico-anatomical analysis. Under these circumstances it is often possible to use more automated video/EEG techniques and frequently to use radio- or cable-telemetered EEG alone. If the patient or attending nurse, relative, etc. is aware of all the seizures that occur, a signal marker makes the retrospective analysis easy and reliable. If this is not the case, some way of rapidly reviewing all of the record is mandatory. Although technically feasible, it is highly impractical to write out days and days of EEG on paper and look at each page.

Role in Surgical Evaluation

For the evaluation of patients for surgery, the role of video/EEG is crucial (11,14,15,19,27,33,34; J.R. Gates, *this volume*). The possibility of doing major harm to the patient by inappropriate surgery is, unfortunately, all too real. Unnecessary paralysis, difficulties with speech, and the catastrophic inability to retain new learning from creating lesions in both temporal lobes can all occur. Different types of monitoring are required at different stages. The question of whether the patient has multiple seizure types must be answered. There is substantial controversy as to whether or not all patients undergoing temporal lobectomy require depth electrodes. In any case, those patients who do require depth electrodes require the closest monitoring.

Stereo EEG (SEEG), chronic recording from stereotactically placed multicontact depth electrodes, is carried out to survey mesial, temporal, and other forebrain limbic structures (15). It is the most commonly employed technique for intracranial recording. The main indications for SEEG are: (a) to determine the side of epileptogenic lesion when bilateral, independent, frontotemporal interictal spikes are present, and clear lateralization of ictal EEG onset has not been obtained; (b) to differentiate between temporal and extratemporal epileptogenic lesions when EEG recorded onsets are well lateralized but equally prominent in well defined extratemporal and temporal regions; (c) to confirm the presence of an epileptogenic lesion in one temporal lobe when EEG recorded ictal onsets are well localized to this area, but evidence of focal functional deficit is missing or conflicting, or other data, including characteristics of the behavioral seizures, suggest a contralateral extratemporal lesion; and (d) to determine whether an epileptogenic lesion localized to one temporal lobe might extend beyond the limits of the standard *en bloc* anterior temporal lobectomy.

Indications for placement of a multi-electrode grid or other cortical surface electrodes are still being developed, but include: (a) to precisely identify the site of a neocortical epileptogenic lesion when interictal and ictal EEG recordings localize the abnormality to a relatively broad cortical zone on one side; (b) to delineate the limits of a neocortical epileptogenic lesion when it has been well localized by interictal and ictal EEG recordings, but its extent is not certain; (c) to determine if there is a single primary epileptogenic lesion when interictal and ictal EEG recordings have localized two or more neocortical areas of epileptogenicity; and (d) to map areas of primary cerebral function adjacent to an identified epileptogenic lesion in order to determine the safe boundaries of the resection. This last functional mapping technique may become the most useful application of chronic multi-electrode grid recording, particularly in children who are unable to cooperate during long procedures carried out under local anesthesia in the operating room. Because placement of the multi-electrode grid requires a craniotomy, it is preferable to use this technique unilaterally when the suspected epileptogenic lesion is well lateralized by noninvasive studies. Bilateral grid placements can be used, however, in exceptional situations.

Intensive neurodiagnostic monitoring with intracranial electrodes should never be undertaken as a "fishing expedition." It is inappropriate when prior noninvasive evaluation has failed to limit potential locations of a resectable epileptogenic lesion to a number that can be reasonably explored by the technique to be used.

Epilepsy in Children

It is particularly difficult to come to a precise diagnosis of epilepsy in infants and children (25; P. Kellaway, *this volume*). They are commonly subject to behavioral and subjective symptoms that may be misconstrued as epileptic. Descriptions of the critical events are often vague and distorted. Positive diagnosis is critical in this period, probably more so than any other time of life. The determination that a child does not have epilepsy is as important as establishing that he does. Because the diagnosis must often be made with only vague and limited historical information, the physician is often forced to rely unduly on the routine EEG to provide definitive information. This age group is particularly prone to show normal or nonspecific EEG findings that may be misinterpreted as supporting a diagnosis of epilepsy. Conversely, the yield of routine EEG in providing specific epileptiform findings in infants and young children who do indeed have epilepsy may be disappointing. Even with provocative techniques, detection of a specific EEG abnormality may be less than 50%. Video/EEG is a particularly valuable tool in this age group. Especially in this age group, casual recording without the presence of a highly trained technologist and the frequent involvement of the electroencephalographer is likely to lead to false diagnoses.

Ambulatory Cassette and Telemetered EEG

If the events have been tightly characterized and need only be counted, or the lateralization confirmed, an ambulatory cassette recorder can be used on an inpatient basis for quantification. It may be necessary to perform this test on an inpatient basis if the patient has had anticonvulsant drugs withdrawn. It is unsafe to allow such a patient out of the hospital because of the likelihood of frequent generalized seizures or other injury occurring.

Ambulatory cassette-recorded EEG has the advantage of providing full patient mobility and one can use it on outpatients. Telemetered EEG limits the patient to the hospital setting, but provides the opportunity for continuous monitoring of the EEG by the technologist and/or electroencephalographer. In addition, specially trained hospital personnel are available to correlate electrical events with behavioral changes.

The following listing of recommended clinical indications for mobile and ambulatory EEG monitoring is not all inclusive, since special circumstances may warrant additional considerations (13). These tests can only be carried out on responsible, cooperative patients who will not abuse the equipment.

1. Documentation of clinically suspected, paroxysmal electrographic abnormalities in patients with normal or equivocal routine EEG studies.
2. Documentation of clinically suspected, non-EEG, paroxysmal electrographic abnormalities. These include cardiac arrhythmias via ECG, abnormalities of sleep or sleep-related respiration via EEG, EMG, EOG, ECG, and/or respiration parameters.
3. Characterization (lateralization, localization, distribution) of EEG abnormalities, both ictal and interictal, associated with seizure disorders. The extent of characterization is dependent on the number of EEG channels available. Lateralization, but not localization, is possible with four-channel ambulatory EEG systems.
4. Characterization of the relationship of seizures to specific precipitating circumstances or stimuli (e.g., nocturnal, catamenial, situation-related, activity-related). Verification and/or characterization of periodic seizure patterns.
5. Quantification of the number or frequency of seizures and/or interictal discharges and their relationship to naturally occurring events or cycles, or to therapeutic intervention or modification (e.g., drug alteration).

There are, however, several areas where ambulatory cassette EEG recording is not adequate because of spatial sampling restrictions and technical limitations. These are in the final evaluation of patients for possible seizure surgery and in the documentation of electrocerebral silence in those patients with possible brain death. Additionally, a negative ambulatory cassette recording (ACR), i.e., no electrographic changes or definite epileptiform activity during a spell, cannot by itself establish a diagnosis of a nonepileptic seizure or psychiatric disturbance. The limited number of channels may have missed a highly restricted discharge, and true complex partial seizures may have no surface EEG manifestations. Video/EEG monitoring is recommended for these differential diagnoses. Sixteen-channel epoch recordings are also not appropriate in the evaluation of interictal features or seizures for which the patient has no aura, or is too confused to push the marker button.

Outpatient Intensive Neurodiagnostic Monitoring

Some investigations are best carried on outside of the hospital. Patients with frequent minor seizures (at least three per week) may simply come in to an outpatient recording suite for video/EEG. The same is true of patients who have had frequent minor seizures who are being checked for the efficacy of anticonvulsant drugs. Patients with frequent generalized motor or prolonged complex partial seizures are at serious medical risk and require hospitalization for treatment even if INDM is not available.

Ambulatory cassette recorders play a particularly useful role in outpatient evaluations. The studies must be very carefully performed by experienced personnel. Artifacts are potential major problems, and misinterpretations are easily made. On the other hand, seizures may actually be recorded in a substantial number of patients, and the information obtained if an 8- or 16-channel recorder is used is often adequate to make a diagnosis. This information, however, is not adequate for anatomical localization for surgical work-up. Ambulatory cassette recorders are particularly useful in outpatient studies of selected patients with psychogenic seizures, sleep disturbances, frequent absence attacks, and those in whom the events appear only at unusual times and circumstances that cannot be duplicated in the protected atmosphere of an inpatient service.

Nonepileptic Seizures

Video/EEG has become absolutely essential in dealing with patients with nonepileptic seizures (10,12,17,21,23,30–32). Some of these are organic events, such as cardiorespiratory problems and vertigo. The ability to perform polygraphic recording while recording the patient on video is helpful. Often, equally helpful is polygraphic recording with ambulatory cassettes.

The second major subgroup of nonepileptic seizures are psychogenic seizures. These are events which resemble epileptic seizures, but which are found to be unaccompanied by a disturbance in the EEG that is compatible with epilepsy, or are precipitated, modified, or stopped by a simple command.

In the most flagrant cases, it is possible to record the patient on an EEG, preferably with combined video/EEG, and determine that there is no epileptic activity when the patient is going through bizarre, generalized motor activity. However, in patients with both psychogenic seizures and genuine seizures, or with less bizarre psychogenic seizures, it is usually necessary to hospitalize the patient, withdraw anticonvulsants, and proceed with intensive monitoring. Intensive monitoring in this context includes behavioral observation, serum anticonvulsant level monitoring, the use of simultaneous video and EEG recording, and the adjunctive use of radiotelemetered EEG and/or ambulatory cassette recorders. The indications for intensive monitoring are to confirm the diagnosis of psychogenic seizures, to determine if real seizures also exist, and to define the relationship between both real and psychogenic seizures when they coexist. Unless this is done, it is impossible to treat the patient appropriately.

GENERAL COMMENTS

Intensive neurodiagnostic monitoring is not a thing or a procedure that stands alone. Rather, it is an additional tool for the neurologist to greatly reduce the rate of error, and thereby minimize the number of patients who are in a state of uncertain diagnosis. Patients present with a wide range of severity and complexity of problems. The type of tool we use depends on the situation.

Intensive neurodiagnostic monitoring ceased to be experimental 10 years ago. It is now ready to move from a very few highly specialized centers into a larger number of units if they possess the necessary expertise. In order to avoid the mistakes of the past that led to overutilization and overpricing of highly technical procedures, we must learn from the experience of those who have developed these techniques.

Certain problems can readily be handled on an outpatient basis. For example, frequent events, those occurring or precipitated outside the hospital, those requiring polygraphic sleep analysis, and those in which a problem occurs at a stated time each day (for example, toxicity following a noon dose of an anticonvulsant drug) are appropriately handled on an outpatient basis. The patient may come to the EEG/monitoring suite, or ambulatory cassette recording can be used, depending on the clinical problem.

Certain problems require prolonged combined video/EEG in an inpatient setting. Whether the EEG needs to be written out continuously, and whether the physician, nurse, or EEG technologist needs to be in constant attendance will vary. Characterization of less frequent events, quantification of events, the recognition of subclinical or subtle events, and lateralization and localization of interictal and ictal activity fall into this category.

A smaller group of patients require the most intense involvement by the physician-nurse-technologist team. These include patients with intracranial electrodes (in which a search is being made for exact seizure localization), clinical correlation with subcortical activity, polysomnography, patients in whom antiepileptic drug withdrawal is needed to precipitate events, patients in status epilepticus, or those in whom minute-to-minute analysis of the EEG activity must be compared with drug levels and efficacy studies.

Although intensive neurodiagnostic monitoring generally uses an EEG machine in some form at some point, it is very different from what goes on in a routine EEG laboratory. Properly performed, INDM requires much more physician time and much more involvement of the physician during the carrying out of the procedures than does EEG. EEG examinations are largely a technologist-performed activity, with an interpretation of the written record provided by the physician at some later point in the day. INDM requires the ongoing presence of the physician in many instances, and his ready availability in all. The amount of time spent interpreting the lengthy records is considerable. For this reason, INDM will necessarily be more costly than EEG. Furthermore, at least for the moment, the equipment costs are substantially greater.

The quality of EEG interpretation in the United States (and elsewhere in the world) leaves much to be desired. The average patient receiving an EEG test in the average hospital is not in the hands of a board-certified technologist or of a board-certified electroencephalographer. Indeed, in the United States there are two sets of boards and questions have been raised about whether or not the applicants for certification by the two groups are held to equal standards. So far, INDM has largely been used in a few major universities and teaching hospitals where the quality of the technologist and electroencephalographers has been good. However, even the finest equipment cannot make up for deficiencies in quality of the technical and professional personnel. Unless carried out with consistently high technical standards and provided with interpretations that are clinically reliable, INDM is simply an expensive waste of time.

A primary indication, at present, for intensive neurodiagnostic monitoring is to answer the question of whether or not a patient is having seizures. In other words, is the presenting complaint an epileptic event (i.e., a paroxysm of electrical activity brain cells) or is it something else? However, more than a simple yes or no answer is required. We need a definitive diagnosis of the event. Is it cardiovascular, rhythm disturbance, hypertension, hypotension, respiratory disturbance, etc.? Perhaps it is vertigo. Is it psychologically determined? Mistaken interpretation, conversion reaction, or whatever? One must be in a position to make a positive psychiatric diagnosis. The absence of an EEG abnormality during the event is helpful, but unless the patient presents the rest of the psychological constellation, the physician must be careful not to jump to the conclusion that the problem is psychological in nature.

Is it a seizure? If so, which kind? Is there only one type of seizure? Is it the type of seizure that is amenable to surgery? Have the anticonvulsant drugs that have been prescribed done anything to reduce the frequency of seizures? Especially in the case of intractable seizures, while a monitoring unit is a necessary component, it is not sufficient to create an epilepsy center. The treatment of epilepsy involves a precise diagnosis, selection of appropriate anticonvulsant medications, surgery at times, and management of the concomitant psychological and social problems.

Does intensive neurodiagnostic monitoring have a role in the selection of anticonvulsant drugs? Patients with frequent small seizures, such as classic absence attacks, may be usefully monitored to see if the anticonvulsant prescribed has reduced or brought about a complete cessation of spells. Quantification is particularly important in this kind of problem (16). Can the EEG pattern predict the type of anticonvulsant drug to be prescribed? This is an empirical question that is yet to be answered. However, there is ample evidence that combined video/EEG monitoring is particularly helpful in evaluating the efficacy of a given anticonvulsant drug in a specific patient. Many experts have noted that it is only by identifying the precise type of seizure that has been controlled by a drug that one can determine which drug is effective in a given patient. It is a common observation in specialized epilepsy centers that patients who are alleged to be intractable to all anticonvulsants really are responsive, but have different kinds of seizures that are responding differentially to the different medications.

It is necessary to use these tools wisely. Except to answer the simplest questions, it appears that a multispecialty team is needed. If the full range of services is to be available, the unit must be busy enough to be practical from a cost basis. It is unlikely that one physician working in a simple milieu will be able to provide the range of services that four specialists can at Yale, or six at Minnesota.

A monitoring unit requires full-time attention. It cannot be run from the hip pocket of the busy practitioner. The contributors to this symposium all emphasized the close involvement and supervision required by the physician. At the risk of being redundant, it is not something that can be turned over to a technician to run and to provide the physician with a report at the end of the day. This type of approach is being attempted in certain sleep laboratories and is failing there. It will certainly fail in the complex cases requiring intensive neurodiagnostic monitoring.

As intensive neurodiagnostic monitoring is introduced around the country, much resistance has been encountered. There is a definite policy on the part of Medicare and many commercial insurance companies to resist recognizing new techniques in order to reduce the outflow of dollars. It is a tedious and frustrating task to work from company to company, and from state to state, convincing the lay administrators (and often the medical directors) of the usefulness and cost-effectiveness of a new technique and how best to use it. The changes occurring in Medicare regulations and the development of Health Maintenance Organizations (HMOs) and Preferred Provider Organizations (PPOs) definitely discriminate against the patient with chronic disease. Much of the discussion at the conference revolved around the problems created when payment schemes and reimbursement tables do not recognize the time involvement and expense required to care for patients with chronic disease such as epilepsy.

What many fail to recognize is the enormous cost to the patient (in terms of disability, anxiety, and misery) and to the insurance industry (in terms of unnecessary and useless expense) when patients are not properly treated. There are a large number of patients who require repeated hospitalizations because their seizures have not been adequately controlled. Others run up large bills going from doctor to doctor and repeating expensive diagnostic tests that are not helpful. The basic principles of medical treatment hold. We must come to the correct diagnosis, and properly evaluate the outcome of treatment. Intensive neurodiagnostic monitoring is a powerful tool with which to achieve this aim.

Our welfare system places patients with chronic seizure disorders in a bizarre situation. Most of them are started on Supplemental Security Insurance (SSI) disability payments because this is a federal, rather than a state, expense. SSI recipients are covered under Medicare rather than Medicaid. The Medicare Diagnostic Related Group (DRG) prospective payment system does not recognize the high cost of these few patients. However, they can only be cared for in specialized centers. The specialized centers can provide the care only at a great loss (because of the large number of expensive patients treated). Some centers have closed their units because they cannot afford it. Thus, the patients are denied the care they need to get off the welfare role and back to work.

Any new technique that is an expensive procedure invites abuse. The way to deal with abuse is not to deny the use of the technique, but rather to directly and quickly punish the thieves. All practitioners can be held to nationally accepted standards (3) and to the indications of intensive neurodiagnostic monitoring outlined here and which are presented in greater detail by the various authors.

ACKNOWLEDGMENTS

This work was supported by funds from the National Institutes of Health; grants P50-N516308 and R13-NS20816-01.

REFERENCES

1. Aarts, J.H.P., Binnie, C.D., Smith, A.M., and Wilkins, A.J. (1984): Selective cognitive impairment during focal and generalized epileptiform EEG activity. *Brain,* 107:293–308.
2. Ajmone-Marsan, C. (1984): Electroencephalographic studies in seizure disorders: Additional considerations. *J. Clin. Neurophysiol.,* 1:143–157.
3. American Electroencephalographic Society Guidelines for Long-Term Neurodiagnostic Monitoring in Epilepsy. (1985): *J. Clin. Neurophysiol.,* 2(4):419–452.
4. Binnie, C.D. (1983): Telemetric EEG monitoring in epilepsy, In: *Recent Advances in Epilepsy,* edited by T.A. Pedley and B.S. Meldrum, pp. 155–178 Churchill Livingstone, New York.
5. Binnie, C.D., Rowan, A.J., Overweg, J., Meinardi, H., Wisman, T., Kamp, A., and Lopes da Silva, F. (1981): Telemetric EEG and video monitoring in epilepsy. *Neurology (New York),* 31:298–303.
6. Blumhardt, L.D., and Oozeer, R. (1982): Problems encountered in the interpretation of ambulatory EEG recordings. In: *Mobile Long Term Recording,* edited by H. Stefan and W. Burr, pp. 37–53. Fischer, Stuttgart.
7. Bridgers, S.L., and Ebersole, J.S. (1984): The clinical utility of ambulatory cassette EEG monitoring. *Neurology (Cleveland),* 35:166–173.

8. Delgado-Escueta, A.V. (1979): Epileptogenic paroxysms: Modern approaches and clinical correlations. *Neurology (Minneapolis)*, 29:1014–1022.
9. Delgado-Escueta, A.V., Envile-Bascal, F. and Treiman, D.M. (1982): Complex partial seizures on closed-circuit television and EEG: A study of 691 attacks in 79 patients. *Ann. Neurol.*, 11:292-300.
10. Delgado-Escueta, A.V., Mattson, R.H. King, L., Goldensohn, E.S., Spiegel, H., Madsen, J., Crandall, P., Dreifuss, F.E., and Porter, R.J. (1981): Special report. The nature of aggression during epileptic seizures. *N. Engl. J. Med.*, 305:711–716.
11. Delgado-Escueta, A.V., Nashold, B., Freedman, M., Keplinger, C., Waddell, G., Miller, P., and Carwille S. (1979): Videotaping epileptic attacks during stereoelectro-encephalography. *Neurology (Minneapolis)*, 29:473–489.
12. Desai, B.T., Porter, R.J. and Penry, J.K. (1982): Psychogenic seizures: A study of 42 attacks in six patients, with intensive monitoring. *Arch. Neurol.*, 39:202–209.
13. Ebersole, J.S. (1985): Ambulatory cassette EEG. *J. Clin. Neurophysiol.*, 2(4):397–418.
14. Engel, J. (editor) (1986): *Surgical Management of the Epilepsies*. Raven Press, New York (*in press*).
15. Engel, J., Crandall, P.H., and Rausch, R. (1983): The partial epilepsies. In: *The Clinical Neurosciences, Vol. 2,* edited by R.N. Rosenberg, R.G. Grossman, S. Schochet, E.R. Heinz, and W.D. Willis, pp. 1349-1380. Churchill Livingstone, New York.
16. Frost, J.D. (1986): Automatic recognition and characterization of epileptiform discharges in the human. *EEG J. Clin. Neurophysiol.* (*in press*).
17. Gates, J.R., Ramani, V., Whalen, S.M., and Loewenson, R.B. (1985): Ictal characteristics of pseudoseizures. *Arch. Neurol.*, 42:1183–1187.
18. Gloor, P. (1975): Contributions of electroencephalography and electrocorticography to the neurosurgical treatment of the epilepsies. In: *Advances in Neurology, Vol. 8, Neurosurgical Management of the Epilepsies,* edited by D.P. Purpura, J.K. Penry, and R.D. Walter, pp. 59–105. Raven Press, New York.
19. Gotman, J. (1982): Automatic recognition of epileptic seizures in the EEG. *Electroencephalogr. Clin. Neurophysiol.*, 54:530–540.
20. Graf, M., Brunnei, G., Weber, H., Auinger, C., and Joskowicz, G. (1982): Simultaneous long-term recording of EEG and ECG in 'syncope' patients. In: *Mobile Long Term Recording,* edited by H. Stefan and W. Burr, pp. 67–76. Fischer, Stuttgart.
21. Gulick, T.A., Spinks, I.P., and King, D.W. (1982): Pseudoseizures: ictal phenomena. *Neurology,* 32:24–30.
22. Gumnit, R.J., and Gates, J.R. (1986): Psychogenic seizures. *Epilepsia* (*in press*).
23. Holmes, G.L., Sackellares, J.C., Ragland, M., and Dreifuss, F.E. (1980): Pseudoseizures in childhood: A clinical appraisal using prolonged EEG telemetry and videotape monitoring. *J. Pediatr.*, 97:554–558.
24. Kamp, A., and Lopes da Silva, R. (1982): Special techniques of recording and transmission. In: *Electroencephalography—Basic Principles, Clinical Applications, and Related Fields,* edited by E. Niedermeyer and F. Lopes Da Silva, pp. 639–654. Urban and Schwartzenberg, Baltimore.
25. Kellaway, P., and Frost, J.D. (1985): Monitoring at the affiliated hospitals of Baylor College of Medicine, Houston. In: *Long-term Monitoring in Epilepsy* (*EEG Suppl., No. 37*), edited by J. Gotman, J.R. Ives, and P. Gloor, pp. 397–408. Elsevier, Amsterdam.
26. King, D.W., Gallagher, B.B., Murvin, A.L., Smith, D.B., Marchs, D.J., Hartlage, L.C., and Ward, L.C. (1982): Pseudoseizures: Diagnostic evaluation. *Neurology,* 32:18–23.
27. Lieb, J.P., Walsh, G.O., Babb, T.L. Walter, R.D., and Crandall, P.H. (1976): A comparison of EEG seizure patterns recorded with surface depth electrodes in patients with temporal lobe epilepsy. *Epilepsia,* 17:137–160.
28. Mattson, R.H. (1983): Closed-circuit-televised video tape recording and electroencephalography (CCTV/EEG) in convulsive status epilepticus. In: *Advances in Neurology, Vol. 34, Status Epilepticus,* edited by A.V. Delgado-Escueta, C.G. Wasterlain, D.M. Treiman, and R.L. Porter, pp. 37–46. Raven Press, New York.
29. Perry, T.R., Gumnit, R.J., Gates, J.R., and Leppik, I.E. (1983): Routine vs. intensive monitoring in the evaluation of intractable epilepsy. *Public Health Rep.* 98:384–389.
30. Ramani, V., and Gumnit, R.J. (1981): Intensive monitoring of epileptic patients with a history of episodic aggression. *Arch. Neurol.*, 38:570–571.

31. Ramani V., and Gumnit, R.J. (1982): Intensive monitoring of inter-ictal psychosis in epilepsy. *Ann. Neurol.,* 11:613–622.
32. Ramani, V., Quesney, L.F., Olson, D., and Gumnit, R.J. (1980): Diagnosis of hysterical seizures in epileptic patients. *Am. J. Psychiatry,* 137:705–709.
33. Spencer, S.S. (1981): Depth electroencephalography in selection of refractory epilepsy for surgery. *Ann. Neurol.,* 9:207–214.
34. Spencer, S.S., Williamson, P.D., Bridgers, S.L., Mattson, R.H., Cicchetti, D.V., and Spencer, D.D. (1985): Reliability and accuracy of localization by scalp ictal EEG. *Neurology,* 35:1567–1575.
35. Sutula, T.P., Sackellares, J.C., Miller, J.Q., and Dreifuss, F. (1981): Intensive monitoring in refractory epilepsy. *Neurology (New York),* 31:243–247.
36. Williamson, P.D., Spencer, D.D., Spencer, S.S., Novelly, R.A., and Mattson, R.H. (1985): Complex partial seizures of frontal lobe origin. *Ann. Neurol.,* 18(4):497–504.

Subject Index